MRCP 2
Success in PACES

Second Edition

Douglas C Macdonald BM(hons) BSc(hons) MRCP
Specialist Registrar in Gastroenterology and Hepatology
University College Hospital
London

Philip Kelly MBBS MRCP
Department of Diabetes and Metabolism
Whipps Cross Hospital
London

Thomas Powles MBBS MRCP MD
Senior Lecturer and Consultant in Medical Oncology
St Bartholomew's and the London NHS trust
London

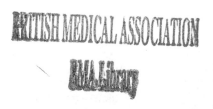
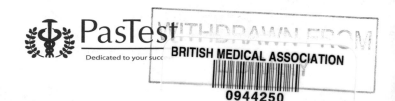

© 2009 PasTest Ltd
Egerton Court
Parkgate Estate
Knutsford
Cheshire WA16 8DX

Telephone: 01565 752000

First edition 2003
Second edition 2009

ISBN: 1 90462782X
ISBN: 9781904627821

A catalogue record for this book is available from the British Library.

The information contained within this book was obtained by the authors from reliable sources. However, while every effort has been made to ensure its accuracy, no responsi-bility for loss, damage or injury occasioned to any person acting or refraining from action as a result of information contained herein can be accepted by the publisher or the authors.

PasTest Revision Books and Intensive Courses
PasTest has been established in the field of postgraduate medical education since 1972, providing revision books and intensive study courses for doctors preparing for their professional examinations. Books and courses are available for the following specialties:

MRCGP, MRCP Parts 1 and 2, MRCPCH Parts 1 and 2,
MRCPsych, MRCS, MRCOG Parts 1 and 2, DRCOG, DCH,
FRCA, PLAB Parts 1 and 2

For further details contact:

PasTest, Freepost, Knutsford, Cheshire WA16 7BR
Tel: 01565 752 000   Fax: 01565 650 264
Email: enquiries@pastest.co.uk   Web site: www. pastest.co.uk

---

Typeset by Saxon Graphics Ltd, Derby
Printed and bound in the UK by Page Bros (Norwich) Ltd

Contents

Acknowledgements

I would like to thank Hristina for her patience throughout the many Sundays this book devoured.

Preface to the second edition

The second edition of Success in PACES bears at most a passing resemblance to its predecessor. The reader will find a totally new chapter on history taking – the format itself is also novel and we believe that it conveys the approach to history taking for any observed examination more completely than any other text – a totally rewritten section on communication and ethics – the edges of our moral, social, professional and legal framework continue to move – and hugely expanded and rewritten sections on all the clinical cases.

The authorship has evolved and expanded: Paul Jenkins – the kernel around which the flesh of the first edition formed – has taken on a more supervisory role and Douglas Macdonald has joined the team, a gastroenterologist and general physician at the Hammersmith Hospital, and you can particularly see his influence in the marvellous, completely new chapters on abdominal and musculoskeletal examination and the ground-breaking history section.

The whole profession is becoming much more familiar with guidelines and protocols that, where carefully designed, can assist in the ever more complex work that we do; where these may help in the diagnosis, classification, investigation or management of the patient they have been mentioned. One must, however, remember your duty to the patient in front of you; a guideline or protocol could never envisage the diversity of human behaviour, disease, understanding and interaction. Important trials, about which you might wish to know, have also been mentioned throughout the text.

Clinical images have been added throughout where we believe that they aid understanding of the cases. There has been extensive use of clinical figures, particularly in the sections on neurology and examination of the eyes. Neurology has a special place in most candidates' memories of PACES. Clinical neurosciences form a minor part of undergraduate education and the presence of a neurologist on the acute ward is uncommon. If you have not done a neurology post, or perhaps, as second best, worked on an acute stroke or a rehab ward, you may have had a comparatively sparse exposure to clinical neurology. Furthermore, in the exam, it has perhaps the broadest 'number' of cases that you can reasonably be expected to face and the techniques to face those cases are varied. Hence, we have made free use of line drawings to assist the understanding of this difficult topic.

Philip Kelly
Douglas Macdonald
Thomas Powles

About this book

The PACES exam covers a potentially enormous range of clinical cases and topics. As such, it is almost impossible to know everything that the examiners may wish to ask. The secret to success is to have a thorough basic knowledge of clinical examination and communication skills, which can then be applied to almost any situation that you will encounter. Experience has shown that, in all three areas of the exam, a number of scenarios are tested time and time again.

In each clinical section the introduction goes into more detail about the likelihood of various scenarios appearing and the relative weight that must be attached to various clinical cases. For instance, you must give more time to the preparation of dystrophia myotonica compared with hereditary lipodystrophy, otherwise that lack of insight might best be rewarded by re-sitting the exam. When you are on-call or in the clinic think about the clinical problems that you are dealing with and tie this together with the key clinical cases that we have outlined in the book and you will have a strong foundation with which to pass.

This book is divided into the same five sections as the PACES. Each section begins with guidance on generic skills applicable to that particular area, before covering the essential cases commonly encountered by candidates. It is to be expected that, once proficient in all these skills and cases, you are unlikely to be surprised in the exam.

THE CASES AND SCENARIOS

The demands of the various stations are different and we have written the clinical scenarios solely with the aim of getting the information across for that clinical problem. In some stations it is a question of finding the murmur or the lump – the technique of doing this might be fairly standard. However, when one is asked to examine someone who cannot raise him- or herself from a chair, the clinical problem is really quite different and the approach to that case must take a different form. Some cases are included because they illustrate important practical clinical considerations that enhance the framework of our clinical skills.

We have endeavoured to provide a framework for likely or possible discussions on the clinical scenarios, which may include, where appropriate, the aetiology, differential diagnosis, symptoms, investigations and management.

This renders the book ideally suited for PACES, where you may be asked to examine a patient with hemiparesis, take a history from him or her, perhaps explain what is the likely cause and differential diagnosis or finally convey information about outlook and prognosis to him or her or the family. Thus, these are not cases solely for clinical examination; rather you must think 'how can this case appear in the history or the communication and ethics station?'.

In exactly the same frame of mind the history-taking stations can often be turned round to communication scenarios; again, consider the legal and ethical issues around each case as they arise. Think what information you might gather from examining this patient whom you are discussing in the ethics station.

Hopefully, after reading this book, candidates will realise that the list of things to know in order to pass the exam is not quite endless. When you go into the exam you will be at the peak of your ability. The signs will be simple to elicit and the examiners will be impressed not only with your technique but also with your manner to the patient. The patients will want you as their doctor and the relatives will never have spoken to someone so understanding, authoritative yet approachable.

In critical and baffling situations, it is always best to return to first principle and simple action

Winston Spencer Churchill

Introduction

The Diploma of Membership of the Royal College of Physicians of the United Kingdom – MRCP (UK) – is a considerable peak on the road to becoming a physician of any description. Even on the other side it is no less formidable a challenge and holds a special place in the memory of every practising physician. Its worth is recognised all over the world; each stage of the examination has been extensively validated and it provides reliable evidence of attainment in knowledge, clinical skills and behaviour.

The clinical part of the Practical Assessment of Clinical Examination Skills (PACES) is the most difficult challenge of the MRCP, but it is, overall, a very fair examination of your skills. The required skills are passed down from one generation of physicians to the next, the same skills that enable us to be confident in our handling of clinical cases in the middle of the night in the receiving room, at the tail end of a Friday afternoon clinic, on a busy ward with competing demands for our attention, at the end of the bed when we can confidently say that a critical corner has been turned or in a quiet office as we explain the enormity and perhaps uncertainty of a dreadful situation to a scared patient or relative, the skills that we recognise internally as being necessary to start on the long road to becoming a physician. The need to keep an internal standard of our clinical behaviour is increasingly important because there are more outside influences on our standards than ever before – not every outside influence will want us to be so thorough. There are compelling reasons to 'dumb down' physicians and we must always remain vigilant that we do not allow it to happen to ourselves or to those whom we teach.

The examiners are not looking for the next professor of medicine, but rather a safe and competent doctor, who is suitable for higher specialist training. Examiners say, time and time again, that their criteria for passing are based on whether they would entrust the care of one of their relatives to the candidate. Alternatively, would they be able to have a sensible and practical conversation if the candidate, as the on-site senior physician, rang in the early hours of the morning about a patient? However, as with the previous parts of the examination, a pass is the result of successful examination technique *together* with clinical skills and knowledge. Communicating to the examiners that you are safe, competent and knowledgeable is a vital component of the examination. Careful preparation is therefore essential because you are being tested on both examination technique and presentation skills. All too often the candidates fail themselves through lack of self-belief that they are able to pass the exam and adopt the 'rabbit caught in the headlights' stance. It is vital to remember the key words 'confidence' and 'competence'.

GENERAL APPROACH

Remember that the examiners are trying to find out what you know and are not trying to catch you out. Their brief is to determine whether you are suitable for specialist training.

Approach the examiners in a friendly and confident manner, although obviously over-familiarity and arrogance are a sure way to antagonise. When discussing the patient do so in an interested manner, as you would when talking to your consultant or another senior colleague and not as a first-year medical student talking to the professor. Dress smartly and conservatively – a suit is ideal. Do not smell of cigarettes, aftershave, strong perfume or alcohol. Eye contact is an important part of communication and should be appropriately maintained with the examiners. Far too many candidates enter the 'victim mode', with arms folded, eyes downcast, almost expecting to fail; do not do this. Keep your hands by your sides or behind your back, where fidgeting or finger twisting will not be noticed. Remember, people all too often fail themselves in this exam, despite being good clinicians in their normal hospitals. The exam is easy to pass *and* easy to fail.

Treat the patients with consideration and respect at all times. Remember, they have given their time freely. There is no easier way of failing than inadvertently hurting a patient during clumsy examination of a limb or abdominal system. Always ask patients if they have any pain or tenderness before you put 'hands on'.

Finally, prepare for the exam carefully. If you have failed the exam previously, make sure that you know the reason why. Identify those areas in which you are weak and make sure that you see as many cases as you can, preferably under an exam environment.

ABOUT THE EXAM

The PACES examination consists of a carousel of five stations, each of 20 minutes' duration, but with 5 minutes of rest/preparation between stations. Candidates start at any one of the stations and then move round the carousel at 20–minute intervals until they have completed the cycle.

Station 1:	Respiratory examination	10 minutes each
	Abdominal examination	
Station 2:	History taking – 20 minutes	
Station 3:	Cardiovascular examination	10 minutes each
	Neurological examination	
Station 4:	Communication skills and ethics – 20 minutes	
Station 5:	Skin	5 minutes each
	Locomotor	
	Eyes	
	Endocrine examination	

Each station is assessed by two independent examiners, and each has a structured mark sheet; the two examiners will thus examine each candidate in turn at that one station only.

Clinical Station 2: History Taking

Candidates are given 5 minutes before the station begins in which to review the written instructions, usually in the form of a letter from the patient's GP (see box) and to prepare themselves. They are encouraged to make preparatory notes during this period but this is not assessed.

Dear Doctor

This 25–year-old man has been increasingly troubled by back pain these last few months. He has Crohn's disease, which is not clinically active at present. I would be grateful for your assessment and advice on investigation and management.

Yours sincerely

The consultation with the patient or individual lasts 14 minutes. This is followed by 1 minute to collect your thoughts and then 5 minutes of discussion with the examiners.

The 'history-taking skills station' aims to assess the ability of the candidate to gather data from the patient, to assimilate these data in a structured manner, and then to discuss the case in a coherent manner with the examiners. Although most candidates may regard this station as perhaps the easiest, in the exam situation many find that this is not the case. A common reason for failure is inadequate preparation and approach, leading to missing out whole sections of a medical history, eg drugs, family or social history. The examiners place great emphasis on a careful and thorough social/occupational history. Imagine yourself as the patient and how the illness would affect all the daily activities that you might take for granted, eg how does a dialysis patient cope with changing the peritoneal bags, or a rheumatoid arthritic patient cope with dressing and eating?

Try to cultivate a friendly rapport with your patient and remember that, at the end of the history, you should ask: 'Is there anything else that you think I ought to know, or that we have not covered?' Often the patient may mention an aspect of the case that is of particular importance that you have overlooked.

You must use the 1 minute after the consultation to collect your thoughts and organise the history in a logical and thoughtful manner. This is not your final MB and the examiners will become irritated by a sloppy presentation with irrelevant negative findings. 'Ums' and 'uhs' and long pauses do not convey the best image and can be to your detriment. Think and speak clearly, be certain in both your uncertainty and your certainty. You should be prepared to discuss the case in relation to the normal presentation of the condition and to discuss subsequent investigation and treatment. The examiners will expect a considered and mature approach to the case, using a problem-oriented method.

In all aspects of the exam do not start your discussion with the esoteric and obscure in the belief that you will impress the examiner – the reverse is likely to be true. Any discussion about investigation and management should start with the simple and practical issues, eg a full blood count or chest radiograph, and quickly work through to the more sophisticated and elaborate investigations/treatments. However, when there is one specific diagnostic test that will give the diagnosis, say it straight away. For example, in a case of spastic paraparesis in a young woman with nystagmus and optic neuritis, say that you wish to do an MRI of the brain and brain stem, not a full blood count. Do not use abbreviations, eg TPR and BP, U&Es – even though we all use them in our daily work. It is preferable to use the full term in the exam. If you do not understand what the examiner is getting at, ask politely to repeat the question. This is perfectly acceptable and much better than launching into an inappropriate answer.

Clinical Stations 1, 3 and 5: Examination of Systems

For each case at the clinical stations the candidate will receive written instructions as to what is required of him or her, eg at the neurological station:

This 48–year-old man has been having difficult getting up the stairs for the last few weeks. Please would you examine the neurology in the lower limbs, and tell the examiners what signs you find, and discuss your proposed management.

Many candidates find this to be the most difficult and stressful part of the examination. However, with adequate preparation and practice, this should not be the case. Remember that most cases will be patients with chronic stable disease, often encountered in a hospital setting. There are eight clinical examination stations. Be sure that for each system you have your own well-rehearsed method of examination. This is vital so that, if the examiner says, 'Examine the cardiovascular system', or 'Examine the hands', you do not have to think about what to do. The detail of your examination routine should be absolutely automatic and look slick and well practised, so that you can concentrate on whether the signs are abnormal or normal. Although there is no completely 'right' examination technique, there are accepted standard methods that one should learn and broadly adhere to.

Most of the patients whom you will encounter will have common pathology, eg valvular heart disease, diabetic retinopathy, bronchiectasis, arthritides, rather than obscure rarities of tertiary referral centres. It is a common misconception of candidates that esoteric cases are over-represented, but the following cannot be stated enough:

> *Imagine that you are the registrar calling patients up, and whom you might find available with good, stable signs and who is well. If a patient fails to turn up on the day what cases are likely to be available in the hospital, who might be amenable to helping with the examination? Who will be well enough? What conditions have stable, predictable signs?*

Do your thinking while you are examining the patient because otherwise, when you lift your head from listening to the patient's heart/looking at a fundus and the examiner says, 'Diagnosis?', you will be in difficulty. If you know the diagnosis, it is preferable to continue your presentation by stating it, followed by the *relevant* supporting clinical findings, eg 'This patient has mitral stenosis. The relevant findings are a mitral valvotomy scar; she is in atrial fibrillation with a tapping apex and has a low-pitched mid-diastolic rumbling murmur …'. If you do not know what the diagnosis is, then describe what you see, eg 'A rash with plaques involving the trunk and extensor aspects of the elbows', and then give your diagnosis 'consistent with psoriasis'. Take charge of the situation and try not to be pressurised. Once you have decided on your findings, stick with them. The examiners may ask you if you are sure: indecision and changing your mind can all too easily lead to floundering and digging a hole with subsequent dire consequences. However, if there is uncertainty, state it and proceed to say how you would resolve the uncertainty. Present the examiners and thus the patient with a solution, not a problem, and they will be happy.

Concentrate on the current station and the task in hand, rather than perceived mistakes made in previous stations. Although coming up with the right answer is obviously important, most of the marks are awarded for overall technique, approach, ability to discuss your findings and clinical judgement, as well as being able to solve clinical problems.

The only way to be confident about the systems examinations is practice, practice and more practice. You should enter the systems examinations as a finely honed diagnostic machine.

Station 4: Communication Skills and Ethics

The 'communication skills and ethics station' aims to assess the ability of the candidate to guide and organise an interview with the subject in a clear and structured manner, provide emotional support and discuss further management issues. There are no marks specifically awarded for medical knowledge, and the ability of the candidate to discuss issues in an open and non-prejudiced manner rather than simply imparting information is of paramount importance.

The written instructions will provide a framework for the start of the consultation but its subsequent direction will depend on your interaction with the patient. The consultation should ideally start with relatively 'open' questions before focusing on specific points – 'closed' questions. It is important to assess the patient's knowledge and expectations of the condition before imparting new information, and patients should be allowed sufficient time to digest information and to ask any questions. Examiners will field questions ranging from 'How do you think you did?', 'What did you do well and badly?', 'What do you think the patient will remember from the consultation?' to more detailed questions about legal issues: 'How long after a fit can you start driving again?'

As a third of the allocated marks are for legal and ethical issues, it is vital to consider these during the 5 minutes of preparation at the beginning. These are discussed in detail in the relevant section in the book.

Finally, as always, practise your technique with colleagues – many people make the mistake of failing to prepare for this important part of the exam.

Marking

Each candidate will receive 14 structured marking sheets before the start of the examination. One sheet is given to each examiner at Stations 2, 4 and 5 and two sheets are given to each examiner at Stations 1 and 3. Examiners record their marks, independently of each other, and place them into a box at the end of the station. There are four possible marks:

Clear fail = 1 mark
Fail = 2 marks
Pass = 3 marks
Clear pass = 4 marks.

A total of 56 marks is possible. The pass mark is usually set at 42 marks, allowing a pass rate of 45–50%.

Any candidate receiving three 'clear fails' automatically fails the examination.

Exam statistics

PACES is designed to test your suitability for specialist training, not the completion of that training. You must be sure that you have a thorough knowledge of the basics. As such consider the following: being able to pass PACES and being a good clinician are not one and the same.

- If your whole aim is to pass PACES, you might not have the required skills to be a good clinician; the examiners should find this out quite quickly.
- If your aim is to be a thorough, rounded, general physician you will more than likely have the skills to pass PACES; the examiners should find this out quite quickly.

The number of cases that you are *likely* to see in PACES is quite small, as we shall show. Therefore you must direct your preparation so that you have a thorough knowledge of the clinical problems that you are likely to face.

Your preparation must also reflect a broader base of clinical knowledge and clinical skills that might be tested in the exam. The reason that they are tested in the exam is that the College – made up of practising clinicians – think that these cases/clinical scenarios:

- test those skills
- are common
- are uncommon but of such clinical importance that it is core knowledge because their prompt recognition may:
  - allow lifesaving treatment
  - prevent life-threatening treatment
- will be available for the exam, have predicable signs and be comfortable being examined.

Furthermore the examination ought to be *fairly* standardised across the country for all the candidates. That is not to say that every candidate will see the same cases as every other one but that the pool of potential cases is relatively small.

However, the examination has got to be run, the cases have to be available, and the clinical centre that runs PACES is putting on a show for the candidates, the internal examiners and the external examiners – there must be cases there and they have got to have someone or something to examine!

It is worth putting yourself in the shoes of the person who does the leg work getting the patients – the medical registrar; on the day, if the person with diabetic retinopathy or myotonic dystrophy does not turn up, what are they going to do? They are going to phone up the admitting team, and the ward teams and the neurologists, oncologists, general surgeons, ENT, etc on the wards and in clinic, and ask what patients are available at short notice who fulfil some of these above qualities. If someone is in with a jugular foramen syndrome they will come over for the exam – if the signs are good and easy you will be expected to be able to elicit them and have a reasoned discussion about the case. It will not matter to the examiner that you may not have done much anatomy as an undergraduate; if you do not possess the skills to get on with the case in a sensible manner you had better learn them before re-sitting the exam.

So, learn the common things very well, but have a rounded knowledge by knowing what else might come up.

The following section deals with the cases that you might see in a little more detail.

ABDOMINAL CASES

Four cases account for over two-thirds of cases encountered: polycystic kidney disease, renal transplantation/dialysis, hepatosplenomegaly and chronic liver disease. The six cases below account for about 95% of cases encountered. Other cases that have occurred include scars on the abdomen, hereditary haemorrhagic telangiectasia, isolated lymphadenopathy and a liver transplant (Mercedes' sign scar on the abdomen).

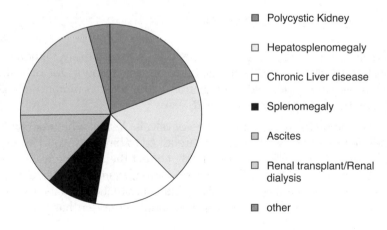

- Polycystic Kidney
- Hepatosplenomegaly
- Chronic Liver disease
- Splenomegaly
- Ascites
- Renal transplant/Renal dialysis
- other

RESPIRATORY CASES

Four cases account for over 75% of respiratory cases. These are pulmonary fibrosis, chronic obstructive pulmonary disease, bronchiectasis (usually associated with cystic fibrosis) and unilateral pneumonectomy/fibrosis. Other cases include pleural effusion, lung cancer, lung transplant and Cushing syndrome.

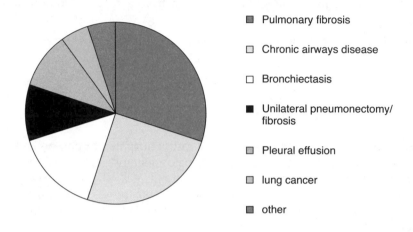

■ Pulmonary fibrosis

☐ Chronic airways disease

☐ Bronchiectasis

■ Unilateral pneumonectomy/ fibrosis

▨ Pleural effusion

▨ lung cancer

▨ other

CARDIOVASCULAR CASES

A broad spectrum of cardiovascular cases occurs in this exam, although the combination of either aortic or mitral value disease accounts for over three-quarters of all cases. Tricuspid regurgitation is the most common right-sided valve lesion but this occurs in only 1 in 20 cases.

It is more common to encounter one type of valvular lesion rather than multiple valvular lesions (see below). Candidates are asked to have a 'second listen' in a third of cases. No one who was completely correct the first time was asked to have a 'second listen'. When having a second listen, examiners often ask candidates to reconsider their diagnosis. This is a difficult situation and the examiners are not always helpful in this situation. You should consider that your original diagnosis was not completely correct.

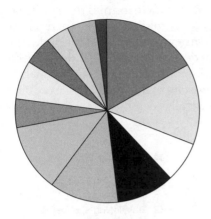

- Mitral regurgitation
- Aortic stenosis
- Mixed aortic valve disease valve disease
- Aortic regurgitation
- Congenital valve disease
- Prosthetic valve
- ASD or VSD
- Mitral stenosis
- Mixed mitral valve disease
- Tricuspid regurgitation
- Mixed Aortic and mitral valve disease
- other

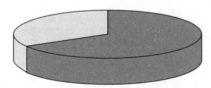

- One valvular lesion
- more than one valvular lesion

LOCOMOTOR CASES

The most common single case perhaps in the whole exam is rheumatoid hands in this section. It alone accounts for over a third of cases. There are a few scenarios that you might not consider *purely* locomotor; these include systemic sclerosis (which is more common in the dermatology station), the diabetic foot (which can rightly occur in the endocrine or neurological stations), abnormal gait (also the neurological station) and wasting of the small muscles of the hand (again the neurological station or occasionally seen but rarely the focus of the respiratory station).

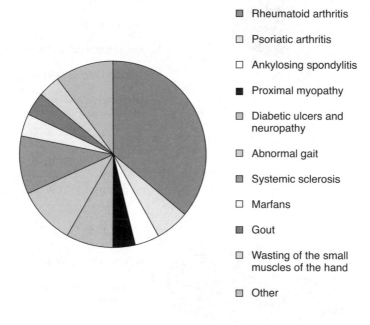

- Rheumatoid arthritis
- Psoriatic arthritis
- Ankylosing spondylitis
- Proximal myopathy
- Diabetic ulcers and neuropathy
- Abnormal gait
- Systemic sclerosis
- Marfans
- Gout
- Wasting of the small muscles of the hand
- Other

ENDOCRINE CASES

Four cases account for three-quarters of the scenarios encountered.

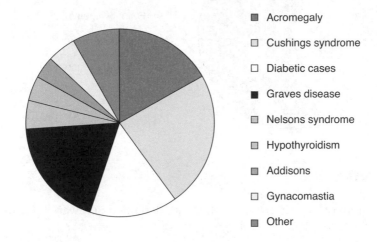

- Acromegaly
- Cushings syndrome
- Diabetic cases
- Graves disease
- Nelsons syndrome
- Hypothyroidism
- Addisons
- Gynacomastia
- Other

EXAMINATION OF THE EYE

The diagnosis depends on performing fundoscopy in over 50% of cases. The four most common fundoscopy cases appearing in the exam are diabetic eye disease, retinal pigmentation, hypertension and optic atrophy.
If you cannot perform fundoscopy, competently, with both eyes, looking at both the patient's eyes, you should not be sitting the PACES.

Laser-treated diabetic retinopathy is by far the most common case in this station.

Ophthalmoplegia is most commonly Graves' ophthalmopathy with ophthalmoplegia, an isolated nerve III palsy, a nerve VI palsy, myasthenia gravis/ocular myopathy or an internuclear ophthalmoplegia; cavernous sinus syndrome may occur in this station or the neurology one.

Visual field defects are most commonly bitemporal hemianopia or homonymous hemianopia/quadrantanopia, or anterior causes such as a patch of retinitis or retinal vein occlusion.

Pupillary abnormality is most commonly Holmes Adie pupil or Horner syndrome.

Orbital abnormality is usually exophthalmos in the context of Graves' disease and rarely because of a retro-orbital tumour.

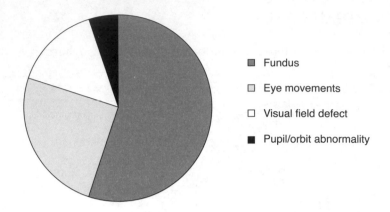

Legend:
- Fundus
- Eye movements
- Visual field defect
- Pupil/orbit abnormality

SKIN CASES

A wide spectrum of cases is possible, which are described herewith. Only four cases occur more that 10% of the time:

1. Systemic sclerosis: scleroderma
2. Diabetic skin changes: necrobiosis lipoidica diabeticorum, granuloma annulare, ulcers
3. Lupus: malar rash with follicular plugging, scaring alopecia, ulcers
4. Xanthoma.

Of the other cases, psoriasis, eczema, hereditary haemorrhagic telangiectasia, vasculitis, neurofibromatosis, lichen planus, dermatitis herpetiformis, dermatomyositis and gout occur frequently.

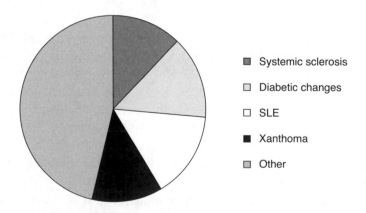

Legend:
- Systemic sclerosis
- Diabetic changes
- SLE
- Xanthoma
- Other

NEUROLOGY

A broader spectrum of cases may occur in the neurology station than in any other.

The cases that stand out are spastic paraparesis, myotonic dystrophy, multiple sclerosis (in its legion of presentations), peripheral sensorimotor neuropathy (often diabetic) and parkinsonism.

Candidates are asked to perform specific tasks. Candidates are occasionally asked to examine eye movement and fundoscopy, although there is a separate section for this in the exam (the same applies to gait and the locomotor section).

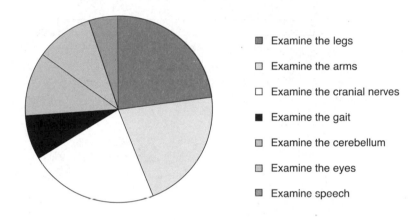

- ▨ Examine the legs
- ▢ Examine the arms
- ▢ Examine the cranial nerves
- ■ Examine the gait
- ▨ Examine the cerebellum
- ▨ Examine the eyes
- ▨ Examine speech

HISTORY SECTION

The number of cases in this section is limitless. The history-taking section in this book addresses a very broad spectrum of cases from every relevant medical specialty.

The history cases that occur in the exam fall into three sections. The main problems are not always apparent from the information given in the test, eg a man with gastrointestinal symptoms may have depression or social problems as his primary problem.

There are three main groups of scenarios that occur:

1. A case that requires questions to come to a diagnosis, ie weight loss
2. A series of medical problems that are known by the patients, need to be assessed and prioritised, eg someone with diabetes, who has complications and is undergoing investigation for bleeding per rectum

3. An interaction of medical and social problems that are of equal importance to the patient.

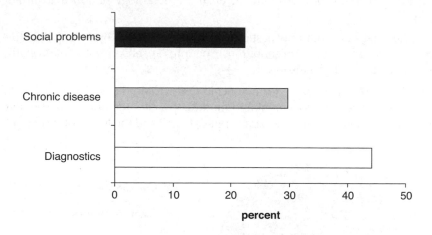

STATION 1

The Abdominal and Respiratory Examinations

THE ABDOMINAL EXAMINATION

Abdominal cases in PACES fall into three main categories:

1. Liver disease: cirrhosis, portal hypertension, encephalopathy, right ventricular failure/tricuspid regurgitation, metastatic disease, chronic viral hepatitis, infiltration or inflammation
2. Splenomegaly/hepatosplenomegaly: myeloproliferative, lymphoproliferative or autoimmune disease
3. Renal disease: renal replacement therapy, renal transplantation.

The examiner's instructions and general inspection will often indicate which of the three categories a case is likely to fall into from the start. Although patterns of organomegaly are almost always present, most candidates will successfully identify these. The key to a clear pass is spotting peripheral stigmata in order to *identify the cause* of disease and to *stage its severity*. Unlike the cardiovascular examination, where most of the important information is gleaned from examination of the precordium, the crucial clues to the abdominal cases are peripheral.

Examination sequence

Although the examination should follow a well-practised and smooth routine, allow the peripheral stigmata and examiner's instructions to focus your attention on particular elements of your examination, eg the finding of an old fistula in the forearm should prompt a careful search for a multitude of signs: gum hypertrophy (ciclosporin immunosuppression), parathyroidectomy scar (tertiary hyperparathyroidism), insulin injection sites (diabetic nephropathy), hearing aid (Alport's disease, Wegener's granulomatosis), small neck scars (from previous haemodialysis catheters), small abdominal scars (previous Tenckhoff's catheters for peritoneal dialysis) and a raised JVP (fluid overload indicating under-dialysis or renal graft failure). All such signs would be easily missed in a 'routine' abdominal examination.

Introduce and expose

- Introduce yourself.
- Ask: 'Do you have pain anywhere?'
- Position the patient so that he or she lies supine, with the head resting on one pillow and the arms by the sides.
- Expose men from the pubic tubercle upwards. Women should be exposed from the pubic tubercle to the xiphisternum,
- Say: 'I'm going to look you over then feel your tummy if that's all right?'

Inspection

General

Many candidates rush this stage (keen to get to the hard signs) and miss important and obvious clues. Stand at the end of the bed and take time to look at the patient.

Ask the patient to take a deep breath in. Look for descending masses, eg liver, spleen or kidneys. Note any obvious scars and their likely significance. Look for muscle wasting, loss of subcutaneous fat and oedema – it is important to demonstrate the ability to recognise poor nutritional status whether or not you successfully identify the underlying diagnosis.

Hands

Ask the patient to stretch the arms out in front of him or her and cock the wrist back as though pressing against a wall. This is not only the means to look for a liver flap but also a good way of positioning the hands for examination. Although the hands are a rich source of potential signs do not waste time examining the hands exhaustively. Examiners will become quickly irritated if you examine each finger in turn for nailbed fluctuance or Dupuytren's contractures.

Skin

Make a close survey of the skin over the legs and thorax on your way to the face.

Face

Ask the patient to look upwards and look at the conjunctivae (only one side is necessary) for anaemia. Examine the iris for the inflammation of uveitis. Palpate the parotid glands. Ask the patient to open the mouth and warn him or her that you are going to use a tongue depressor. Use a pen torch to examine the oral cavity thoroughly.

Neck and chest

Sit the patient forwards at this point and from behind press your fingers firmly into the left supraclavicular fossa, palpating for lymphadenopathy (Virchow's node/Troisier's sign). Examine the neck for scars of multiple haemodialysis catheters or parathyroidectomy.

It is not usually necessary to examine the JVP in the abdominal examination. However, you will not be shot for returning to it at the end if you suspect that fluid balance is relevant to the case (ie end-stage renal failure, dialysis or renal transplant recipients) or you have detected hepatomegaly in the absence of stigmata of chronic liver disease (suggesting possible right ventricular failure or tricuspid regurgitation).

While the patient is sitting forwards, glance down the back looking for far lateral/posterior nephrectomy scars. These are easy to miss on anterior inspection alone.

Examine the breast tissue in men for gynaecomastia and look in the axillae for loss of hair.

Abdomen

Make a closer inspection of the abdomen kneeling at the patient's side.

Palpation

If the patient has pain, begin at the segment furthest from its location.

Look at the patient and not at your hand to ensure that you are not causing discomfort.

Palpate with the wrist in a neutral position and the hand flat on the abdomen, flexing at the metacarpophalangeal joints in a 'dipping' action. You should begin with quick, light palpation to determine if there is any tenderness or obvious masses or organomegaly, and then use deeper palpation in each region in turn.

Liver

Start in the right iliac fossa with the hand parallel to the subcostal margin, using the radial border of the index finger to detect any liver edge. Ask the patient to take deep breaths, pressing the fingers firmly inwards as he or she does so. Rather than pushing the hand up against the liver edge, you are anticipating the sensation of the edge sliding under the radial border of the hand and gently pushing the hand upwards with inspiration. Avoid the temptation to press more deeply and 'follow' the liver upwards because you feel less resistance with expiration. Advance your hand towards the costal margin 2 cm at a time.

If you feel a liver edge, ask yourself the following:

- Is it smooth or nodular?
- Is it soft, firm or hard?
- Is it pulsatile?
- Is it tender?
- Is there a Reidel lobe (a tongue-like projection from the right lobe that can extend as far as the right iliac fossa).

Spleen

Start in the right iliac fossa and move diagonally to the left subcostal region. Place your left hand behind the left lower ribs and apply sustained anterior pressure. Ask the patient to take deep breaths and palpate as you would for a liver edge. Finding the spleen is a difficult and often unrewarding experience. If you suspect mild-to-moderate splenomegaly try the following to confirm it:

- 'Tipping' the spleen: roll the patient towards you on the right side. Place your left hand over the patient's left ribs while palpating under the costal margin with your right hand. A mildly enlarged spleen may drop below the costal margin and be more readily palpable with this manoeuvre.

- Percuss for dullness between the lower border of the ninth rib and the costal margin in the midaxillary line.
- Percuss the space of Traube. This is over the stomach medial to the left costal margin. It is usually resonant as a result of a gas bubble in the stomach, but dullness might indicate that the stomach is displaced medially by an enlarged spleen.

All your examiners will have been taunted by many a phantom spleen – a foray into percussion before completion of the palpation sequence is forgivable if you suspect splenomegaly.

Kidneys

Place your left hand under the patient's flank below the twelfth rib lateral to the long strap muscles of the spine and place your right hand anteriorly. Push the bottom hand firmly upwards – an enlarged kidney should be palpable.

If not palpable the kidney may be ballottable. Ask the patient to breathe in deeply and at maximal inspiration flex the fingers posteriorly and attempt to 'flick' the kidney upwards against the right hand anteriorly.

Distinguishing between a liver/spleen and a kidney:

- Cannot get above the spleen.
- The spleen has a notch.
- The spleen moves inferomedially on inspiration, whereas the kidney moves inferiorly.
- The spleen is not ballottable.
- The spleen is dull to percussion; the kidney is often resonant as a result of overlying bowel.
- A friction rub may be heard over a spleen but not over a kidney.

Other Masses

Palpate the aorta bimanually with the tips of the fingers on the midline above the umbilicus. The normal diameter is up to 3 cm.

The bladder and bowel may be felt in normal individuals. Pressure on the bladder, which rises out of the pelvis, may induce a desire to micturate. Pressure on a faecally loaded bowel may leave an indentation.

Percussion

Liver and spleen

A number of studies have investigated the accuracy of percussion in determining liver and spleen size compared with radiological techniques. A recurrent finding is that light percussion is more discriminatory than generating the loudest possible sound. Firm percussion seems consistently to underestimate liver size, for example. Also, percussion of the liver and spleen is best performed in inspiration.

Percussion should follow a similar pattern to palpation. Define the upper border of the liver (around the sixth rib). This determines whether the liver is truly enlarged or displaced inferiorly by a hyperexpanded chest. The normal lower border of the spleen is the ninth rib in the midaxillary line and dullness below this indicates mild splenomegaly. Enlargement of the spleen by 40% or less may be detectable only by this means.

Ascites

Compared with ultrasonography, the sensitivity and specificity of the clinical examination for ascites are very wide ranging and highly dependent on the examiner's experience (50–94% and 29–82% respectively in one survey).

Percuss horizontally across and through the umbilicus. If an area of dullness is found in the left flank, ask the patient to roll towards you keeping the finger in the same position. Wait 20 seconds then percuss again – if it is resonant this is indicative of shifting dullness. Only perform this test if there is definite dullness in the flanks or obvious abdominal distension, otherwise it is a waste of precious time. The absence of dullness in the flanks excludes ascites with 90% accuracy. If there is tense ascites a fluid thrill may be demonstrable. Ask the patient to place the side of his or her hand in the midline of the abdomen and press down firmly. With the left hand pressed against the left side of the abdomen flick the near side. This creates a percussion wave that can be felt by the left hand.

Auscultation

Listen with the diaphragm over the abdomen for 30 seconds. A succussion splash may be demonstrated in gastric outlet obstruction by vigorously shaking the abdomen back and forth between both hands.

Bruits may be detectable over an enlarged liver or spleen, over the renal arteries (posteriorly, at the sides of the long strap muscles below the twelfth rib) or over an abdominal aortic aneurysm (in the epigastrium).

Finally

Palpate the hernial orifices.

Tell the examiner you would wish to examine the external genitalia, perform a per rectum examination, test the urine with a dipstick and look at the observations chart.

Thank the patient and re-cover them.

Abdominal Scenarios

1. Transplanted kidney
2. Polycystic kidney disease
3. Chronic liver disease
4. Primary biliary cirrhosis
5. Hereditary haemochromatosis
6. Alcohol-induced liver disease
7. Chronic viral hepatitis
8. Autoimmune hepatitis
9. Isolated hepatomegaly without stigmata of chronic liver disease
10. Ascites without stigmata of chronic liver disease
11. Hepatosplenomegaly/splenomegaly without stigmata of chronic liver disease
12. Polycythaemia rubra vera
13. Hereditary spherocytosis

SCENARIO 1. TRANSPLANTED KIDNEY

Examination

Face

- Cushingoid
- Anaemia
- Gum hypertrophy
- Hearing aid (Alport's disease, Wegener's granulomatosis).

Neck and chest

- Parathyroidectomy scar
- Haemodialysis catheter scars
- Dilated superficial veins (stenosis of central veins secondary to multiple previous lines).

Hands

- Forearm fistula
- Nailbed vasculitis
- Half-and-half nails.

Fluid status

- Raised JVP
- Sacral or ankle oedema
- Hypertension.

Abdomen

- Peritoneal dialysis scar (midline)
- Mass in iliac fossa
- Hepatomegaly (adult polycystic kidney disease or APKD)
- Bilateral renal masses (APKD)
- Nephrectomy scar.

Other

- Skin tumours (immunosuppression)
- Insulin injection sites
- Amputation (diabetes/renovascular disease)
- Rashes (autoimmune disease).

A good candidate

The good candidate will assess and comment on:

- The likely aetiology of end-stage renal failure (ESRF)
- Evidence of previous or current renal replacement therapy

- Current function of any transplanted kidney
- Evidence of immunosuppressive therapy.

The examiner's subsequent questions will usually relate to one or more of these individuals.

Likely aetiology of ESRF

Diabetes

Insulin injection sites, visual impairment, diabetic foot, BM sticks/glucometer at bedside.

Glomerulonephritis

Features of multisystem disease (eg butterfly rash of SLE, purpura of vasculitides or cryoglobulinaemia, scleroderma, rheumatoid arthritis and vasculitis, alopecia, vitiligo, cushingoid in the absence of a renal graft), hearing impairment (Alport's disease, Wegener's granulomatosis), stigmata of infective endocarditis (rare in PACES).

Renovascular disease

Signs of extrarenal embolisation or advanced atherosclerosis (eg focal neuro-logical deficits, previous amputation, ischaemic foot ulcer), stigmata of hyper-cholesterolaemia or hyperlipidaemia.

Pyelonephritis

Nephrectomy scar.

Hypertension

Usually no specific stigmata.

APKD

Hepatomegaly (50–70% will have liver cysts but hepatomegaly is much more common in women and usually present only in the context of severe renal cystic disease), focal neurological deficit (associated intracranial aneurysms in 8%) and nephrectomy scars (20% undergo nephrectomy pre-, post- or during transplan-tation for recurrent infection, haematuria or chronic pain caused by renal bulk).

If you cannot find any stigmata that might indicate the aetiology of ESRF (or there are none) keep in mind the frequency chart in Figure 1.1. These figures were derived from the 2005 Renal Registry Report and indicate the underlying cause of ESRF in 4767 patients started on dialysis that year in the UK. ESRF of unknown cause and renovascular disease is much more common in patients aged over 65.

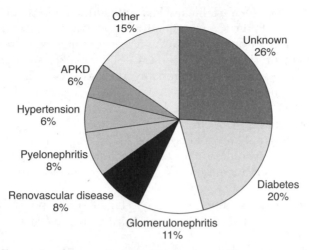

Figure 1.1   Underlying causes of endstage renal failure 2005.

Questions

1. *What investigations would you perform on patient presenting with renal failure for the first time?*

- **Establish severity:**
  - urea and creatinine
  - potassium
  - arterial blood gas (pH) } Indications for urgent dialysis: symptomatic uraemia, hyperkalaemia, acidosis, fluid overload
  - bicarbonate
  - chest radiograph (fluid overload)
    In chronic renal failure approaching dialysis, the most accurate measure of glomerular filtration rate (GFR) is a ^{51}Cr-labelled EDTA (ethylenediaminetetraacetic acid) clearance study. The 24-hour creatinine collection and clearance calculation is unreliable and often less accurate than estimates derived by the Cockroft–Gault formula (1976) or the MDRD (Modification of Diet in Renal Diseases) study equation (Levy et al. 2000).
- **Establish cause:**
  - **24-hour urine collection** (microalbuminuria – 30–300 mg/day; macroalbuminuria – 300–3000 mg protein/day; nephrotic: > 3 g/day proteinuria; nephritic: haematuria and proteinuria)
  - **urinalysis** (red casts – glomerular disease; myoglobinuria – rhabdomyolysis)

- **ANA and ENA (extractable nuclear antigen)**: double-stranded DNA (dsDNA) – SLE; pANCA (anti-neutrophil cytoplasmic antibody) – microscopic polyarteritis; cANCA – Wegener's granulomatosis
- **complement**: decreased C3 and C4 – SLE, vasculitis, membranous glomerulonephritis, IgA nephropathy; decreased C4 and normal C3 – cryoglobulinaemia (and angio-oedema in C1 esterase inhibitor deficiency)
- **creatine kinase**: rhabdomyolysis
- **chest radiograph**: renopulmonary disease (Wegener's granulomatosis, Goodpasture syndrome, microscopic polyarteritis), malignancy, sarcoid; more rarely polyarteritis nodosa, SLE, HUS [haemolytic uraemic syndrome])
- **infectious causes**: anti-streptolysin O titre (ASOT) – post-infectious glomerulonephritis; thick/thin film – malaria; blood cultures – infective endocarditis
- **anti-glomerular basement membrane (anti-GBM) antibody**: Goodpasture syndrome
- **cryoglobulinaemia**: must be transported at body temperature to lab
- **renal ultrasonography**: Doppler studies to detect renal artery stenosis or thromboembolism; large kidneys in diabetes, hydronephrosis, amyloidosis, renal vein thrombosis; small kidneys in chronic renal failure (CRF)
- **renal biopsy**: light and electron microscopy with immunofluorescence.
- **Establish chronicity:**
  - **renal ultrasonography**: small in CRF
  - **calcium and phosphate**: unreliable but hyperphosphataemia and hypocalcaemia usually associated with CRF
  - **parathyroid hormone**: raised in CRF
  - **haemoglobin**: normochromic/normocytic anaemia secondary to failure of erythropoietin synthesis in CRF
  - **chest radiograph**: annular calcification of mitral or aortic valves.

2. *How may prerenal failure be distinguished from acute tubular necrosis?*

In the early stages of renal failure resulting from prerenal causes, tubular concentrating power is retained, whereas in acute tubular necrosis (ATN) it is lost. Prerenal insults will eventually result in ATN, making this distinction impossible.

Prerenal	ATN
Urine sodium < 10 mmol/l	Urine sodium > 10 mmol/l
Urinary osmolality > 500 mosmol/l	Urinary osmolality < 400 mosmol/l
Urine:plasma osmolality > 1.1	Urine:plasma osmolality < 1.1

3. How does diabetes cause renal failure?

- **Genetic factors**: the Wisconsin cohort study demonstrated that metabolic control did not differ between patients with diabetes and patients without nephropathy. Furthermore a high number of patients with diabetes did not develop the nephropathy, despite long-term, severe, chronic hyperglycaemia. It is becoming increasingly evident that genetic factors are important in the development of renal failure in diabetes, although these are not yet clearly characterised.
- **Microvascular disease**: diffuse or nodular glomerulosclerosis may result from high glucose indirectly stimulating an increase of *TGF-β1* gene expression (TGF-β is transforming growth factor β), thus modulating both human mesangial cell proliferation and mesangial matrix production. Once glomerular damage has occurred, tubulointerstitial injury ensues as a direct consequence of proteinuria.
- **Macrovascular disease**: haemodynamic dysfunctions in patients with diabetes are represented by blood arterial hypertension, glomerular hypertension and hyperfiltration, renal artery atherosclerosis and thromboembolic renal disease (leading to papillary necrosis).
- **Infection**: recurrent pyelonephritis results in a stepwise decline in renal function and infection is thought to contribute to diabetic papillary necrosis.

4. What is papillary necrosis and what causes it?

The papillae of the medulla are the regions of the kidney most anatomically vulnerable to ischaemia. These necrose with a clearly demarcated line between viable and non-viable tissue, and eventually fall off. This gives rise to characteristic appearances on intravenous urogram (IVU) of a filling defect in the pelvic-alyceal system (the detached papilla) and forniceal widening and calyceal clubbing, where papillae have detached. In advanced disease interstitial fibrosis develops with accompanying renal insufficiency.

Although the final common pathway is probably ischaemia, the exact mechanism of necrosis is unclear and varies according to cause (*mnemonic*: postcard):

- **p**yelonephritis
- **o**bstruction
- **s**ickle cell disease
- **t**uberculosis
- **c**irrhosis
- **a**nalgesic nephropathy (paracetamol and aspirin)
- **r**enal vein thrombosis
- **d**iabetes.

Evidence of previous or current renal replacement therapy

Dialysis patients (and transplant recipients) bear a storybook of scars from previous dialysis access and its complications. The good candidate will elicit this history from the examination:

- **Arteriovenous (AV) fistulae**: these are placed, in order of preference, in the wrist of the non-dominant arm > cubital fossa of the non-dominant arm > wrist of the dominant arm > cubital fossa of the dominant arm. A thrill can be felt over a functioning fistula and a bruit should be easily heard.
- **Permanent cuffed tunnelled catheters**: the right internal jugular is the preferred site for haemodialysis catheters. Left-sided catheters follow a more tortuous route to the SVC and this can affect flow rates. Look for multiple scars at both exit sites (over the upper chest) and incisions at the base of the neck.
- **Subcutaneous 'buttonhole' ports**: these recently invented dialysis catheters have terminals lying just beneath the skin. The skin re-grows over the port between sessions, reducing the likelihood of infection.
- **Dacron/PTFE (polytetrafluoroethylene) grafts**: these have a more uniform shape and a less distensible texture on palpation compared with AV fistulae. They are often sited in the groin, if arm sites have been exhausted by multiple previous fistulae.
- **Tenckhoff catheters**: these are usually sited just above the umbilicus in the midline. Look for the scars of previous lines in all patients with evidence of renal disease – continuous ambulatory peritoneal dialysis (CAPD) is used in the UK to a much greater degree than in the USA.

Signs of complications of access and long-term dialysis

- **Horner syndrome**: patients who have had multiple lines inserted are at risk of Horner syndrome as a result of damage to the cervical sympathetic chain.
- **Dilated superficial veins**: multiple central venous stenoses or thromboses are not uncommon in long-term haemodialysis patients reliant on central venous tunnelled catheters. This can result in unmistakeable superficial varicosities over the chest wall.
- **Digital ischaemia**: radiobrachiocephalic steal syndromes may occur after an AV fistula is fashioned in the arm. Patients with diabetes are particularly vulnerable to impaired blood supply to the fingers if this occurs.
- **Abdominal hernias**: about 15% of patients on long-term CAPD develop abdominal wall hernias. Umbilical hernias occur more commonly than inguinal ones. High-volume exchanges and APKD are key risk factors for herniation.
- β_2-**Microglobulin amyloidosis**: the earliest manifestation is often carpal tunnel syndrome – look for the scars of a previous carpal tunnel release or wasting of the thenar eminence. It may then progress to amyloid arthropathy, which manifests initially in the shoulders followed by the

knees, wrist and small joints of the hands. Chronic joint swelling or evidence of joint destruction may be seen.
- **Malnutrition**: protein loss through peritoneal dialysis is a significant problem. Make a subjective global assessment of nutritional status (estimate BMI, subcutaneous fat and extent of muscle wasting).

Questions

1. What is the preferred form of access for haemodialysis?

AV fistulae are the optimum means of access because they carry a low risk of infection and provide good blood flow rates. Permacath tunnelled lines are usually effete by 5 years because of infection or reduced flow secondary to intraluminal build-up of bacterial microfilm. They also impose limitations on a patient's lifestyle such as no swimming or bathing.

2. What are the complications of peritoneal dialysis?

- **Bacterial peritonitis**: peritonitis is the most common cause of CAPD failure. Each patient has about a 50% chance of developing peritonitis each year. The earliest warning is often the patient reporting clouding of the drained peritoneal fluid. A white cell count and culture of peritoneal dialysate fluid confirm the diagnosis. Recurrent episodes of peritonitis reduce the efficiency of the peritoneum as a dialysis exchange membrane and the efficacy of dialysis. Recurrent or chronic peritonitis can result in sclerosing encapsulating peritoneal disease and secondary obstruction.
- **Abdominal hernias**: see above.
- **Protein loss and malnutrition**: see above.
- **Diabetes**: CAPD relies upon the osmotic pressure exerted by glucose in the dialysate to remove water across the peritoneal membrane. A significant proportion of this glucose is absorbed, which poses a problem for patients with diabetes. New non-glucose peritoneal dialysis solutions may offer the solution to this problem in the near future.
- **Mechanical failure**: kinking of the catheter, leakage at the exit site and pain due to contact with the abdominal viscera can all result in unsuccessful CAPD.

3. What are the advantages and disadvantages of CAPD over haemodialysis?

Advantages	Disadvantages
Simple to learn	Time-consuming exchanges
Ambulatory	Peritonitis
Haemodynamic tolerance	Protein loss
Few dietary restrictions	Excessive glucose load
	Sterile technique needed
	Peritoneum vulnerable to injury

Current function of the transplanted kidney

Clues pointing towards a failing transplant include the following:

- Signs of fluid overload
- Hypertension
- Tenderness over the graft (suggesting chronic rejection)
- A tunnelled line for haemodialysis
- Signs of uraemia (uraemic frost, fetor, distal sensorimotor neuropathy)
- Cushingoid features (evidence of recent high-dose steroid therapy used to manage a period of rejection).

Questions

1. *What are the causes of graft failure?*

- Rejection:
    - **Hyperacute**: this is immediate and antibody mediated. The graft must be removed to prevent a severe systemic inflammatory response (hyperacute rejection is unresponsive to immunosuppressive therapy). The recipient has usually been presensitised to HLA in the donor graft by blood transfusion, pregnancy or previous transplantations. Complement-mediated small vessel thrombosis and graft ischaemia characterise the final common pathway of hyperacute rejection.
    - **Acute**: T-cell-mediated destruction of the graft is mostly interleukin-2 (IL-2) mediated and usually responds to increasing immunosuppressive therapy. A patient may have several episodes of acute rejection.
    - **Chronic**: antibody-mediated graft destruction can continue insidiously despite apparently adequate immunosuppression. The arterial endothelium is involved, resulting in ischaemia and fibrosis.
- Surgical: stenoses at the vascular or ureteric anastomosis and ureteric leaks can occur in the immediate postoperative period or develop later. Haematomas and lymphoceles can exert significant pressure effects and cause vascular and ureteral compromise.
- Disease recurrence: nearly all diseases causing ESRF can recur in the graft with the exception of
    - Alport syndrome
    - polycystic kidney disease
    - hypertension
    - chronic pyelonephritis
    - chronic interstitial nephritis.

    However, only 5% of graft loss is the result of recurrence of the original disease. Diseases that commonly recur are listed in the table on page 19.

High risk of early graft failure contraindicating transplant	High risk of recurrence with shortened graft lifespan	High risk of recurrence but unlikely to cause graft dysfunction within 10 years
Haemolytic uraemic syndrome (idiopathic or inherited)	Primary hyperoxaluria	Diabetes mellitus
Mesangiocapillary glomerulonephritis		Cystinosis
Focal segmental glomerulosclerosis (partially contraindicated)		Amyloidosis
		Anti-GBM disease (Alport syndrome, crescentic glomerulonephritis, vasculitides)
		IgA nephropathy
		SLE
		Membranous glomerulonephritis

2. *What are the absolute contraindications to receiving a renal transplant?*

Clinical guidelines:

British Transplantation Society (BTS) and the Renal Association (RA) guidelines 2006:

- Predicted patient survival < 5 years
- Predicted risk of graft loss > 50% at 1 year
- Patients unable to comply with immunosuppressant therapy
- Immunosuppression predicted to cause life-threatening complications (eg malignancy, chronic viral infection).

However:

- Patients with severe vascular access problems could be considered for transplantation even if their overall prognosis for survival is < 5 years.
- Patients with BMI > 30 have significantly poorer graft and patient survival after transplantation.

---

3. *What are the survival rates after renal transplantation?*

About 80% of cadaveric grafts are functional at 5 years with an associated 85% patient survival rate. Living donor transplants have a slightly better outcome, with 88% of grafts functional at 5 years and 90% of patients alive at 5 years post-transplantation.

Evidence for immunosuppressive therapy

The following are signs that may be evident in PACES.

Ciclosporin and Tacrolimus (Calcineurin Inhibitors)

- Gum hypertrophy
- Sebaceous gland hypertrophy and acne (especially in males)
- Alopecia
- Tremor
- Hirsutism.

Corticosteroids

- Cushingoid appearance
- Proximal weakness
- Recent fracture.

Azathioprine

- Cholestatic jaundice.

Infection

- HSV (herpes simplex virus): shingles
- CMV (cytomegalovirus): lymphadenopathy, pyrexia of unknown origin (PUO), splenomegaly pneumonitis, retinitis (but often clinically silent)
- PCP (*Pneumocystis jiroveci* pneumonia): signs of pneumonia, desaturation < 90% on exercise.

Malignancy

- Skin and lip squamous carcinomas
- Lymphoma
- Post-transplantation lymphoproliferative disorders (PTLD).

Questions

1. What are the mechanisms of action and major toxicities of immunosuppressive agents used after kidney transplantation?

Ciclosporin is a polypeptide of 11 amino acids of fungal origin. It acts through calcineurin inhibition, thus preventing production of IL-2 and T-helper cell recruitment and activation. Adverse effects include the following:

- Nephrotoxicity (dose related)
- Hyperlipidaemia
- Glucose intolerance.

Tacrolimus is a macrolide antibiotic that also works through calcineurin inhibition. Adverse effects include the following:

- Nephrotoxicity
- Neurotoxicity
- Glucose intolerance (worse than with ciclosporin)
- QT prolongation (patients must avoid grapefruit juice).

Azathioprine is an anti-metabolite derivative of 6-mercaptopurine. It reduces DNA and RNA synthesis, thus limiting immune cell turnover. Adverse effects include the following:

- Pancreatitis
- Hepatitis and/or cholestasis
- Myelosuppression: leukopenia, thrombocytopenia.

Corticosteroids inhibit all stages of T-cell maturation and activation. They also prevent IL-1 and IL-6 production by macrophages. Adverse effects include the following:

- Cushing's disease,
- Osteoporosis
- Avascular necrosis
- Glucose intolerance
- Hyperlipidaemia.

Basiliximab and **daclizumab** are humanised monoclonal antibodies that target the IL-2 receptor. Hypersensitivity reactions have been reported with both.

2. How is immunosuppressive therapy used after kidney transplantation?

Clinical guidelines

Adapted from NICE (2007) guidelines.

INDUCTION THERAPY

This is a course of intensive immunosuppression 2 weeks immediately post-operatively that aims (1) to reduce the chance of accelerated rejection and (2) to reduce exposure to nephrotoxic calcineurin inhibitors in the early stages after transplantation, when the graft is most vulnerable.

Agents: basiliximab or daclizumab (usually in combination with ciclosporin).

INITIAL THERAPY (0–3 MONTHS)

This 'triple therapy' is given to all recipients for 0–3 months after transplantation.

Agents: calcineurin inhibitor (traditionally ciclosporin but increasingly tacrolimus), prednisolone, azathioprine.

MAINTENANCE THERAPY (LIFELONG)

The graft becomes immunologically more stable with time as tolerance develops. Maintenance therapy is thus similar to initial therapy but at much reduced doses. The occurrence of side effects and toxicity often presages several alterations in the combination of drugs and dosage.

ACUTE REJECTION THERAPY

The standard strategy for controlling a period of acute rejection is a course of high-dose corticosteroids. If this fails, monoclonal antibody agents may be used at induction. Switching from ciclosporin to high-dose tacrolimus can also be effective.

3. *What is PTLD and how is it treated?*

The term PTLD includes many tumours, ranging from B-cell hyperplasia to immunoblastic lymphoma. The overwhelming majority are B-cell proliferations associated with EBV infection. All cases carry a high mortality. Around 50% of cases occur in the first year after transplantation and have a poorer prognosis. Symptoms and signs are often non-specific and include fever (about 60%), lymphadenopathy (about 40%), gastrointestinal symptoms (about 30%), glandular fever syndrome (about 20%) and weight loss (about 10%). Nearly all organs and systems can be affected. A high index of suspicion is therefore necessary to make the diagnosis.

The cornerstone of treatment involves reduction or cessation of immunosuppression (replacing it with corticosteroid therapy). Further treatment includes radiation for localised disease, CHOP (cyclophosphamide–hydroxydaunorubicin–vincristine [Oncovin]–prednisone) combination therapies and recombinant interferon α (IFN-α).

SCENARIO 2. POLYCYSTIC KIDNEY DISEASE

Examination

Signs similar to 'Scenario 1. Transplanted Kidney' plus the following:

- Bilaterally (or unilaterally) palpable kidneys OR evidence of renal replacement therapy/transplantation and bilateral or unilateral nephrectomy scar
- Irregular hepatomegaly (50% have associated liver cysts but these are only large volume in women with severe renal disease)
- Neurological deficit (5–10% prevalence of intracranial aneurysms versus 1% in general population)
- Hypertension: ask to measure the blood pressure.

A good candidate

The good candidate will assess and comment on the following:

- Other causes of a renal angle mass that they would like to exclude
- The presence or absence of associated features (liver disease, neurological deficit, hypertension)
- The stage of disease (evidence of renal replacement therapy, previous or current transplant).

Other causes of a renal angle mass that they would like to exclude

Make a point of explaining why the mass is not a liver or a spleen:

- Can get above it
- Ballottable
- Is not notched
- Irregular surface
- Minimal movement inferiorly with inspiration
- Resonant to percussion as a result of overlying bowel (ie retroperitoneal).

Other cause of a mass in the same region

- **Renal cell carcinoma**: these patients present with haematuria, flank pain and/or a flank mass. The most common form of presentation is as an incidental finding on ultrasonography or CT. Look for associated lymphadenopathy and cachexia, the latter being a common paraneoplastic finding even in non-metastatic disease.
- **Hydronephrosis**: smooth enlargement is clinically detectable only in severe cases. An associated palpable bladder suggests bladder outlet obstruction.
- **Adrenal mass**: phaeochromocytoma and adrenal carcinoma.
- Retroperitoneal soft tissue tumours.

Questions

1. What are the indications for surgical intervention in polycystic kidney disease?

- Massive cysts > 40 cm
- Recurrent abdominal pain
- Transplant work-up (to make room for the graft)
- Recurrent infection of cysts
- Possible malignancy.

2. What inherited conditions are associated with renal cystic disease?

- **Tuberous sclerosis**: 20% of patients will develop single or multiple renal cysts but fewer than 5% develop severe disease with hypertension and ESRF. Renal angiomyolipomas and renal cell carcinomas are also more common in this condition.
- **Von Hippel–Lindau disease**: inherited mutation of the von Hippel–Lindau (VHL) tumour-suppressor gene gives rise to cyst formation in the kidney, pancreas, liver and epididymis. Of these patients, 70% develop renal cell carcinoma. The oncogenesis of renal cell carcinoma in genotypically normal patients involves somatic mutation of the VHL gene in 50% patients.
- **Autosomal dominant polycystic kidney disease (ADPKD)**: defects in *PKD1* and *PKD2* genes give rise to faulty polycystin proteins, but a 'second hit' acquired mutation is required in the normal allele to give rise to cyst formation (hence the onset in adulthood).
- **Autosomal recessive polycystic disease**: the gene for fibrocystin (*PKHD1*) is defective, resulting in faulty embryogenesis of the collecting tubule (and biliary defects invariably resulting in liver disease). Neonatal presentation is with pulmonary hypoplasia secondary to oligohydramnios. Childhood presentation is similar to adult polycystic disease with hypertension and renal insufficiency.

Acquired forms of cystic disease include simple cysts (benign) and medullary cystic disease (which leads to progressive renal failure).

3. What is the screening process for relatives of patients with ADPKD?

Clinical guidelines

Genetic testing is now available for family members but the *PKD1* and *PKD2* genes are large and mutations at multiple different sites can give rise to cystic disease. Mutations in *PKD1* account for the vast majority (85%) of cases. The genetic test is around 70% sensitive.

The bedrock of screening family members remains ultrasonography after 18 years of age. Over the age of 20 this is 99% sensitive for *PKD1* disease, but lower for the rarer *PKD2*.

The presence or absence of associated features (liver disease, neurological deficit, hypertension)

Expect to find these with the following frequency:

- **Liver cysts** occur in up to 70% of cases but significant involvement and hepatomegaly are almost entirely restricted to female patients with severe renal disease.
- **Intracerebral aneurysms** have up to 15% prevalence but the relative incidence of subarachnoid haemorrhage (SAH) is around four times greater than in the general population.
- Hypertension is almost universal once kidneys are palpable. It is detectable in 70% of adults before cysts can be detected on ultrasonography. Cysts overproduce both renin and angiotensin, and are often removed for this reason during transplantation to prevent hypertensive damage to the graft.
- **Mitral valve prolapse** is present in around 25% of patients; significant mitral regurgitation is present in 13%. *If you suspect polycystic kidney disease, tell the examiner during your summing up that you would like to examine the precordium.*

Question

1. *What are the benefits of screening for intracerebral aneurysms in polycystic kidney disease?*

- The relative increased risk of SAH in polycystic kidney disease is 4.4. However, no studies have identified any clear benefit in screening. Invasive tests (cerebral angiography) and interventional radiological therapies are not without significant risk of causing more harm than benefit.
- Current guidelines (although there is no consensus) are that those patients with a positive family history of SAH should undergo screening.

The stage of disease

Approximately 60% of patients develop ESRF by the age of 70, with a mean age of onset at 57. Of the remaining 40% of patients at least half will have hypertension. Look for:

- Evidence of renal replacement therapy
- Evidence of previous or current transplanted kidney
- Evidence of ESRF (see page 12)
- Evidence of other organ involvement
- Evidence of longstanding hypertension (eg left ventricular hypertrophy).

Question

1. *How is APKD managed?*

- The non-hypertensive patient should have regular monitoring of blood pressure, renal function and regular renal ultrasonography to anticipate local complications.

- Recurrent infections may require antibiotic prophylaxis and infected cysts may require drainage.
- Hypertension should be managed aggressively (dual risk of SAH) with ACE inhibitors or angiotensin II antagonists.
- Liver disease, if severe, can be managed with ultrasonically guided drainage or surgical de-roofing of cysts. In rare cases liver transplantation may be required.
- Intracranial aneurysms require treatment if there is a history of SAH.

SCENARIO 3. CHRONIC LIVER DISEASE

Examination

Face
- Yellow sclerae
- Pale conjunctivae
- Kaiser–Fleischer rings (Wilson's disease)
- Xanthelasmas (primary biliary cirrhosis or PBC)
- Parotid swelling/squaring of face (alcoholic liver disease).

Hands
- Clubbing
- Leukonychia
- Kolionychia
- Palmar erythema
- Liver flap
- Dupuytren's contracture (alcoholic liver disease)
- Needle-track sites (viral hepatitis).

Abdomen
- Hepatomegaly
- Splenomegaly
- Caput medusa
- Venous hum
- Testicular atrophy.

Neck and chest
- Spider naevi
- Scratch marks
- Absence of body hair
- Gynaecomastia
- Tattoos (viral hepatitis)
- Barrel-shaped chest (α_1-antitrypsin deficiency).

Other
- Oedema
- Glove-and-stocking sensory loss
- Slate-grey skin (haemochromatosis).

A good candidate

The good candidate will assess and comment on the following:

- The likely aetiology of liver disease
- Evidence of decompensated liver function.

The likely origin of liver disease

This is frequently discernible from careful attention to the stigmata.

Remember that dual pathology is common and alcohol accelerates any cirrhotic process. Say that you would like to take a full history of alcohol consumption whatever the suspected underlying cause.

Questions

1. *What investigations would you perform on a patient presenting for the first time with evidence of chronic liver disease?*

- **Establish cause**:
    - Viral hepatitis serology:
        - hepatitis B surface antigen (HBsAg)
        - hepatitis C antibody (HCV IgG)
    - Metabolic disorder screen:
        - haemochromatosis (serum ferritin > 500 µg/l, transferrin saturation > 50%, total iron-binding capacity (TIBC), free serum iron, followed by *HFE* genotyping if positive
        - Wilson's disease: serum copper/24-hour urinary copper, caeruloplasmin
        - α_1-antitrypsin deficiency – α_1-antitrypsin level followed by genotyping if low
    - Autoimmune liver disease:
        - PBC – anti-mitochondrial antibodies, ANA
        - autoimmune hepatitis – ANA, anti-smooth muscle antibody (ASMA), anti-liver–kidney microsomal antibody (ALKMA), anti-soluble liver antigen antibody (ASLA), rheumatoid factor
    - Liver biopsy (if cause remains unclear and clotting permits; transjugular liver biopsy may be necessary if prothrombin time [PT] is prolonged).

- **Establish severity**:
  - LFTs:
    - bilirubin, ALT (alanine transaminase), AST (aspartate transami
      GGT (γ-glutamyltransferase), ALP (alkaline phosphatase)
  - FBC:
    - Hb (microcytic anaemia in gastrointestinal blood loss; mean
      corpuscular volume [MCV] raised if ongoing drinking or
      hypersplenism)
    - platelets (low in portal hypertension)
    - WCC (white cell count) (susceptibility to sepsis)
  - Clotting profile: PT measures liver synthetic function
  - Renal function:
    - urea – often low even in renal failure
    - creatinine – hepatorenal failure carries a very poor prognosis
  - EEG/tests for subclinical encephalopathy (five-pointed star, reverse
    counting)
  - Ultrasonography of right upper quadrant (RUQ): establish abnormal
    echotexture (signal compared with right renal cortex – if more
    echogenic suggests cirrhosis); exclude focal lesions (in conjunction with
    α-fetoprotein); establish if portal hypertension present (splenomegaly)
  - OGD (oesophago-gastro-duodenoscopy): surveillance for varices
    (guideline below).

2. *What are the indications for liver biopsy in chronic liver disease?*

Clinical guidelines (Grant et al. 2004)

Note that in those conditions where biopsy is diagnostic, accurate non-invasive tests already exist. The main role of biopsy remains staging of disease and stratifying patients according to risk of end-stage liver failure and thus determining therapy and monitoring.

...ng utility of biopsy)

	...cated in the diagnosis and before cessation of ...pressive treatment in those in remission
	...ndicated in cases with clinical signs of chronic liver disease ...ovious cause on testing
	...ul before initiation of therapy to establish stage of fibrosis
	...ly useful only in clinical trials
	...en that only biopsy can accurately identify steatohepatitis (and ...erefore risk of fibrosis), there is an argument for biopsy in all cases of ...atty liver. This would have major resource implications
Haemochromatos...	Emergence of genetic testing and advanced biochemical markers means biopsy rarely necessary
Wilson's disease	There are no pathognomic histopathological features of Wilson's disease, so biopsy is rarely useful
Primary biliary cirrhosis	AMAs sufficiently sensitive and specific to exclude need for liver biopsy
Primary sclerosing cholangitis	Diagnosis is usually by ERCP or MRCP. Small duct disease may require liver biopsy

AMA, anti-mitochondrial antibodies; ERCP, endoscopic retrograde cholangiopancreatography; MRCP, magnetic resonance cholangiopancreatography; NAFLD, non-alcoholic fatty liver diseases; NASH, non-steatotic hepatitis.

Evidence of decompensated liver function

Any patient with the following is likely to have decompensated liver function:

- Jaundice
- Ascites
- Encephalopathy.

Many candidates wrongly interpret evidence of portal hypertension (splenomegaly, caput medusa) as a sign of decompensation. Liver size is an unreliable indicator of the severity of underlying cirrhosis or liver function – remember, almost any combination of normal or enlarged liver and spleen can occur in cirrhosis.

Questions

1. How is chronic liver disease classified according to severity?

The Child–Pugh classification is important in determining prognosis and fitness for treatment – particularly antiviral therapies. It was initially devised in the context of fitness for surgery

The individual scores are summed and then grouped as:

Score	1	2	3
Bilirubin (μmol/l)	< 34	34–50	> 50
Albumin (g/l)	> 35	28–35	< 28
PT – control PT (ie seconds prolonged)	< 4	4–6	> 6
Encephalopathy	Subclinical/none	Grade 1	Grade 2–3
Ascites	None	Moderate	Severe/diuretic resistant

- < 7 = A – associated 10% perioperative mortality rate
- 7–9 = B – associated 30% perioperative mortality rate
- > 9 = C – associated 82% perioperative mortality rate.

Class A patients have a greater than 90% 6-month survival rate, whereas class C patients with a score > 12 have a 40% 6-month survival rate. Although several of the scores are biochemical the good candidate can make conclusions as to the minimum Child–Pugh score according to clinical features, eg a jaundiced patient with ascites and a liver flap must have at least Child–Pugh class B disease.

2. *What are the guidelines for varices surveillance and treatment in chronic liver disease?*

Clinical guidelines (Jalan and Hayes 2000)

The two most important factors that determine risk of a variceal bleed are the Child–Pugh class severity and size of varices on endoscopic examination.

Grading of varices:

Grade 1: varices that collapse to inflation of the oesophagus with air
Grade 2: varices between grades 1 and 3
Grade 3: varices that are large enough to occlude the lumen.

- Following successful eradication of the varices at the index presentation, endoscopy should be repeated at 3 months and every 6 months thereafter. In case of recurrence of varices, they should be treated with variceal banding. If banding is not available, sclerotherapy should be used.
- β Blockade with propranolol (irrespective of the success of eradication therapy) is recommended.
- Patients who re-bleed despite these measures should be considered for transhepatic portosystemic shunting (TIPSS). This reduces the risk of re-bleeding to a much greater degree than banding but is associated with an approximately 30% risk of encephalopathy.

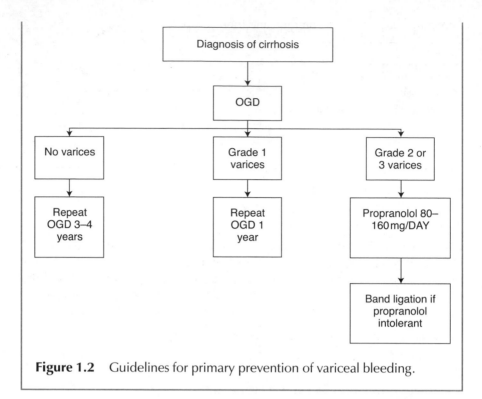

Figure 1.2   Guidelines for primary prevention of variceal bleeding.

3. How is ascites in chronic liver disease treated?

Clinical guidelines (Runyan 2004)

An initial therapeutic paracentesis (with salt-poor human albumin replacement) should be performed in patients with tense ascites and then the following:

- Salt restriction (refer to dietician) to < 2 g/day.
- Spironolactone to induce sodium excretion of more than 78 mmol/day (a spot urine sample can be taken and, if the sodium level is greater than the potassium level, this corresponds to adequate natriuresis). If this is achieved and ascites persists, furosemide should be added.
- Fluid restriction is unnecessary unless serum sodium is < 125 mmol/l.
- Patients should be considered for liver transplantation if appropriate.

Diuretic-resistant ascites occurs when renal impairment prohibits increasing diuretics or ascites simply does not resolve despite maximal therapy. Serial paracentesis and TIPS are potential therapeutic options while liver transplantation is expedited.

SCENARIO 4. PRIMARY BILIARY CIRRHOSIS

Examination

As for chronic liver disease but the following usually apply:

- Middle-aged woman
- Xanthelasma
- Jaundice
- Scratch marks
- Sicca syndrome (xerophthalmia, xerostomia).

Rarely:

- Kaiser–Fleischer rings.

A good candidate

The good candidate will assess and comment on the following:

- The factors favouring PBC over other aetiologies and how to confirm the diagnosis
- Evidence of decompensated liver function/estimate of minimum Child–Pugh score
- Efficacy of disease control, ie scratch marks as evidence of insufficient anti-pruritic therapy, xanthelasma as evidence of inadequate cholesterol control.

Factors favouring PBC over other aetiologies and how to confirm the diagnosis

State that you would request AMAs to confirm the diagnosis of PBC and AMA subtype analysis to determine prognosis. Liver biopsy is not necessary if these are positive because their specificity and sensitivity are greater than 95%.

Anti-gastric parietal cell antibodies are positive in 60% of cases, ANAs in 20% and ASMAs in 50%.

It is also worth mentioning that you would have a low threshold for testing for other associated autoimmune conditions:

- Hashimoto's thyroiditis
- Systemic sclerosis
- Sjögren syndrome
- Coeliac disease.

All these share 'lethargy' as part of their symptom complex with PBC.

Question

1. What are the pathological hallmarks of PBC and what is the aetiology?

The aetiology remains obscure. Researchers are divided into several camps, broadly separated into those who believe that the AMAs play a pathogenic role and those who believe that these antibodies are an irrelevant epiphenomenon. The existence of an almost identical disease entity, 'autoimmune cholangitis', that is histologically and clinically inseparable from PBC, but lacks AMAs, suggests that the latter group may be correct. The pathological hallmark is cholestasis (caused by destruction of small intrahepatic bile ducts), eventually leading to fibrosis and cirrhosis.

Evidence of decompensated liver function: see above.

Note that, in estimating the Child–Pugh score in patients with PBC, the relative contribution of jaundice is de-emphasised by an upward shift in the ranges that attract 1, 2 or 3 points.

Efficacy of disease control

Treatment of PBC

- **Cholestasis** is treated with ursodeoxycholic acid, which delays the progression to cirrhosis, improves biochemical markers of cholestasis (bilirubin, ALP, GGT) and can improve symptoms of lethargy and pruritus.
- **Pruritus** is treated initially with cholestyramine (bile acid sequestrant) and antihistamines but for many patients this is inadequate. Oral naltrexone (an opiate antagonist) is effective second-line therapy. Rifampicin may be of benefit but may cause deterioration in liver function. Plasmapheresis and MARS (molecular adsorbent recycling system) have been used with varying efficacy in severe cases. Finally, severe uncontrollable pruritus in PBC is an indication for liver transplantation.
- **Hypercholesterolaemia** can be safely treated with statins (while monitoring for a deterioration in LFTs). Xanthelasma may regress if cholesterol is successfully lowered.
- **Osteoporosis** occurs in PBC independently of vitamin D malabsorption. The mechanism seems to involve reduced bone deposition rather than more rapid bone resorption. Calcium supplements and bisphosphonates are the mainstays of treatment.
- **Fat-soluble vitamin deficiency** resulting from poor bile salt excretion (or depletion caused by cholestyramine) is present in 20% and treated with oral vitamin supplements. Coeliac disease should be excluded in the presence of steatorrhoea or fat-soluble vitamin deficiency.

Question

1. What investigations are useful in determining prognosis?

A poorer prognosis can be expected in the following:

- Patients with a high bilirubin level
- Women compared with men
- High anti-M2 and anti-M4 AMA subtype concentrations
- PBC in patients with only anti-M9 AMA subtype tends to run a benign, non-progressive course.

SCENARIO 5. HEREDITARY HAEMOCHROMATOSIS

Examination

As for chronic liver disease but the following may also be present in hereditary haemochromatosis (HH):

- Middle-aged (or older) men (twice as common in men as in women)
- Slate-grey skin pigmentation
- Evidence of arthritis
- Evidence of diabetes: look for insulin injection sites
- Evidence of cardiomyopathy: displaced apex, signs of congestive cardiac failure
- Venesection marks in the cubital fossa.

A good candidate

The good candidate will assess and comment on the following:

- The signs favouring haemochromatosis over other aetiologies and how they would go about confirming the diagnosis
- Evidence of extrahepatic manifestations of haemochromatosis
- Evidence of decompensated liver function/estimate of minimum Child–Pugh score.

Signs favouring haemochromatosis and how to confirm the diagnosis

Indirect serological markers of iron stores – state that you would initially request the following:

- Fasting serum free iron
- TIBC
- Ferritin level.

The fasting free iron and TIBC determine the transferrin saturation; a value > 50% has a sensitivity of 92% and specificity of 93% for HH. If the cut-off is lowered to 45% the sensitivity increases to 100%, but this also detects liver disease associated with secondary iron overload such as alcohol-induced liver disease, hepatitis C and NASH.

A raised (> 50%) transferrin saturation and/or raised ferritin (> 1000 ng/ml) warrant *HFE* gene status testing. Of all patients with iron overload:

- 90% will be homozygous for the *C282Y* mutation
- 5–6% will be compound heterozygotes for the *C282Y* and *H63D* mutations
- the remainder will have 'non-*HFE*'-associated iron overload.

Note that half of cirrhotic patients with HH will have normal LFTs. Liver biopsy was therefore previously indicated in patients either aged over 40 (fibrosis is rarely present before this age) or with raised transaminases in order to rule out other causes of liver disease and assess the degree of hepatic iron concentration and fibrosis (both useful prognostic indicators). However, the role of biopsy is increasingly being supplanted with MRI (magnetic resonance imaging) which can assess both fibrosis and iron content.

In patients with the *HFE* gene mutations, a fasting glucose, luteinising hormone (LH), follicle-stimulating hormone (FSH), testosterone level, AP radiology of both hands and echocardiography are crucial screening tests for extrahepatic manifestation of the disease (see below).

Questions

1. Which groups of patients should be tested for haemochromatosis?

Clinical guidelines (Tavill 2001)

- Symptomatic:
    - unexplained liver disease or a known cause of liver disease with abnormality of one or more indirect serum iron markers
    - type 2 diabetes mellitus with hepatomegaly or elevated liver enzymes, atypical cardiac disease or early onset sexual dysfunction early onset atypical arthropathy, cardiac disease and male sexual dysfunction.
- Asymptomatic:
    - first-degree relatives of confirmed cases
    - patients with abnormal serum iron markers discovered by chance
    - asymptomatic disordered LFTs or hepatomegaly.

HFE mutations (compound heterozygotes or homozygotes) have a population incidence of 1 in 200. There is a compelling case for screening of the general population.

---

2. What is the treatment for HH?

- Regular phlebotomy (once or twice a week) is the mainstay of treatment, removing 1 unit of blood on each occasion (about 250 mg iron) and aiming for a target ferritin level of 50 ng/ml. This may take many years. Maintenance phlebotomy (up to 1 unit a month) then continues lifelong, monitoring carefully for iron deficiency.
- Hypogonadism and arthropathy tend not to improve with phlebotomy, whereas insulin requirements may fall and cardiac function improve.

- Fibrosis does not reverse after phlebotomy and the risk of HCC (hepatocellular carcinoma) remains. HCC accounts for 30% of all deaths in haemochromatosis, so regular surveillance (ultrasonography and α-fetoprotein levels) is necessary.
- Decompensated liver disease and early HCC are indications for liver transplantation. The survival rates are lower than transplantation for other forms of liver disease, coexistent cardiomyopathy and susceptibility to infection.
- Cardiac dysrhythmias are a common cause of death in HH and preventive measures should be taken when there is evidence of cardiomyopathy (eg anti-arrhythmics and/or ICD [implantable cardiac defibrillator]).

Evidence of extrahepatic manifestations of HH

These are common and (with the exception of arthropathy and cardiac arrhythmias) usually occur in tandem with cirrhosis.

Skin hyperpigmentation	70%
Hypogonadism	50%
Amenorrhoea	15%
Diabetes mellitus	50%
Arthropathy	70%
Cardiomyopathy	15–30%
ECG abnormalities/arrhythmias	35%

Question

1. *What distinguishes the arthropathy of HH from other causes of arthritis?*

- HH arthropathy typically begins at the first metacarpophalangeal (MCP) joint causing a characteristic squaring of the joint.
- Chondrocalcinosis (calcium pyrophosphate deposition) is seen in the menisci and articular cartilage on radiograph and distinguishes HH arthropathy from osteoarthritis.
- Unlike osteoarthritis, the arthropathy is usually difficult to control with non-steroidal anti-inflammatory drug (NSAID) therapy.
- Joint deformity is rare.

Evidence of decompensated liver function/estimate of Child–Pugh score

See chronic liver disease (p. 27).

SCENARIO 6. ALCOHOL-INDUCED LIVER DISEASE

Examination

As for chronic liver disease but look for the following:

- Parotid swelling and squaring of the jaw
- Dupuytren's contractures
- Peripheral neuropathy (tell the examiner that you would like to exclude this)
- Facial flushing
- Three to four times more likely to be a man than a woman.

A good candidate

The good candidate will assess and comment on the following:

- The factors favouring alcohol as the aetiology of liver disease and how they would confirm the diagnosis
- Any evidence of decompensated liver function/estimate of minimum Child–Pugh score
- Other alcohol-related pathologies that must be excluded
- Nutritional status.

Factors favouring alcohol as the aetiology of liver disease

State that you would like to take a full alcohol history (see page 192) and send a liver screen (see above) to exclude dual pathology. This is crucial not only because viral hepatitis is more prevalent among people with alcohol problems but also because alcohol will dramatically accelerate other cirrhotic processes.

Questions

1. What are the current department of health guidelines on safe weekly alcohol consumption?

Clinical guideline

The Department of Health recently stated that 3–4 units a day for men and 2–3 units a day for women were probably safe. This raised the weekly recommended limit from 21 to 28 for men and from 14 to 21 for women respectively. The previous limits of 21 and 14 units were recommended by a joint committee from the Royal Colleges of Physicians, GPs and Psychiatrists.

---

2. What pharmacological treatments are available for alcohol dependence?

Treatment for alcohol dependence is a two-stage process involving detox-ification followed by rehabilitation. Traditionally the former was pharmacologi-cally managed (chlordiazepoxide) and the latter the domain of support workers and psychotherapists.

However, naltrexone and acamprosate have been shown in several trials and meta-analyses to be useful adjuncts to traditional rehabilitative methods:

- Naltrexone is an opioid receptor antagonist and is thought to reduce the reward effect of alcohol. Its major drawback is dose-related hepatotoxicity, making it contraindicated in those with active hepatitis or decompensated liver disease.
- Acamprosate normalises the altered *N*-methyl-D-aspartate (NMDA)-mediated glutamatergic excitation that occurs in alcohol withdrawal and early periods of abstinence.

The COMBINE trial is currently under way to assess the efficacy of both agents together.

Evidence of decompensated liver function and estimate of minimum Child–Pugh score

See Chronic liver disease, pages 30–31.

Other alcohol-related pathologies that must be excluded

Cardiac

- **Dilated cardiomyopathy**: an impaired ejection fraction can be demonstrated in a third of patients drinking 70 g or more alcohol each day for more than 20 years. A third of all cases of dilated cardiomyopathy are alcohol related.
- **Hypertension**: drinking 4 units of alcohol a day doubles the risk of hypertension compared with teetotallers. There is a dose-related increase in blood pressure above this level of consumption.

Gastrointestinal

- **Acute/chronic pancreatitis**: alcohol increases the viscosity of luminal secretions, resulting in ductal obstruction with upstream inflammation, fibrosis and atrophy. Some 5–10% of people with alcohol problems develop chronic pancreatitis, accounting for 60% of all cases.
- **Peptic ulcer disease**: alcohol has been shown to increase the risk of developing ulcers and to delay ulcer healing
- **Oral, oesophageal and gastric cancers** are all more common in those who drink heavily.

Nervous system

- **Cerebellar atrophy**: increased sway is found in up to 70% of people with chronic alcohol problems and ataxia in around a third. There seems to be little correlation with peripheral neuropathy, suggesting a different pathogenesis in the loss of cerebellar Purkinje cells compared with peripheral neurons.
- **Polyneuropathy**: using DSM-IV (*Diagnostic and Statistical Manual of Mental Disorders*, 4th edn) criteria to define chronic alcoholism, one study found that 58% of patients had some form of polyneuropathy. Typical features include:
  - reduced sensation to pinprick stimulation in stocking-and-glove distribution
  - reduced tendon reflexes, especially the ankle
  - reduced distal power, eg plantar flexion
  - gait ataxia.
- **Marchiafava–Bignami disease**: the pathological hallmark of this disease is necrosis of the corpus callosum. The key sign is apraxia of the non-dominant hand, indicating interhemispherical disconnection.
- **Wernicke's encephalopathy**: alcohol reduces thiamine absorption by up to 50%, which combined with malnutrition can lead to negligible thiamine levels and myelin degeneration in the brain stem. The incidence can be as high as 12% in patients with alcohol dependence. Only a minority of patients (10%) present with the classic triad of global confusion, ophthalmoplegia and ataxia.
- **Korsakoff syndrome**: permanent anterograde and retrograde memory loss may remain after the initial confusion characterising Wernicke's encephalopathy has resolved. Patchy retrograde memory loss results in confabulation, whereas anterograde formation of memories is often severely impaired.

Nutritional status

The evidence that malnutrition is a major factor in the morbidity and mortality of alcoholism is vast. Indeed, only 30 years ago it was thought to be the principal mechanism of liver cirrhosis.

Look for muscle wasting, subcutaneous fat loss and oedema. If any of these is present, state that you suspect malnutrition and would like to:

- take a full dietary history (or refer to dietician!) and determine if there is a history of weight loss and its time-scale
- calculate the BMI.

Question

1. What is re-feeding syndrome?

This was first described in severely malnourished prisoners of war in the Far East. It was observed that resumption of feeding after prolonged starvation was associated with the development of heart failure.

During prolonged periods of starvation insulin levels drift very low as the body switches from carbohydrate metabolism to protein and fat metabolism. This can result in intracellular phosphate depletion (while serum levels may remain normal). On re-introduction of carbohydrates there can be rapid cellular uptake of phosphate, resulting in hypophosphataemia. Levels < 0.5 mmol/l can result in disruption of crucial phosphorylation cascades and ATP metabolism, resulting in cardiac dysfunction, arrhythmias, respiratory failure and sudden death.

Monitoring serum phosphate and magnesium levels (and replacing deficiencies) after commencing nasogastric feeding is crucial in any high-risk patient. This includes all patients with alcohol dependence.

SCENARIO 7. CHRONIC VIRAL HEPATITIS

Examination

As for chronic liver disease but look for the following:

- Signs of current intravenous drug use
- Tattoos/piercings
- Age and nationality (see below).

A good candidate

The good candidate will assess and comment on the following:

- The factors favouring a viral aetiology of liver disease
- Any evidence of decompensated liver function/estimate of minimum Child–Pugh score
- Further tests that they would like to confirm the diagnosis and assess disease stage and prognosis.

Factors favouring a viral aetiology

Three distinct epidemiological trends in hepatitis C are evident world wide. In developed western countries, the peak prevalence is among patients aged 30–49, consistent with the greatest risk of exposure among intravenous drug users 15–20 years ago. In developed countries in the Far East (eg Japan) the hepatitis C-positive population is far older, consistent with exposure some 50 years ago – probably as a result of re-use of medical equipment without sterilisation. Ongoing hepatitis C infection is observed in all age groups in developing countries, caused primarily by healthcare-related procedures rather than intravenous drug use or high-risk sex.

In hepatitis B, country of birth is the most significant risk factor.

A significant (and rapidly rising) proportion of hepatitis B and C in this country is therefore a result of immigration rather than the stereotypical groups with high risk factors. Be wary, therefore, of the traditional tattoo/piercing/injection mark doctrine of hepatitis risk.

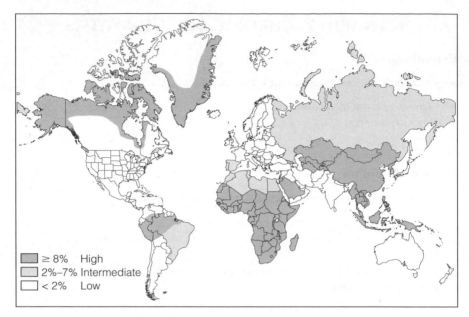

Figure 1.3   Hepatitis B surface antigen prevalence.

Question

1. What are the principal modes of transmission of chronic hepatitis?

Hepatitis B (similar to HIV but higher rates of transmission for equal exposure)	Hepatitis C
Vertical transmission	Blood products
Sexual contact	Needle sharing
Needle sharing	
Blood products	

Evidence of decompensated liver function/estimate of Child–Pugh score

See Chronic liver disease, pages 30–31.

Further tests that would confirm the diagnosis, assess stage and prognosis

Note that with improved EIA (enzyme immunoassay) tests for hepatitis C, the false-positive rate has dropped, thus rendering the RIBA (radioimmunoblot assay) test less useful.

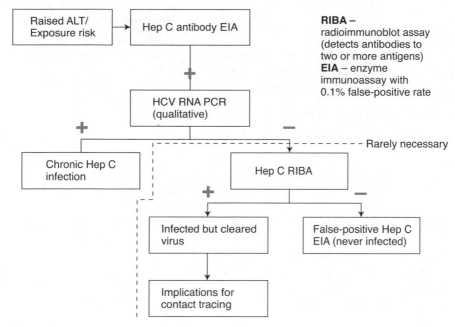

Figure 1.4 Hepatitis C diagnosis and staging: algorithm.

Figure 1.4 ensures the most rapid and cost-effective means of differentiating false positives, chronically infected patients and those who have been infected but have cleared the virus. Once the diagnosis of chronic infection is established, disease must be staged to assess whether treatment is indicated.

The decision of who, when and how to treat is complex. Treatment is unpleasant and associated with serious side effects, and around half of patients with chronic hepatitis C will not progress to cirrhosis. The following are the key factors in the initial assessment:

- Liver histology and liver function tests
- Presence of contraindications
- Quantitative HCV (hepatitis C virus) level by PCR (polymerase chain reaction) testing
- Genotype.

Liver histology (assessing inflammation and fibrosis) and the presence or absence of contraindications assess suitability, genotype and viral load, and determine the duration of therapy.

Contraindications to combination therapy with pegylated interferon and ribavarin:

- Depressive illness or psychosis
- Untreated autoimmune thyroid disease

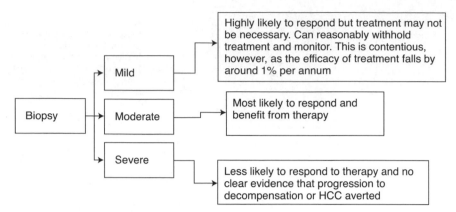

Figure 1.5   Decision-making in hepatitis C therapy by disease stage.

- Neutropenia and/or thrombocytopenia
- Organ transplantation other than liver
- Symptomatic heart disease
- Decompensated cirrhosis
- Uncontrolled seizures
- Evidence of ongoing alcohol or intravenous drug abuse.

All such guidelines are controversial, eg some clinicians believe that all the patients with hepatitis C and mild inflammation (including ongoing intravenous drug users) should be treated to reduce the risk of infecting others.

Treatment for hepatitis C

The mainstay of therapy is pegylated interferon (P-IFN) and ribavarin. The pegylation of IFN results in sustained therapeutic levels and a more convenient one-a-week injection. The addition of ribavarin has markedly increased the rates of sustained viral response (SVR) – the goal of therapy. This is defined as a negative HCV PCR test 6 months after cessation of treatment.

In brief, genotype 1 or high-level viraemia HCV is treated for 12 months but often terminated at 6 months if quantitative HCV PCR indicates ongoing viraemia (ie treatment failure). Other genotypes can be treated for 6 months alone. Female patients must have a pregnancy test before therapy and use contraception for at least 6 months after combination therapy. Monitoring during therapy involves regular psychological assessment, urinalysis, serum chemistry, FBC and thyroid function tests.

This is a rapidly changing field with new protease inhibitors (eg telapravir) set to dramatically increase response rates. Management in a specialist viral hepatitis clinic is essential.

Hepatitis B diagnosis and staging

After an acute hepatitis B infection (which may rarely lead to fulminant liver failure) 90% of patients will become HBsAg negative and HBsAb positive (hepatitis B surface antigen and antibody, respectively) by 6 months (ie permanently clear the virus and attain immunity from further infection). The remainder will go on to have chronic hepatitis B, which may be active or inactive.

Phases of infection may last many years and include:

- Immunotolerance, in which viral replication is high but the inflammatory response is negligible. This usually occurs in childhood infection or vertical transmission. Patients will go on to develop active disease in adulthood.
- Active disease ('e' antigen positive) in which both viral replication and the immune response is active.
- Carrier state ('e' antigen negative) which follows development of anti-HBeAb (hepatitis B 'e' antibody) and suppression of viral replication. This should not be considered 'inactive' disease because most patients will reactivate at some stage and therefore require close monitoring.
- The 'e' antigen-negative active disease (precore mutant), which occurs when the virus loses the ability to secrete 'e' antigen but maintains a high degree of replication. This may result from primary infection with a precore mutant virus or by mutation of a wild-type virus. A number of carriers may develop reactivated disease by this mechanism.

Treatment for hepatitis B

Knowing a patient's phase of infection is crucial to determining whether treatment is needed and the aim of treatment, which, on the whole, is to prevent progression to cirrhosis or HCC.

In 'e' antigen-positive hepatitis B the aim of treatment is to encourage HBeAg seroconversion to the inactive carrier state with its associated benign prognosis.

In 'e' antigen-negative hepatitis (precore mutants) this is not possible, and the desired end-point is to keep HBV replication as low as possible.

Treatment consists initially of short-term therapy with pegylated IFN-α. About a third of patients with HBeAg-positive disease will undergo HBeAg seroconversion to the 'e' antigen-negative inactive carrier state with this therapy. Those who fail short-term therapy may seroconvert with long-term nucleoside analogue therapies, which are rapidly improving.

IFN therapy is contraindicated in decompensated cirrhosis, hence oral nucleoside analogue therapy is the only treatment option in this scenario. Use of these drugs before liver transplantation (in addition to HBsAb IgG infusion perioperatively) has dramatically reduced the rates of reinfection in the donor liver, to the extent that the subsequent prognosis is as good as liver transplantation for any other indication.

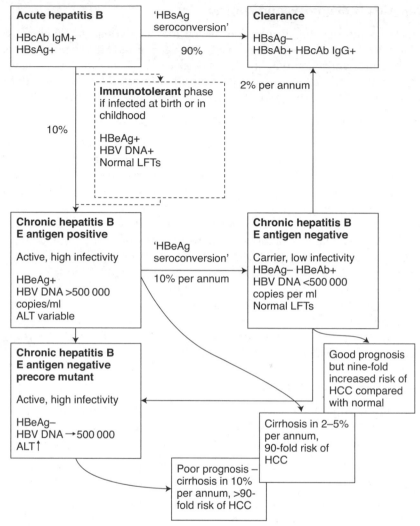

Figure 1.6   Infectivity status (commonly seen in hepatitis B).

This should not be considered 'inactive' disease because most patients will reactivate at some stage and therefore require close monitoring.

Questions

1. What advice would you give a patient who has just been diagnosed with hepatitis C?

Clinical guideline (Booth et al. 2001)

- The natural history is slowly progressive (median time to cirrhosis is about 30 years).
- They should not donate blood, organs, tissues or semen.
- The risk of sexual transmission is small – maximum of 5%, but possibly much less. Barrier contraception advised.
- Transmission from mother to child is rare.
- Breast-feeding is not contraindicated.
- Excess alcohol consumption (50 g/day) hastens progression.
- Avoid third party contact with blood by not sharing toothbrushes and razors and by covering open wounds.

---

2. What are the success rates of treatment?

Genotype 1, treatment-naïve patients have around 50% SVR rate after 48 weeks of combination therapy. This is likely to improve to 70% with telapravir if this drug attains full FDA (US Food and Drug Administration) and NICE approval. Genotype 2 or 3 patients have around 80% SVR rate after 24 weeks of combination therapy.

3. What are the adverse effects of treatment?

Some 75% of patients experience at least one side effect:

- Interferon: bone-marrow suppression, neuropsychiatric disorders, autoimmune disorders (particularly thyroid) and flu-like symptoms are the principal complications.
- Ribavirin: haemolysis and teratogenicity are the principal complications. Patients are at greater risk of gout.

4. What are the extrahepatic manifestations of viral hepatitis?

- **HBV:**
  - polyarteritis nodosa
  - glomerulonephritis and nephrotic syndrome
  - 'arthritis–dermatitis' syndrome
  - palpable purpura.
- **HCV:**
  - essential mixed cryoglobulinaemia
  - lymphoma
  - glomerulonephritis
  - porphyria cutanea tarda
  - diabetes mellitus
  - autoimmune phenomena
  - peripheral neuropathy.

SCENARIO 8. AUTOIMMUNE HEPATITIS

Examination

As for chronic liver disease but look for the following:

- Usually a middle-aged woman
- Signs of thyroid disease
- Signs of rheumatoid arthritis
- Signs of scleroderma.

A good candidate

The good candidate will assess and comment on the following:

- The factors favouring an autoimmune aetiology of liver disease and how you would confirm the diagnosis
- Any evidence of decompensated liver function/estimate of minimum Child–Pugh score
- Other autoimmune conditions that he or she would like to exclude.

Factors favouring autoimmune hepatitis and how to confirm the diagnosis

Autoimmune hepatitis (AIH) may present as one of the following:

- Acute hepatitis: tender hepatomegaly, fever and jaundice
- Chronic hepatitis: serendipitous finding of abnormal LFTs
- Cirrhosis: presents with decompensation (ascites, jaundices, variceal bleed, encephalopathy).

The last presentation is the most likely to be encountered in PACES. Such patients are likely to be or have been on corticosteroid therapy so look for:

- cushingoid features,
- evidence of previous fractures
- steroidal skin purpura.

Diagnosis of AIH

Liver biopsy is the most important test when AIH is suspected. There is a high degree of overlap with other conditions (PBC, PSC [primary sclerosing cholangitis], autoimmune cholangitis) which can be differentiated only histologically. Autoantibodies help differentiate between three main types of AIH.

Type 1	ANA, anti-smooth muscle antibody (ASMA)
Type 2	Anti-liver–kidney microsomal (ALKM)
Type 3	Anti-soluble liver antigen (ASLA)

Type 2 is rare in adults. Types 1 and 3 have similar responsiveness to steroids, female predominance (80%), rates of other autoimmune disease (40%) and raised polyclonal γ-globulin. Type 3 is, however, more likely to progress to cirrhosis.

Serum electrophoresis and immunoglobulins will detect a polyclonal expansion of IgG.

Transaminases are crucial to the monitoring of response to therapy, although it must be noted that up to 50% of patients with normal LFTs have ongoing inflammation on histology. Histological resolution tends to lag behind biochemical remission by 3–6 months.

Questions

1. What is the aetiology of AIH?

Autoimmune cell-mediated hepatocyte destruction is caused by aberrant expression of normal liver cell membrane constituents on HLA class II surface molecules of hepatocytes. The triggers for such aberrant expression may be viral infection (HAV, HBV, EBV) or medications (eg nitrofurantoin, melatonin, methyldopa). HLA-DR3 predisposes patients to more aggressive disease, whereas HLA-DR4 appears to increase the likelihood of extrahepatic manifestations.

2. How is AIH treated?

Clinical guidelines (Czaja and Freese 2002)

Indications for Treatment

- AST more than tenfold upper limit of normal or more than fivefold with an IgG level more than twofold normal
- Bridging or multiacinar necrosis on liver biopsy
- Raised AST below criteria but symptomatic (fatigue, arthralgia, jaundice).

Steroids and azathioprine are the principal agents used. A reducing dose of steroids is used to initiate therapy followed by maintenance on low-dose steroids with azathioprine or monotherapy, depending on tolerance and side effects. Approximately 65% of patients respond to initial therapy and enter histological remission; however, 80% of these patients relapse after drug withdrawal within 3 years. Some clinicians thus advocate long-term maintenance therapy on azathioprine.

---

3. What is the prognosis in AIH?

Remission is rarely achieved in the first year of treatment. Of patients 80% achieve remission within 3 years. However, with immunosuppressant therapy the prognosis is good with 10-year survival rates of around 90% irrespective of the presence of cirrhosis at presentation.

Any evidence of decompensated liver function/estimate of minimum Child–Pugh Score

See Chronic liver disease, pages 30–31.

Other autoimmune conditions that he or she would like to exclude

AIH should be regarded as a multisystem disorder associated with a plethora of autoimmune diseases. These can be divided into intrahepatic ('overlap') and extrahepatic.

Intrahepatic 'Overlap' Conditions
- PBC about 7%
- PSC about 6%
- Autoimmune cholangitis
- Antibody-negative AIH.

Extrahepatic Associations
- Rheumatological:
  - rheumatoid arthritis
  - Sjögren syndrome
  - systemic sclerosis
- Endocrine:
  - Graves' disease
  - autoimmune thyroiditis
  - juvenile diabetes mellitus
- Gastrointestinal:
  - coeliac disease
  - inflammatory bowel disease
- Haematological:
  - haemolytic anaemia
  - pernicious anaemia
- Cardiological:
  - pericarditis
  - myocarditis
- Renal: glomerulonephritis.

SCENARIO 9. ISOLATED HEPATOMEGALY WITHOUT STIGMATA OF CHRONIC LIVER DISEASE

Examination

- Face:
  - flushing – carcinoid
  - pale conjunctivae – anaemia of chronic disease (amyloid, sarcoid) or malignancy
- Hands: clubbing
- Neck:
  - JVP raised/giant V waves
  - lymphadenopathy, Virchow's node
- Precordium: S3 or murmur of tricuspid regurgitation
- Abdomen:
  - hepatomegaly
  - pulsatile? – tricuspid regurgitation
  - smooth? – sarcoidosis, amyloidosis,
  - irregular? – malignant infiltration, polycystic, hyatid cysts
  - tender ? – acute hepatitis, Budd–Chiari syndrome
  - lymphadenopathy – malignancy
  - ascites (malignant, congestive cardiac failure [CCF], Budd–Chiari syndrome)
  - Sister Mary Joseph nodule
- Other:
  - cachexia – malignancy
  - fever – amoebiasis
  - ankle oedema – CCF.

Note that primary liver tumours are extremely rare in the absence of cirrhosis.

A good candidate

The good candidate will assess and comment on the following:
- The most likely aetiology
- How they would confirm the diagnosis.

The most likely aetiology

Hepatomegaly without stigmata of chronic liver disease (ie cirrhosis) has a narrow differential diagnosis. The most common causes (in the UK and in PACES) are the following:

- CCF (± tricuspid regurgitation)
- Metastatic malignancy.

Note that primary liver tumours are extremely rare in the absence of cirrhosis.

Rarer causes of isolated hepatomegaly include:

- Budd–Chiari syndrome
- Hydatid cyst
- Riedel's lobe
- Polycystic liver disease (usually with accompanying renal enlargement)
- Sarcoidoisis
- Amyloidosis
- Carcinoid.

Acute hepatitis is rarely encountered in PACES.

Questions

1. Is liver failure likely in CCF?

No. Liver biopsy rarely reveals signs of cirrhosis. Only 10% of patients become jaundiced and encephalopathy is extremely rare. Signs and symptoms of cardiac failure dominate the clinical picture, varying according to whether the underlying cause of hepatic congestion is CCF, cor pulmonale, pericardial disease or tricuspid incompetence.

2. What is the mechanism of jaundice in metastatic liver disease?

Obstructive jaundice is surprisingly rare. Jaundice is usually a consequence of massive infiltration and carries a very poor prognosis.

3. What is hydatid cyst disease?

Hydatid disease is a parasitic infestation by a tapeworm of the genus *Echinococcus*. In the UK the most common intermediate host is the sheep, hence the higher incidence of the disease in farming areas. Cysts grow most commonly in the liver (and lung) over many years. **Sequelae** include painful hepatomegaly, obstructive jaundice or rarely acute rupture with an associated anaphylactic response. Secondary infection can also occur. **Diagnosis** is by abdominal CT, which has the highest sensitivity and specificity. Serological tests have a sensitivity of 90% for hepatic echinococcosis and are a useful initial screening test. Treatment is with a 6-month course of albendazole and mebendazole.

4. What is Riedel's lobe?

This is a normal anatomical variant. It is not a true accessory lobe but a tongue-like projection of the right lobe of the liver that may extend downwards as far as the right iliac fossa. In one CT-based study that defined Riedel's lobe as a protuberance of the right lobe below the costal margin, the prevalence was 33% rising to 65% in patients aged over 50.

How the candidate would confirm the diagnosis

The initial investigation should be led by the clinical picture.

Cardiac disease

If there are signs of cardiac failure, initial tests should include:

- echocardiography
- chest radiograph
- liver ultrasonography (to exclude other pathology).

Irregular hepatomegaly

In the absence of cardiac signs liver ultrasonography is the best initial investigation. Further imaging may well be needed to distinguish benign from sinister lesions. Biopsy risks upstaging and seeding a malignant lesion in the biopsy tract, and should be undertaken only if tumour markers are negative and imaging has failed to distinguish the nature of the lesion.

CT, MRI and laparoscopy with intraoperative ultrasonography are all useful modalities in further characterising hepatic lesions.

Smooth Hepatomegaly

Budd–Chiari syndrome often presents with ascites and jaundice. Ultrasonography with Doppler flow examination of the hepatic veins reveals thrombus with a high sensitivity and specificity (90%). MRI with pulsed sequencing may clarify venous anatomy.

Sarcoidosis rarely presents with hepatomegaly alone, yet liver granulomas are present in up to 70% of patients with sarcoidosis *post mortem*. CT may reveal the coalescing granulomas apparent as multiple hypointense or hypoattenuating nodules. In the context of other clinical features of sarcoid (eg pulmonary involvement) no further investigation is necessary to confirm hepatic sarcoid. However, multiple nodules in hepatic sarcoidosis are easily mistaken for metastases or lymphoma and screening for malignancy may be required.

Secondary amyloidosis caused by excessive serum amyloid A (AA) secretion in chronic inflammatory conditions is the most common form affecting the liver. By the time that there is hepatomegaly there are usually signs of renal impairment (anaemia, hypertension and oedema). The presence of macroglossia, CCF, peripheral neuropathy or carpal tunnel syndrome suggests AL amyloid. Rectal biopsy with Congo red staining (displaying apple-green birefringence on polarised light examination if amyloid is present) has an 80% sensitivity. Liver biopsy is rarely undertaken because of the high risk of bleeding or rupture.

Carcinoid syndrome is suggested by irregular hepatomegaly in combination with skin flushing and telangiectasias. Liver metastases must occur before symptoms develop. A dietary history may reveal specific foods that induce flushing. Investigations:

- Elevated urinary 5-hydroxyindole acetic acid (5HIAA)
- Elevated plasma chromogranin A

- Octreotide scanning (scintigraphy with labelled octreotide) is the gold standard diagnostic test. It is highly sensitive and specific and also predicts the degree to which a patient will respond to octreotide treatment.

Question

1. *What benign lesions of the liver may be confused with malignancy on ultrasonography or CT?*

- Haemangiomas
- Focal nodular hyperplasia
- Complex liver cysts
- Focal fatty infiltration/focal fatty sparing
- Hepatic adenomas
- Biliary hamartomas.

MRI with gadolinium contrast enhancement is often the best means of distinguishing these lesions from primary or secondary liver malignancies.

SCENARIO 10. ASCITES WITHOUT STIGMATA OF CHRONIC LIVER DISEASE

Examination

Non-cirrhotic ascites, similar to isolated hepatomegaly, is usually the result of either CCF or intra-abdominal malignancy. The signs that you should look for are thus very similar to those in the previous scenario. In younger patients consider nephrotic syndrome (look for ankle oedema, hypertension, evidence of hypercholesterolaemia, evidence of DVT).

A good candidate

The good candidate will assess and comment on the following:

- The most likely aetiology
- The speediest and most efficient sequence of investigations for determining the cause.

The most likely aetiology

Rare causes include the following:

- Budd–Chiari syndrome: look for jaundice and hepatomegaly
- Tuberculous peritonitis: look at ethnic origin and lung signs
- Chylous ascites resulting from lymphatic obstruction.

Question

1. *What are the most common primary tumours leading to malignant ascites?*

- Ovarian (most common)
- Endometrial
- Breast
- Colon
- Gastric
- Pancreatic.

The speediest and most efficient sequence of investigations for determining cause

A diagnostic tap is the key investigation, requesting the following:

- **The plasma–ascites albumin gradient (PAAG):** this is calculated by subtracting the ascitic fluid albumin level from the plasma value. Values > 1.1 g/dl indicate portal hypertensive ascites. Values < 1.1 g/dl indicate non-portal hypertensive causes (infection or malignancy). This has almost 100% accuracy in discriminating between these two aetiological categories.

- **Cell count**: lymphocytic infiltrate suggests tuberculous or carcinomatous peritoneal disease, whereas neutrophils suggest bacterial peritonitis.
- **Culture/Gram stain** and stain for acid fast bacillis.
- **Cytology**: if an adequate sample is taken for centrifugation (about 500 ml) cytology has up to 75% sensitivity in detecting malignant cells.

Other useful investigations include the following:
- Echocardiography if CCF is suspected
- Abdominal CT if malignancy is suspected
- Breast examination ± mammography
- Diagnostic laparoscopy
- Ultrasonography: useful for tapping small-volume or loculated ascites.

Question

1. What are the therapeutic options for management of ascites?

The management of ascites in CCF is similar to that of chronic liver disease (see pages 27–32) with salt restriction and diuretics.

Malignant ascites is often painful and difficult to treat because of its resistance to chemotherapy and rapid reaccumulation after drainage. The usual life expectancy is less than 4 months, although this varies according to the underlying causes. Serial paracentesis is an appropriate means of controlling symptoms but care are must be taken to ensure adequate dietary protein replacement. Permanent exteriorised catheters and peritoneovenous shunts are other therapeutic options in patients with a longer life expectancy. These often become infected or blocked within 6 months.

SCENARIO 11.
HEPATOSPLENOMEGALY/SPLENOMEGALY
WITHOUT STIGMATA OF CHRONIC LIVER DISEASE

Examination

- **Head and neck:**
  - lymphadenopathy
  - alopecia (recent chemotherapy)
  - pale conjunctivae (anaemia caused by bone marrow failure)
  - tunnelled catheter (for chemotherapy)
  - jaundice (haemolysis)
  - butterfly rash (SLE)
- **Abdomen:**
  - smooth enlargement of liver and spleen
  - lymphadenopathy
- **Hands:** rheumatoid arthritis (Felty syndrome)
- **Other:**
  - petechial rash
  - shingles
  - bruises
  - evidence of bone marrow biopsy over iliac crest?

A good candidate

The good candidate will assess and comment on the following:

- The likely aetiology and differential diagnosis
- First-line investigations to confirm the diagnosis.

The likely aetiology

The differential diagnosis is vast and examiners are principally concerned that the candidate has a good grasp of the diagnostic possibilities and their categorisation. It is therefore imperative to have a clear diagnostic algorithm in your mind in order to determine the most likely differential diagnosis. A suggested schema is outlined below.

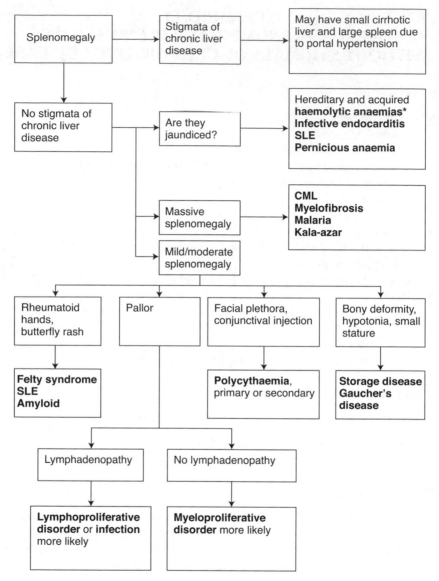

Figure 1.7   Suggested flow chart for determining cause of splenomegaly by clinical type. *All entries in bold are diagnosis.

There is rarely time for in-depth discussion about a particular aetiology but knowledge of basic investigations to confirm the diagnosis must be demonstrable.

The principal causes of hepatosplenomegaly or isolated splenomegaly without cirrhosis are usually:

- haematological
- infectious
- storage disorders
- inflammatory.

Haematological (Look for Anaemia)

- **Myeloproliferative:**
  Chronic myeloid leukaemia (CML):
  - massive spleen ± hepatomegaly
  - pallor
  Acute myeloid leukaemia (AML):
  - mild/moderate splenomegaly ± hepatomegaly
  - pallor
  - petechiae
  - tunnelled line for chemotherapy ± alopecia
  Myelofibrosis:
  - massive spleen ± hepatomegaly
  - pallor
  - evidence of gout
  Essential thrombocytosis (often no physical signs):
  - mild spenomegaly
  - bleeding diathesis
  - DVT
  - digital gangrene/ischaemia
  Polycythaemia rubra vera (PRV) – see page 65.
- **Lymphoproliferative:**
  CLL:
  - lymphadenopathy
  - mild/moderate splenomegaly ± hepatomegaly
  - pallor
  - petechiae
  Acute lymphoblastic leukaemia (ALL):
  - lymphadenopathy
  - mild/moderate splenomegaly ± hepatomegaly
  - pallor
  - purpura, petechiae
  - skin rash
  - fever
  - tunnelled line for chemotherapy ± alopecia
  Lymphoma:
  - lymphadenopathy
  - mild/moderate splenomegaly ± hepatomegaly
  - skin rashes (mycosis fungoides/Sézary syndrome)
  - abdominal mass (Burkitt's lymphoma).

Acute leukaemias are understandably rare in PACES. Note that, in the presence of marked lymphadenopathy, an underlying lymphoproliferative disorder is more likely than a myeloproliferative one.

The presence of splenomegaly, anaemia and jaundice in the absence of stimagata of chronic liver disease suggests a haemolytic disorder such as hereditary spherocytosis (see page 68).

Infectious

The most common causes of hepatosplenomegaly world wide are vanishingly rare in PACES:

- Malaria
- Kala-azar (abdominal leishmaniasis)
- Schistosomiasis
- TB.

In the UK more common infectious causes of hepatosplenomegaly are the following:

- Brucellosis (agriculture worker, neurological signs, skin rash)
- Leptospirosis with Weil's disease (jaundice, fever, muscle tenderness, positive Murphy's sign)
- Toxoplasmosis (cervical lymphadenopathy)
- Infectious mononucleosis (lymphadenopathy).

Storage disorders

- Gaucher's disease (bony deformity, previous fractures)
- Glycogen storage disease (small build, hypotonia, muscle atrophy).

Inflammatory

- Felty syndrome (look for rheumatoid features)
- Amyloid (look for evidence of chronic inflammatory disease).

Questions

1. *How does the extent of splenomegaly help differentiate the underlying cause?*

Mild (spleen just palpable)	• Infectious mononucleosis • Infective endocarditis	• Myeloproliferative disorders • Lymphoproliferative disorders • Cirrhosis and portal hypertension	• CML • Myelofibrosis • Malaria • Kala-azar*
Moderate (up to four finger breadths)			
Massive			

*These cases can also be listed under mild and moderate splenomegaly

2. What investigation would you perform to confirm the diagnosis?

Haematological	Myeloproliferative disorders	CML	Bone marrow sampling (BMS) cytogenetics: Philadelphia chromosome
		Myelofibrosis	Peripheral blood smear – leukoerythroblastosis with teardrop poikilocytosis BMS – reticular fibrosis
		AML	BMS > 20%blasts
		Essential thrombocytosis	Raised platelets BMS – hypercellular with giant megakaryocytes
		PRV	Increased red cell mass
	Lymphoproliferative disorders	CLL	Sustained WCC > 50 with lymphocytosis Lymph node/BMS required if transformation to lymphoma suspected
		Lymphoma	Lymph node biopsy, CT and BMS staging
		ALL	BMS > 30% lymphoblasts Cytogenetics for typing
Storage disorders	Glycogen storage disease		Liver/muscle biopsy
	Gaucher's disease		Reduced acid β-glucosidase activity in peripheral blood leukocytes Plain radiology to detect flask deformity of the distal femur
Inflammatory	Amyloid		Rectal biopsy
	Felty syndrome		Presence of rheumatoid arthritis, positive rheumatoid factor
Infectious	Schistosomiasis		Urine/stool egg count; serology cannot distinguish past from active infection
	Brucellosis		Serum tube agglutination test (developed in 1887!), blood cultures, PCR
	Toxoplasmosis		Detection of *Toxoplasma gondii* antigen in blood by ELISA (enzyme-linked immunosorbent assay)
	Kala-azar		Detection of antibodies to recombinant K39 antigen (ELISA) or PCR test for leishmaniasis DNA
	Malaria		Thick and thin blood films
	Infectious mononucleosis		Monospot test followed by EBV serology if negative
	Weil's disease		Blood cultures, microscopic agglutination test

3. What is the Philadelphia chromosome?

Chromosomal translocation of the *c-abl* oncogene, which encodes for a tyrosine protein kinase from chromosome 9 to the *bcr* locus of chromosome 22, resulting in markedly increased tyrosine kinase activity. This is the basis for malignant clonal expansion. The fusion gene mRNA can be detected extremely sensitively by PCR, which is useful for monitoring residual disease after therapy.

4. What is imatinib?

Imatinib (Glivec) is a tyrosine kinase inhibitor that has revolutionised the treatment of CML (and gastrointestinal stromal tumours or GISTs). It works by inducing apoptosis in cells with the *bcr/abl* fusion gene. It induces complete cytogenetic response in almost all patients in the chronic phase with 3-year survival rates around 95%. The results in the accelerated phase of CML are less impressive (30% complete response) but still a vast improvement over combination chemotherapy. Imatinib is also far better tolerated than older treatments.

SCENARIO 12. POLYCYTHAEMIA RUBRA VERA

Examination

- Middle-aged/elderly patient
- Splenomegaly/hepatosplenomegaly
- Facial plethora
- Scratch marks, hypertension
- Enlarged conjunctival vessels
  (dilated retinal veins on fundoscopy)
- Evidence of venesection
- Gout.

A good candidate

The good candidate will assess and comment on the following:

- How to diagnose PRV
- Evidence of complications or progression.

How to diagnose PRV

The following are common pitfalls in understanding and diagnosis of PRV:

- Although it takes its name from its associated erythrocytosis it is an expansion of three cell lineages including platelets and leukocytes. These result from the clonal expansion of a multipotent haematopoietic progenitor cell. The cause of this is unknown.
- Measuring red cell mass (with ^{51}Cr or chromium-51) is now rarely necessary since the discovery that JAK2 (janus kinase 2) mutations underlie nearly all cases of PRV.
- Bone marrow examination is not diagnostic.

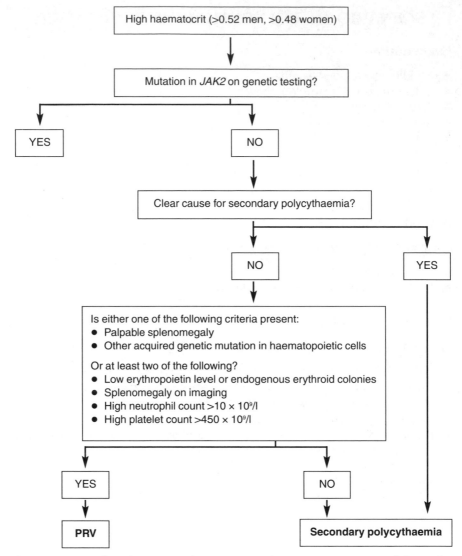

Figure 1.8   Polycythaemia Rubra Vera Study Group (PVSG) guidelines for diagnosis of PRV.

Questions

1. What is the treatment for PRV?

Phlebotomy is the mainstay of therapy, aiming to reduce red cell mass and viscosity. A haematocrit < 45% is the usual goal of therapy (this may require twice-weekly phlebotomy initially).

Hydroxyurea, in addition to phlebotomy, has been shown to reduce the risk of thrombosis compared with phlebotomy alone and is recommended in patients aged over 40.

2. *What is the prognosis in PRV?*

The grim prognosis of 50% survival rate at 18 months if untreated is largely drawn from poorly designed studies in the 1960s. Although referral for treatment should be immediate, PRV generally follows an indolent course. Some groups have presented data that, with adequate treatment and follow-up life expectancy, are not dissimilar to normal.

Evidence of complications or progression

- The principal complication of increased red cell mass and hyperviscosity is thrombosis. As a rule of thumb:
  - 40% present with a thrombotic episode
  - 40% of those who present by other means will eventually experience thrombosis
  - 40% die from a thrombotic complication.
- Arterial thrombosis is more common than venous and the central nervous system is most commonly affected (ie stroke).
- PRV is the leading cause of hepatic vein thrombosis (Budd–Chiari syndrome) in the UK.

Look for evidence of previous cerebrovascular accidents (CVAs; asymmetrical weakness, facial droop, inattention). Other complications include the following:

- Painful organomegaly
- Hyperuricaemia and gout (caused by increased cell turnover)
- Haemorrhage: counterintuitively, this probably occurs as a result of sequestration of von Willebrand's factor by an expanded platelet population.

Question

1. *What conditions can PRV progress to?*

Myelofibrosis occurs in approximately 5% of patients treated with phlebotomy alone and 8.4% in those treated with chemotherapy or radiotherapy. Cases of spontaneous resolution of myelofibrosis have been documented.

Acute leukaemias are probably a consequence of therapy rather than a natural progression of the disease, although this is controversial. Patients treated with radioactive phosphorous and chlorambucil are at greatest risk. Long-term hydroxyurea may also increase the incidence of acute leukaemia.

SCENARIO 13. HEREDITARY SPHEROCYTOSIS

Examination

Look for the triad of:

- splenomegaly
- jaundice
- pallor (anaemia).

The patient is usually of north European origin. Other features include:

- cholecystectomy scar
- splenectomy scar
- leg ulcers.

A good candidate

The good candidate will assess and comment on the following:

- Confirming the diagnosis and estimating the severity of disease
- Other causes of anaemia, jaundice and splenomegaly that he or she would like to exclude.

The severity of disease

Hereditary spherocytosis (HS) has mild, moderate and severe phenotypes:

- **Mild HS** occurs in 20% of cases but is rare in PACES because patients are asymptomatic and rarely have signs. These patients may present either with an aplastic crisis precipitated by infection or through family screening.
- **Moderate HS** accounts for three-quarters of all HS cases. These patients display the classic triad of splenomegaly, jaundice and anaemia. The inheritance is autosomal dominant.
- **Severe HS** occurs in only 5% of all patients. Patients have usually undergone splenectomy but the response is usually incomplete, so they may present in PACES with jaundice and anaemia. This is recessively inherited.

Initial investigations for HS should include the following:

- Reticulocyte count and haptoglobins
- Lactate dehydrogenase
- Split bilirubin
- Peripheral blood smear: may show megalocytosis and Howell–Jolly bodies (if the spleen has been removed).

The diagnosis is confirmed with an osmotic fragility test, which involves incubating blood in saline for 24 h at 37°C.

If there is evidence of an aplastic crisis:

- Vitamin B$_{12}$ and folate stores should be assessed to ensure that recovery is possible
- HSV, EBV and human papillomavirus (HPV) type 19 should be tested for as potential aetiological agents.

Questions

1. What is the pathogenesis of HS?

A number of red cell membrane proteins may be deficient or inadequately integrated. The most common defect in autosomal dominant HS is β-spectrin deficiency. This results in a characteristic spherical structure of erythrocytes, which are rapidly cleared in the spleen leading to (extravascular) haemolysis and splenic hypertrophy.

2. What are the complications of HS?

- Anaemia is the principal concern in HS and may require serial transfusions.
- Gallstones are found in 50% of patients with HS. Biliary colic and obstruction are frequent complications.
- Aplastic crises occur when bone marrow suppression (caused most commonly by infection or drugs) means that the high rate of destruction of erythrocytes can no longer be compensated by increased production.

3. How is HS treated?

Although splenectomy is clearly indicated in severe cases, the treatment of asymptomatic moderate HS is less straightforward. Splenectomy is curative in such cases but must be balanced against the associated 200-fold increase in mortality risk from sepsis. Partial splenectomy may offer a compromise between sustained immunoprotection and minimal ongoing haemolysis.

Post-splenectomy prophylaxis should include the following:

- Immunisation for pneumococci
- Immunisation for *Haemophilus influenzae* type b
- Immunisation for meningococci C
- Flu vaccine yearly
- Lifelong oral penicillin prophylaxis.

Other causes of anaemia, splenomegaly and jaundice to exclude

These are unusual but include the following:

- Infective endocarditis
- SLE
- Pernicious anaemia
- Infectious mononucleosis.

Normally you would expect associated stigmata of these systemic conditions to be apparent.

THE RESPIRATORY EXAMINATION

Data from previous candidates show that the following three cases account for over 65%:

1. Chronic airway disease with or without steroid use
2. Pneumonectomy (any cause)
3. Pulmonary fibrosis.

It is therefore essential to know these cases well. Remember that acute cases such as symptomatic pleural effusion, pneumothorax and acute asthma will not occur in the exam for obvious reasons. Despite this, pleural effusion should always be considered where there is dullness to the lung bases and a case is described below. Other cases that occur in < 10% include bronchiectasis, lung cancer and a thoracotomy scar.

In PACES, most of the respiratory cases involve chronic conditions that can be identified before auscultation. Therefore it is important to practise your observational skills, including of both the patient and the surrounding environment. As the chest is a relatively symmetrical structure, a careful inspection will usually reveal the side with pathology.

Approach to the patient

- Introduce yourself to the patient
- Ask if the patient has any pain
- Position the patient correctly (sitting up at 45°)
- Expose the chest, completely if possible
- Explain what you are going to do: 'I would like to examine your chest and lungs, if that is alright with you.'

Observation

- Observation alone will usually give clues to the origin of the pathological process.
- Look carefully around the bed for paraphernalia of respiratory disease, eg oxygen cylinders, inhalers, nebulisers, peak flow machines, steroid cards or sputum pots.
- Look at the patient – is he or she well/unwell, dyspnoeic at rest? Look for cyanosis, surgical scars (pneumonectomy, previous chest drains), steroids, failure to thrive (cystic fibrosis), cachexia (malignancy), productive cough (bronchiectasis), rashes (autoimmune disease and sarcoidosis), arthropathy (rheumatoid arthritis), bony abnormalities (pectus excavatum/carinatum).

- Stand at the end of the bed, with the patient's chest exposed, and watch the patient breathe. Note the respiratory rate, and the length of the inspiratory and expiratory phases of respiration. Inspiration is usually longer than expiration; this is reversed in emphysema.
- Are there signs of respiratory distress – tracheal tug, intercostal recession, use of accessory muscles?
- Ask the patient to take a deep breath in and out and look carefully for asymmetry.

Noting the presence of asymmetry at this stage immediately gives an advantage. You know that there is likely to be unilateral pathology on the side with reduced ventilation, eg pleural effusion, consolidation, collapse or pneumonectomy. If symmetry is maintained, consider pulmonary fibrosis, bronchiectasis or airway disease.

Hands

- Look for tar stains: COPD (chronic obstructive pulmonary disease) and malignancy
- Clubbing: idiopathic, fibrosis, malignancy and bronchiectasis
- Clubbing and swelling of the wrist: hypertrophic pulmonary osteoarthropathy (a rare paraneoplastic manifestation of lung cancer, with classic radiological changes)
- Warm vasodilated peripheries: carbon dioxide retention
- Cyanosis: central or peripheral
- Tremor: β-agonist therapy
- Asterixis/flap: dorsiflexed wrists with fingers spread out (carbon dioxide retention).

Pulse

- Bounding: carbon dioxide retention
- Tachycardia: infection and β-agonist therapy.

Face

- Conjunctival pallor
- Cushingoid facies
- Meiosis: Horner syndrome
- Plethora
- Lips/tongue: central cyanosis.

Neck

- Lymphadenopathy

- Jugular venous pulse (JVP) elevated with 'v' waves – right ventricular hypertrophy – cor pulmonale; if suspected examine for right ventricular heave and tricuspid regurgitation.

Inspection of the chest

Shape of the chest

- Barrel: an increase in the anteroposterior (AP) diameter (emphysema)
- Pigeon chest (pectus carinatum): outward bowing of the sternum (chronic childhood respiratory illness or rickets)
- Funnel chest (pectus excavatum): developmental defect with depression of the sternum
- Kyphoscoliosis: idiopathic or secondary to polio.

Trachea

- Place the index and ring fingers on the sternal notch
- Place the middle finger on the trachea. It should rest equidistant from the index and ring fingers if the trachea is central. The trachea may be slightly deviated to the right in normal people as a result of the straightness of the right main bronchus.

Causes of tracheal displacement

- Towards the lesion: upper lobe collapse, fibrosis or pneumonectomy/lobectomy
- Away from the lesion: large pleural effusion or tension pneumothorax.

Cardiac apex

- Displaced by pleural effusion/pneumothorax, although may be impalpable; also difficult to feel in patients with hyperexpanded chest
- Pulled towards side of collapse/pneumonectomy.

The chest

It may seem obvious that either the front or the back of the chest should be examined completely before proceeding to the other side. A full respiratory examination is quite tiring, especially with respiratory pathology, and thus the patient should not be moved unnecessarily.

Palpation

Palpate any deformity or lump.

Expansion

Assess the upper and lower chest separately:

- Upper chest: place hands lightly on the upper chest just below the clavicles. The hands should be felt to rise anteriorly. Feel for any asymmetry.
- Lower chest: place the hands on the lateral side of the lower ribs, with the thumbs pointing towards the midline. The thumbs may touch lightly in the midline, but this will depend on the size of your hands and the patient's chest. The thumbs should move symmetrically apart during inspiration. Normal expansion is 4–5 cm.

Percussion

Percuss the clavicles and then the lung fields. Compare left with right at each point, moving down the chest. Do not forget specifically to percuss in each axilla; it is the only place where the upper, middle (lingula on the left) and lower lobes can be examined together.

Tactile Vocal Fremitus (TVF)

Assess fremitus by asking the patient to say '99' while placing the border of the little fingers on the chest wall. Compare the left and right lungs simultaneously by using both hands; move down the chest wall from the top to the bottom.

Auscultation

Once again move down in a zigzag manner, asking the patient to breathe quietly through the mouth. Use the diaphragm of the stethoscope on the chest wall, but the bell for the supraclavicular area because it is smaller.

Breath sounds

One should be familiar with the following terms:

- Normal, ie vesicular
- Bronchial: noise transmitted to the chest wall from a large airway, eg consolidation or along the top of an effusion
- Decreased, eg emphysema
- Wheeze: always expiratory: mono-/polyphonic
- Stridor: always inspiratory and indicates extrathoracic obstruction
- Crackles: fine/coarse; inspiratory/expiratory
- Pleural rub: pleurisy secondary to a pulmonary embolus (PE) or pneumonia.

Vocal Resonance (VR)

This is analogous to TVF and can be performed as an alternative. Bronchophony is heard over consolidation or fibrosis as well as at the top of an effusion, because the large airway noise is transmitted directly to the chest wall. It sounds as if the words are spoken directly into your ear. However, it does provide additional information vis-à-vis bleating aegophony and whispering pectoriloquy above an effusion.

Summary of clinical findings in common respiratory cases:

	Collapse Local fibrosis Pneumonectomy	Consolidation	Effusion	COPD	Pneumothorax (large)	Bilateral fibrosis
Trachea	Deviated towards lesion	No change	No change; away if very large	No change	Usually central; may be deviated away	No change
Expansion	Reduced unilaterally	Reduced unilaterally	Reduced unilaterally	Reduced bilaterally (hyper-expanded)	Reduced unilaterally	No change
Percussion	Dull	Dull	Stony dull	No change	Hyperresonant	No change
TVF/VR	Reduced	Increased	Reduced (aegophony above)	No change	Reduced	No change
Breath sounds	Quiet	Bronchial breathing	Absent/ reduced	Variable Quiet ± wheeze	Absent/reduced	Fine end-inspiratory crackles

To finish

- Measure the peak expiratory flow rate
- Examine any sputum in a pot – quantity, colour (and traditionally smell)
- Thank the patient and help him or her dress.

Respiratory Scenarios

1. Idiopathic interstitial pneumonias
2. Pleural effusion
3. Bronchiectasis
4. Unilateral pulmonary fibrosis
5. Chronic obstructive pulmonary disease
6. Lung cancer
7. Thoracotomy scar

SCENARIO 1.
IDIOPATHIC INTERSTITIAL PNEUMONIAS

This 45-year-old man complains of worsening shortness of breath over the past 3 years. Please examine his respiratory system.

Idiopathic interstitial pneumonias (IIPs) are a group of conditions characterised by the expansion of the interstitial compartment of the lungs with inflammatory cells. Idiopathic pulmonary fibrosis (IPF; formerly known as cryptogenic fibrosing alveolitis) is the most common example of this and accounts for 60% of cases; however, there are six other types (see below). The cause is unknown although environmental factors (such as Epstein–Barr virus, EBV) and genetic factors (such as polymorphisms of tumour necrosis factor α, TNF-α) are thought to play a role. IPF is associated with a classic pathological pattern called usual interstitial pneumonia. It is a debilitating disease and the results of immunosuppressive therapy have been disappointing. Overall, patients have a median survival of 3 years. The pathological pattern described as usual interstitial pneumonia is not unique to IIP and occurs with asbestos exposure, connective tissue disease, hypersensitivity pneumonitis and drugs (see below).

There are seven forms of the IIPs, including the following:

1. IPF (most common, > 60%)
2. Non-specific interstitial pneumonia
3. Respiratory bronchiolitis interstitial lung disease
4. Desquamative interstitial pneumonia
5. Acute interstitial pneumonia (AIP; formerly Hamman–Rich syndrome)
6. Cryptogenic organising pneumonia
7. Lymphoid interstitial pneumonia.

Candidates will be asked to examine a patient's chest. The following findings will be consistent with a diagnosis of IIP, or other forms of lung fibrosis that cause a pathological picture consistent with usual interstitial pneumonia (such as connective tissue disease):

• There is an oxygen cylinder and mask with the patient.
• Does the patient have steroid purpura or Cushing syndrome?
• Finger clubbing is evident and the patient has central cyanosis; on examination of the chest the expansion is symmetrically reduced. TVF is increased (say if it is and with what distribution), and the percussion note is normal.
• On auscultation there are fine end-inspiratory crackles.

A good candidate

Will look for cardiac complications:

- Cor pulmonale: refers to right ventricular hypertrophy as a consequence of pulmonary disease; need to look for:
  - left parasternal heave
  - elevated JVP
  - prominent 'v' waves
  - peripheral oedema.

Conditions associated with IIP

- Autoimmune hepatitis: cirrhosis ± hepatomegaly
- Sjögren syndrome: dry eyes and mouth.

Other conditions associated with Usual Interstitial Pneumonia excluding the diagnosis of IIP

- Connective tissue disorders:
  - rheumatoid arthritis: deforming arthropathy (Caplan syndrome is fibrosing alveolitis associated with exposure to coal dust in patients who tend to be rheumatoid factor positive)
  - systemic sclerosis: typical appearance of the hands and face, telangiectasia
  - Sjögren syndrome
  - systemic lupus erythematosus (SLE)
  - ankylosing spondylitis
  - dermatomyositis: heliotrope rash, Gottren's patches and proximal myopathy
  - Behçet's disease
- Vasculitis: Goodpasture syndrome, Wegener's granulomatosis
- Neoplastic: lymphoma, micrometastases, lymphangitic carcinoma
- Sarcoidosis: lupus pernio and erythema nodosum
- Pneumoconiosis: asbestosis, silicosis, berylliosis and coal dust
- Extrinsic allergic alveolitis, eg bird fancier's or farmer's lung
- Radiation exposure
- Drugs, eg amiodarone, cytotoxics (bleomycin)
- Toxins: toxic gases (chlorine).

Patient's background

- A good occupational history as well as patient's hobbies/activities to exclude types of pneumoconiosis and extrinsic allergic alveolitis
- Family history: IPF and sarcoidosis are rarely familial
- Smoking history: Goodpasture syndrome is almost always associated with smoking
- Drug history: to exclude drug-induced DPLD (Diffuse Parenchymal Lung Disease).

Symptoms and signs

- Progressive dyspnoea with chronic unproductive cough
- Pleurisy: rare in IIP, more common in connective tissue disorders (SLE and rheumatoid arthritis)
- Haemoptysis: rare in IIP, more common in vasculitis
- Haematuria: vasculitis
- Arthritis: connective tissue disorders, sarcoidosis, vasculitis, Goodpasture syndrome
- Rash: connective tissue disorders, sarcoidosis, vasculitis
- Raynaud's phenomenon: IIP, systemic sclerosis
- Bilateral fine end-inspiratory crackles: common in IIP, asbestosis and connective tissue disorders; much rarer with sarcoidosis and extrinsic allergic alveolitis.

Investigations

Guidelines have been written for making the diagnosis of IPF in the absence of an open lung biopsy (which does not always need to be taken). If biopsies are performed (via open biopsy), several should be taken from different lobes.
The following four criteria are required to make the diagnosis of IPF in the absence of biopsy:

1. Exclusion of the known causes of interstitial lung disease (see above)
2. Restrictive pattern on spirometry
3. Reticular abnormalities on high-resolution computed tomography (HRCT)
4. Negative biopsy via bronchoscope.

Other investigations

- Chest radiograph: in early IPF the chest radiograph is often normal. Otherwise, reticulonodular shadowing, 'honeycomb lung' or reduced lung volumes can be seen. The chest radiograph can also point to other causes such as pleural plaques – asbestosis, bilateral hilar lymphadenopathy (BHL), joint changes in shoulder or dilated oesophagus.
- Respiratory function tests: restrictive defect with decreased gas transfer; sarcoidosis may show airflow obstruction.
- HRCT: essential for diagnosis if open lung biopsy is not performed; can detect fibrosis in presence of normal chest radiograph.
- Bronchoscopy and bronchoalveolar lavage: increased cells (lymphocytes carry better prognosis).
- Open lung biopsy: transbronchial or percutaneous biopsy may be required for histology and multiple sites should be biopsied.
- Serum precipitins to environmental allergens (eg avian proteins), full blood count or FBC (eosinophilia for extrinsic allergic alveolitis), renal and liver function tests (multiorgan-affecting systemic diseases).

- Serum ACE (angiotensin-converting enzyme) levels (diagnostic sensitivity of only 60% and poor specificity) and autoantibodies (e.g. antinuclear factor [ANF] and rheumatoid factor [RF]).
- Echocardiography (systemic sclerosis to assess pulmonary hypertension) and ECG (in patients with sarcoidosis).

Management

- The guidelines of the British Thoracic Society (BTS) stipulate that treatment of IPF and other types of IIP should be tailored to individual patients, taking into account the patient's informed wishes and with a respiratory physician being involved in the patient's care.
- There is a debate as to the usefulness of immunosuppressive drugs in this setting, which are of no clear proven benefit. Oral steroids may provide benefit; retrospective reviews show symptomatic improvement in 41–57% of patients. Female gender, less advanced disease, young age and biopsy samples showing increased cellularity show a positive correlation with response to steroids.
- Other immunosuppressant therapy has been used in the treatment of IIP patients who are unresponsive to steroids. There is no evidence to demonstrate that cyclophosphamide or azathioprine alone is effective. Only one study has been carried out comparing low-dose prednisolone and cyclophosphamide with high-dose prednisolone in the treatment of IPF, and no benefit was found. A controlled trial showed an increase in survival in IPF patients being treated with azathioprine and high-dose prednisolone, compared with just high-dose steroids. Other drugs include cholchicine, methotrexate, ciclosporin and penicillamine.
- The BTS recommend that management for IPF should begin with oral prednisolone 0.5 mg/kg coupled with azathioprine 2–3 mg/kg, with a slow or fast tail of prednisolone dependent on the patient's response. If the patient cannot tolerate steroids azathioprine should be used alone. If azathioprine cannot be tolerated cyclophosphamide must be used instead.
- Supplemental oxygen for advanced disease.
- Lung transplantation is an option in younger patients, with rapidly progressive disease having a 60% 1-year survival rate.
- Patients should be regularly followed up with chest radiographs and respiratory function tests under the care of a respiratory physician.

Questions

1. What is Hamman–Rich syndrome?

AIP (formerly known as Hamman–Rich syndrome) is an acute form that responds to steroids (in some series), but overall has a poor outcome.

2. What types of pneumonioses are you aware of?

- Silicosis: upper zone fibrosis, with eggshell hilar calcification that predisposes to TB (tuberculosis) infection
- Berylliosis: granulomatous lesions resulting in fibrosis; similar to sarcoid
- Asbestosis: predominantly affects lung bases; pleural plaques and associated mesothelioma
- Simple coalworkers' lung does not cause pulmonary fibrosis.

3. Describe the main features of sarcoidosis

A multisystemic granulomatous disorder characterised by over-activated T lymphocytes:

- Skin: erythema nodosum, lupus pernio
- Lungs: BHL, pulmonary nodules and fibrosis
- Lymphadenopathy, arthropathy and neuropathy
- Investigation: chest radiograph, serum ACE levels, tissue biopsy (Kveim test is outdated); gallium citrate scan may identify granulomatous disease.

4. Tell me what you know about extrinsic allergic alveolitis

After exposure there is inflammation of the bronchioles resulting in cough, pyrexia and malaise. If exposure becomes chronic it may cause increasing shortness of breath and non-caseating granulomatous disease. Treatment is with steroids in acute disease and long-term avoidance of precipitating factors. Causes of extrinsic allergic alveolitis:

- Bird fancier's lung: pigeons
- Farmer's lung: mouldy hay
- Byssinosis: cotton dust.

SCENARIO 2. PLEURAL EFFUSION

This 72-year-old woman has noticed increased shortness of breath and weight loss. Please examine her chest.

Points on examination

- Tachypnoeic
- Central trachea: a large effusion may push it away
- Apex: impalpable with left-sided effusion or displaced if on the contralateral side
- Expansion: decreased on the affected side
- Percussion: stony dull on the affected side
- Tactile fremitus or VR: decreased on the affected side
- Breath sounds: diminished on the affected side
- There may be whispering pectoriloquy ± bronchial breathing above the effusion
- Above the level of the effusion, 'bleating aegophony' may be heard.

A good candidate

- Will exclude lung collapse or lobectomy as a differential diagnosis and explain these findings to the examiners.
- Will be seen to look for potential causes of the pleural effusion.
- Will describe further investigations fluently.

Clues to the cause

- Malignancy: clubbing, tar staining, cachexia, Horner syndrome and lymphadenopathy
- Mastectomy, colostomy or laparotomy, radiation scars and tattoos
- Chemotherapy: alopecia, mucositis, Cushing syndrome, radiation scars
- TB/lymphoma: lymphadenopathy and fever
- Pneumonia: purulent sputum, tachypnoea, fever
- Cardiac failure: raised JVP, third heart sound, peripheral oedema
- Nephrotic syndrome: generalised oedema and ascites
- Cirrhosis
- Autoimmune disease: characteristic rash or arthritis
- Pulmonary emboli: raised JVP, right ventricular heave, loud P2, deep vein thrombosis (DVT)
- Hypothyroidism: dry skin, bradycardia, characteristic facies, slow relaxing reflexes.

Aetiology

Exudates (see Light's criteria p. 89)

The most common causes are malignancy (primary, eg bronchogenic or mesothelioma) or infection (parapneumonic effusions). Other less common causes include: pulmonary emboli; connective tissue disease (eg rheumatoid arthritis and SLE); pancreatitis; benign asbestos effusion; autoimmune diseases; and post-myocardial infarction syndrome. Rare causes include: drugs (eg amiodarone, methotrexate, phenytoin).

Transudate (see Light's criteria p. 89)

The most common causes are: heart failure; liver cirrhosis; peritoneal dialysis. Other less common causes include: hypothyroidism; pulmonary emboli; nephrotic syndrome; mitral stenosis. Rare causes include: SVC (superior vena cava) obstruction; constrictive pericarditis, ovarian disease (Meigs syndrome and ovarian hyperstimulation).

Note that it is often difficult to differentiate between a transudate and an exudate based on the protein content of the pleural fluid alone, because many samples demonstrate a protein level that lies between 25 g/l and 35 g/l. In these cases 'Light's criteria' are used to distinguish the two.

Differential diagnosis

- Lung collapse – trachea pulled to affected side, percussion note is not stony dull
- Raised hemidiaphragm:
  - phrenic nerve palsy (eg cancer, motor neuron disease)
  - hepatomegaly: the area of dullness moves with respiration, unlike the former.

Symptoms

- Dyspnoea
- Weight loss and lethargy: malignancy
- Productive cough and fever: parapneumonic
- Haemoptysis: malignancy, pulmonary emboli and TB
- Arthritis and rash: autoimmune disease
- Abrupt orthopnoea: phrenic nerve palsy.

Investigations

- Chest radiograph: both PA (posteroanterior) and lateral films should be requested with characteristic changes detectable in the presence of approximately 200 ml plus of pleural fluid.

- Pleural fluid aspiration and analysis: smell and appearance, biochemistry and cell counts, MC&S (microscopy, culture and sensitivity) including acid-fast bacilli (AFB) and cytology:
    - putrid-smelling pleural fluid is indicative of anaerobic infection
    - pleural lymphocytosis is common in malignancy and TB whereas pleural eosinophilia is not always benign
    - low pleural glucose < 2.2 mmol/l is often caused by an exudate secondary to infection (see below), rheumatoid disease, SLE, malignancy, TB or oesophageal rupture
    - pleural and serum amylase should be requested to exclude acute pancreatitis and oesophageal rupture; it is often raised in malignancy, especially adenocarcinomas
    - a low pleural pH is indicative of pleural infection – < 7.2 warrants tube drainage
    - cytology diagnoses 60% of malignant effusions – negative effusions should be repeated at least once more
    - if the fluid is milky triglycerides and cholesterol should be measured for chylothorax and pseudochylothorax (see below)
    - measure complement levels and glucose for rheumatoid disease
    - if the tap is bloody, haematocrit levels are helpful, and positive if the haematocrit of the pleural fluid is more than half the patient's peripheral blood haematocrit.
- Ultrasonography: to guide aspiration if an unguided attempt, based on chest radiograph, has failed. It is successful in 97% of cases and also provides better visualisation of fibrinous separations.
- CT of the chest (contrast enhanced): should be performed with contrast medium to aid in visualising suspected loculated effusions and to differentiate (in most cases) between benign and malignant pleural thickening.
- Percutaneous pleural biopsy: often required to diagnose TB and malignancy. If mesothelioma is suspected then biopsy site is irradiated to prevent local spread. The procedure can be performed blind with an Abrams' needle (requiring four samples from a single site) or by the (enhanced CT) image-guided cutting needle technique which gives a greater yield for malignancy diagnosis.
- Sputum MC&S and cytology.
- Mantoux test.
- Echocardiogram to look for left ventricular failure (LVF).
- Thyroid-stimulating hormone (TSH) and thyroxine (T_4) to exclude hypothyroidism.
- Antinuclear antibody (ANA), rhesus factor, complements C3 and C4 to exclude autoimmune and connective tissue disorders.
- CT pulmonary angiogram/ventilation–perfusion scan to exclude pulmonary emboli.

- Bronchoscopy should be considered when less invasive procedures have failed to yield a diagnosis.

Investigation and treatment guidelines

The BTS released 'key facts' when investigating undiagnosed pleural effusions in 2003:

1. If the pleural fluid protein is between 25 g/l and 35 g/l, then Light's criteria will accurately differentiate exudates from transudates (see p. 89).
2. Pleural fluid pH should be performed in all non-purulent effusions if infection is suspected.
3. When sending a pleural fluid specimen for microbiological examination, it should be sent in both a sterile tube (for Gram stain, AFB and TB culture) and blood culture bottles to increase the diagnostic yield.
4. Only 60% of malignant effusions can be diagnosed by cytological examination. If the first pleural cytology specimen is negative, this should be repeated a second time.
5. Contrast-enhanced CT of the thorax is best performed with the fluid present. This will enable better visualisation of the pleura and can identify the best site for pleural biopsy if cytological examination is unhelpful.

Questions

1. What is the relevance of asbestos exposure in a patient with a pleural effusion?

The incidence of mesothelioma is increasing world wide as a result of previous exposure to asbestos; the lag phase is 20–40 years. The disease is unresponsive to conventional therapy and prognosis is poor.

2. How should a suspected malignant effusion be managed?

In the case of recurrent effusions caused by malignancy, pleurodesis can be attempted. This is usually done with bleomycin; however, pleurodesis via thoracoscopy obtains better results. (Note that tube drainage should be avoided in mesothelioma because of the risk of seeding.)

3. What is the significance of the colour of the aspirated fluid?

- Blood stained points towards malignancy or PE
- Turbid suggests infection
- Milky suggests chylothorax and pseudochylothorax
- It is possible to differentiate between infection and chylothorax by centrifuging the sample. A clear supernatant suggests infection whereas a persistently turbid sample suggests that a chylothorax or a pseudochylothorax is the cause.

4. Chylothorax Pseudochylothorax?

- Chylous effusions are caused by disruption of the thoracic duct, resulting in the presence of chyle in the pleural space.
- Cause: malignancy (50%), trauma (25%), TB, sarcoidosis and amyloidosis.
- Tests: triglycerides, cholesterol levels and cholesterol crystals/chylomicrons in the pleural fluid.
- Pseudochylothorax is a result of accumulation of cholesterol crystals in a long-standing pleural effusion causing fibrosis. Common causes include TB and rheumatoid pleurisy. It can be differentiated from a chylothorax by the absence chylomicrons, reduced triglycerides and raised cholesterol with the presence of cholesterol crystals in pseudochylothoraces.

5. What types of infected pleural effusions are you aware of?

This is a progressive three-stage process.

Simple exudate (simple parapneumonic effusion)

- Features: clear fluid pH > 7.2, LDH (lactate dehydrogenase) < 1000 IU/l, no organisms on culture and glucose > 2.2 mmol/l.
- Treatment: will usually resolve with antibiotics alone. Perform chest tube drainage for symptom relief if required.

Fibrinopurulent stage (complicated parapneumonic stage)

- Features: clear fluid or cloudy/turbid, pH < 7.2, LDH > 1000 IU/l, glucose >2.2 mmol/l, may be positive Gram stain/culture.
- Treatment: requires antibiotics and chest tube drainage.

Empyema (associated with scar tissue formation)

- Features: frank pus, may be positive Gram stain/culture, no additional biochemical tests necessary on pleural fluid (do not measure pH).

Treatment: requires chest tube drainage.

6. How should an infected pleural effusion be investigated and managed?

Clinical guidelines for infected pleural effusions (Thorax 2003)

Pleural fluid should be sampled for diagnostic purposes within 24 hours:

- Pleural fluid pH should be measured with a blood gas analyser.
- Appropriate antibiotics must be given.
- Insert a chest drain where indicated (see above).
- Outcome assessment must take place 5–8 days after starting treatment and patients who have not achieved an effective response should be discussed with a thoracic surgeon

---

- Light's criteria state that, if one or more of the following are present, the fluid is an exudate:
  - pleural fluid protein divided by serum protein > 0.5
  - pleural fluid LDH divided by serum LDH > 0.6
  - pleural fluid LDH more than two-thirds the normal upper limit for serum LDH.

SCENARIO 3. BRONCHIECTASIS

This is permanent thickening and dilatation of the bronchi and bronchioles secondary to chronic infection of these airways. The diagnosis can be made by pathology or radiologically.

Please examine the chest of this 27-year-old woman; she has been suffering from a chronic cough that has not responded to antibiotics.

Examination points

- Clubbing
- Central cyanosis
- Dyspnoeic: increased respiratory rate
- Cachexia and short stature
- Pleuritic chest pain: usually associated with infective exacerbations
- Cough with copious purulent sputum, intermittent haemoptysis and halitosis
- Coarse inspiratory crepitations, often over one or more areas of the lungs.

A good candidate

- Will look for complications and potential causes
- Will not assume that it is CF and investigate for other causes, ie lymphadenopathy or dextrocardia
- Will know about the management of CF including the principles of gene therapy.

Complications

Anaemia, brain abscess, cor pulmonale, amyloid.

Aetiology

- Childhood infection: whooping cough, measles, TB
- Adult infections: severe pneumonia, TB, other mycobacteria
- Cystic fibrosis: young, cachectic, short stature

- Congenital pulmonary sequestration
- Immunodeficiency: chronic lymphocytic leukaemia (CLL), HIV
- Mechanical and chemical damage: intrinsic pressure secondary to tumour, toxic inhalation/aspiration
- Kartagener syndrome: dextrocardia, azoospermia
- Bronchial obstruction: malignancy, TB, lymph nodes
- Hypogammaglobulinaemia (congenital and acquired)
- Allergic bronchopulmonary aspergillosis.

Symptoms

- Asymptomatic
- Recurrent acute bronchitis with no other symptoms
- Recurrent acute bronchitis with mucoid sputum
- Daily purulent sputum ± systemic symptoms
- Haemoptysis with any of the above
- Consider CF (cystic fibrosis) and its symptoms – gastrointestinal disturbance, failure to thrive and male infertility.

Investigations

- FBC, CRP (C-reactive protein) – infective exacerbation
- Sputum MC&S
- Chest radiograph: ring shadows and tramlines (caused by thickening of the airways), gloved finger (consolidation superimposed onto abnormal airways) – only visible in 37% of cases
- HRCT of chest: thickening and dilatation of the bronchi and bronchioles. Signet-ring sign: airways appear thicker than their accompanying blood vessels. Diagnosis made on HRCT
- Pulmonary function tests: often obstructive, test for reversibility component
- Sweat test for CF: those with sweat sodium or chloride levels 70 mmol/l or higher should be checked for the presence of common and rarer genes associated with CF
- Serum immunoglobulins: decreased IgA in hypogammaglobulinaemia
- Aspergillus precipitins, skin tests and RAST (radioallergosorbent test)
- α_1-Antitrypsin levels
- Autoantibodies, eg ANA for associated connective tissue diseases
- Mantoux test
- CF genotyping
- Bronchoscopy and biopsy
- Pulmonary function tests: most patients have an obstructive defect more commonly than a restrictive defect, but the latter may also be present
- Genetic testing: mutations in the cystic fibrosis transmembrane conductance regulator (*CFTR*) gene can be performed.

Treatment

- Postural drainage, breathing techniques, cough augmentation.
- Optimise nutrition.
- Antibiotics: cover *Pseudomonas* and *Haemophilus* species. Short courses are used for acute exacerbations. Antibiotics that reduce purulent sputum volume in short courses can be considered for prolonged use.
- Bronchodilators and steroids: if any reversible component. In the absence of a reversible component, regular inhaled corticosteroids routinely used for patients with CF should be avoided.
- Mucolytics: nebulised recombinant human DNase (rhDNase). The results of randomised controlled studies are contradictory in this area.
- Surgery for localised disease.
- Transplant surgery: individuals with a life expectancy < 2 years and no significant co-morbidity can be considered.
- Gene therapy for CF is experimental (see below).
- Immunisation: against influenza annually and against pneumococci according to Department of Health guidelines.

Questions

1. What do you understand is the genetic basis of cystic fibrosis?

Cystic fibrosis: autosomal recessive disease, chromosome 7 – mutation is present in 1/25 and is thus homozygous in 1/2500. Mutations in *CFTR* are the molecular cause of CF. Many hundred of mutations have been identified. The Df508 mutation is present in 70% of patients and is associated with a poorer prognosis.

2. How might CF present?

CF presents with:

- Meconium ileus: in infants
- Malabsorption/failure to thrive: in children
- Bronchiectasis: as teenagers
- Diabetes develops in 20% of adults as a result of destruction of the islets of Langerhans by mucoid plugging of the pancreatic ducts
- Diagnosis is by sweat testing (sweat chloride > 60 mmol/l); patients and families should be counselled before testing. Genetic testing is helpful for prognosis.

3. What is the prognosis for CF?

In the past, survival has not usually been beyond the third decade. Improved antibiotics, immunisation against *Pseudomonas*, aggressive postural drainage, aerosolised rhDNase and gene therapy have resulted in increased overall survival for these patients, to the fourth decade.

Males are infertile. Pregnant females with a family history can have chorionic villous sampling.

Morbidity and mortality with CF are primarily the result of CF pulmonary sepsis and its associated complications. The most common offending organisms are *Haemophilus influenzae*, *Staphylococcus aureus* and *Pseudomonas aeruginosa*.

With bronchiectasis in general, there tends to be a progression in the types of bacterial organisms that colonise the large airways. In early disease *S. aureus* tends to predominate, followed by *H. influenzae*, *Moraxella catarrhalis* and then, with advanced disease, *Pseudomonas* species.

Gene therapy is based around inhalation of copies of functional *CFTR* genes. Both viral and liposmal vectors are used. The genes act in a complementary manner rather than gene replacement. The two main challenges include getting the genes into the cells more efficiently and enhancing the duration of functional gene expression in the cells.

SCENARIO 4. UNILATERAL PULMONARY FIBROSIS

Please examine this patient who complains of weight loss and a persistent cough.

Points on examination

- Trachea: deviated towards lesion if involving the upper lobes
- Rib resection ± supraclavicular scar (old TB)
- Expansion: decreased on affected side
- Percussion: dullness on affected side
- TVF and VR: increased on affected side
- Coarse inspiratory and expiratory crackles
- If it is caused by malignancy, radiotherapy marks and a thoracotomy scar may be present. In the presence of metastatic disease the primary tumour can be left, causing the above clinical signs. It is unlikely that these patients will appear in examinations.

A good candidate

- Will look for possible aetiology
- Will look for active TB or infection and ask to see a sputum pot
- Will know about multi-drug-resistant TB (MDRTB).

Aetiology of upper lobe fibrosis

- Treated TB: thoracotomy and rib resection with iatrogenic lobar collapse. A supraclavicular scar may indicate prior phrenic nerve crush. Both these procedures render the lung hypoxic and thus have an antituberculous effect before effective chemotherapy. These patients are elderly, because this is a treatment of the past.
- Malignant disease: clubbing, thoracotomy, radiotherapy marks, lymphadenopathy, hepatomegaly, Horner syndrome, wasting of the small muscles – Pancoast's tumour.

Differential diagnosis

- Lobar pneumonia: associated with pyrexia, but unlikely in the exam. However, this is often a point of discussion because it is the most common cause of unilateral coarse crackles.
- Bronchiectasis: productive cough, clubbing cyanosis; coarse inspiratory crepitations, often multifocal.

Symptoms

- With old TB the patient may be asymptomatic, because lung volume is decreased; dyspnoea may occur with exertion – rest and home oxygen if respiratory failure occurs. Respiratory function tests will reveal a restrictive picture.
- With reactivation of TB there may be constitutional symptoms – weight loss, fever, night sweats.
- Malignancy: weight loss, cough/haemoptysis, chest pain, lymphadenopathy, wasting of the small muscles of the hand.

Investigations

- Chest radiograph
- FBC
- U&Es (urea and electrolytes)
- Erythrocyte sedimentation rate (ESR), CRP
- Sputum cytology, smear and culture – if active infection suspected; smear-positive TB warrants isolation
- HRCT
- Respiratory function tests.

Management

- If asymptomatic with unilateral fibrosis, no treatment is required.
- If active TB is suspected investigate and treat along standard lines (see page 106).
- If malignancy is suspected a tissue biopsy and staging should be arranged.

Question

1. *What is MDRTB*

This is TB that is resistant to more than one of the first-line TB chemotherapeutic agents. It accounts for 2% of all TB cases in the UK and is increasing. Although it is no more infectious than other forms of TB, MDRTB can be much more difficult to treat and causes greater morbidity and mortality. Risk factors for MDRTB include immunodeficiency (HIV), previous TB treatment and exposure to MDRTB-infected persons. Patients must be managed in isolation and in close liaison with a microbiologist, and should be started on at least five agents to which the organism will be sensitive. Prophylactic chemotherapy should be given to all those in contact with the patient.

SCENARIO 5. CHRONIC OBSTRUCTIVE PULMONARY DISEASE

This patient has recently commenced home oxygen therapy. Please examine his respiratory system.

Chronic bronchitis and emphysema are two separate diseases that usually coexist, although patients tend to suffer predominantly from one. Chronic bronchitis is a clinical diagnosis relating to chronic cough and sputum production for most days for at least 3 months, recurring in at least 2 successive years, whereas emphysema is a pathological diagnosis characterised by dilatation of the terminal air spaces, with destruction of the alveolar walls. The two diseases are usually described as a single entity – chronic airway/pulmonary disease (CAL, COAD or COPD). COPD is the preferred term and differs from asthma in that there is persistent airflow obstruction with variable reversibility with bronchodilators, and it involves progressively worsening symptoms and an irreversible decline in respiratory function. The aetiology is primarily smoking related but occupational exposures and α_1-antitrypsin deficiency can also contribute.

Points on examination

Clinical signs favouring chronic bronchitis ('blue bloaters')

- Central cyanosis
- Bounding pulse, coarse flapping tremor
- Barrel chest, often moderately obese
- Cough and sputum production, worse in winter
- Wheeze and crackles in the chest – widespread.

A good candidate

- Will look for signs of complications (cor pulmonale, cancer and pneumonia) and treatment associated with the disease (β agonists, steroids and surgery)
- Will discuss the spectrum of emphysema and chronic bronchitis
- Will ask to see a sputum pot
- Will be able to discuss NIV.

Clinical signs favouring emphysema ('pink puffers')

- Tachypnoea
- Hyperinflated chest; patients are often thin
- Reduced suprasternal notch: cricoid cartilage distance
- Decreased chest movement and increased use of accessory muscles

- Hyperresonance
- Decreased breath sounds: particularly over bullae
- Prolonged expiration and pursed lips: to maintain pressure in the lungs and prevent airway collapse (effectively this is positive end-expiratory airway pressure or PEEP)
- Signs of treatment: cushingoid appearance, ecchymoses, fine tremor (β_2 agonist), inhalers, nebulisers and oxygen mask/cylinders.

Associated conditions

- Pneumonia: increased dyspnoea, pyrexia, change in sputum colour, dullness to percussion with increased TVF, crepitations and bronchial breathing over infected area
- Lung cancer: Horner syndrome, cachexia, anaemia, lymphadenopathy
- Pulmonary hypertension leading to cor pulmonale: raised JVP 'cv' waves, peripheral oedema, left parasternal heave, palpable second heart sound and tricuspid regurgitation.

Aetiology

- Cigarette smoking
- Atmospheric pollution
- α_1-Antitrypsin deficiency (emphysema) – predominantly affects the upper lobes.

Investigations

- FBC: to identify anaemia or polycythaemia; secondarily in an acute setting it might suggest infection
- Chest radiograph: to exclude other pathologies
- Diagnostic features:
    - hyperinflated lungs: more than seven posterior ribs, flattened diaphragm
    - black lung sign – attenuated peripheral vasculature
    - apical bullae – may need CT to differentiate from pneumothorax
- BMI (body mass index): should be calculated
- Lung function tests – obstructive picture, $FEV_1 < 80\%$, $FEV_1/FVC < 0.7$, increased residual volume and total lung capacity (FEV_1 is forced expiratory volume in 1 s and FVC is forced vital capacity).

The following investigations can be performed:

- Serial domiciliary peak flow measurements: to exclude asthma if diagnostic doubt remains
- α_1-Antitrypsin levels: if early onset, minimal smoking history or family history

- Transfer factor for carbon monoxide (TLCO): to investigate symptoms that seem disproportionate to the spirometric impairment
- CT of the thorax:
  - to investigate symptoms that seem disproportionate to the spirometric impairment
  - to investigate abnormalities seen on a chest radiograph
  - to assess suitability for surgery
- ECG/echocardiogram: evidence for cor pulmonale
- Pulse oximetry: to assess the need for oxygen therapy if cyanosis, or cor pulmonale, or if FEV_1 < 50% predicted
- Arterial blood gases: type 2 respiratory failure, respiratory acidosis – if severe consider BIPAP (bipositive airway pressure ventilation)
- Sputum culture: to identify organisms if sputum is persistently present and purulent.

Management

- Oxygen (24% until dependence on hypoxic drive is established): long-term oxygen initially as required, but eventually continuous for patients with advanced and end-stage disease.
- Nebulised β_2 agonists, anti-muscarinics and steroids (inhaled and oral) if the disease has a reversible component. This requires lung function tests.
- Start with short-acting β_2 agonists; step up to long-acting or short-acting β_2 agonists in combination with anticholinergic medication if necessary.
- Inhaled steroids should be used if patient's FEV_1 is 50% or less of predicted whereas oral steroids should be prescribed only in severe disease if other therapies are inadequate – in these cases screening for complications of steroid therapy (eg osteoporosis) with prophylactic therapy is warranted.
- Pulmonary rehabilitation should be made available to all appropriate patients with COPD.
- Theophylline: as second-line therapy. Need to monitor plasma levels and interactions with other medication – reduce dose with certain antibiotics (eg macrolides). Caution in elderly people.
- Antibiotics, if infective component.
- Newer treatments:
  - leukotriene-β_4 agonists
  - interleukin-8 (IL-8) antagonists
  - TNF inhibitors.
- Smoking cessation: NICE (National institute for Health and Clinical Effectiveness) guidelines stipulate that all patients, irrespective of age, should be actively encouraged to stop smoking, which should include the use of bupropion or nicotine replacement therapy if necessary, unless either is contraindicated.

- Non-invasive ventilation (NIV): for patients with significant hypercapnia and related acidosis – long-term NIV should be considered in some patients with chronic hypercapnia.
- Surgery: bullectomy, lung volume reduction surgery and lung transplantation are indicated if patients meet certain criteria.

Questions

1. What forms of non-invasive ventilation are you familiar with?

- CPAP (continuous positive airway pressure) ventilation: used in individuals with healthy lungs who require artificial support. It is also used for obstructive sleep apnoea, because it maintains open airways.
- NIPPV (negative intermittent pressure ventilation): used for patients with neuromuscular deficits, eg polio, or in CO_2 retainers. Ventilation is triggered by inspiration.
- BIPAP: used for patients with underlying airway disease. The positive pressure keeps the airways open, allowing oxygen transfer.

2. What are the indications for domiciliary oxygen

- Stable disease
- $FEV_1 < 1.5$ l; FVC < 2 l
- $Pao_2 < 7.3$ kPa
  (Non-smoking: explosion risk)

3. Can you grade the breathlessness?

The Medical Research Council (MRC) dyspnoea scale should be used (adapted from Fletcher et al. 1959):

1. Not troubled by breathlessness except on strenuous exercise.
2. Short of breath when hurrying or walking up a slight hill.
3. Walks slower than peer group on level ground because of breathlessness, or has to stop for breath when walking at own pace.
4. Stops for breath after walking about 100 m or after a few minutes on level ground.
5. Too breathless to leave the house, or breathless when dressing or undressing.

4. What points would you look for in the history?

- Do they smoke cigarettes?
- Calculate the number of pack-years smoked (1 pack-year = 20 cigarettes per day for 1 year)
- Breathlessness
- Cough

- Sputum production
- The presence of the following factors should be noted:
  - weight loss
  - effort intolerance
  - waking at night
  - ankle swelling
  - fatigue
  - occupational hazards
  - chest pain
  - haemoptysis
- A history of multiple exacerbations
- Details of any previous admissions, including to intensive therapy unit (ITU), and treatment, particularly steroids and antibiotics
- Previous arterial blood gases and chest radiographs
- Current treatment
- What is the precipitating factor in this case?

SCENARIO 6. LUNG CANCER

This patient has had haemoptysis for 2 months and is concerned as he is losing weight. Please examine him.

Examination

- Clubbing and tar-stained fingers
- Thoracotomy scar from surgical removal of primary tumour ± radiotherapy marks (see page 105)
- Cachexia and anaemia
- Supraclavicular/cervical lymphadenopathy
- Pleural effusion (see page 84)
- Unilateral collapse and fibrosis (see page 93)
- Evidence of previous chemotherapy: alopecia, nail changes, anaemia, bruising and mucositis.

A good candidate

Once a diagnosis of lung cancer is suspected a good candidate:

- Will look for evidence of locally advanced disease (SVCO and lymphadenopathy)
- Will look for evidence of metastasis, eg examining the liver, cranial nerves, and spine, and looking for spinal cord compression
- Will look for paraneoplastic signs such as finger clubbing, cerebellar signs, skin lesions, hypercalcaemia and Cushing syndrome; it should be remembered that steroids are often used as treatment for these patients, which occurs more commonly than ectopic ACTH production
- Will look for evidence of other treatment such as radiotherapy and chemotherapy. Remember that surgery is rarely performed on SCLC and adjuvant chemotherapy, after surgery, is given for NSCLC.

Associations with lung cancer

Local effects

- SVC obstruction (SVCO): facial oedema, fixed dilatation of superficial neck veins, suffusion and often stridor. This can be caused by lung cancer but is frequently associated with other tumours such as breast cancer, colon cancer or lymphoma. It is treated by either primary stenting or radiotherapy. This is not the case for chemosensitive tumours, such as testicular cancer or lymphoma, where primary chemotherapy is used.
- Horner syndrome and wasting of the small muscles of the hand; Pancoast's tumour (see also page 294).
- Recurrent laryngeal nerve palsy: hoarse voice.

Metastatic effects

- Spinal cord compression: sensory level, weakness, brisk reflexes, upgoing plantars, urinary and bowel symptoms
- Focal neurology (especially cranial nerve lesions): brain or bone metastases, especially small cell lung cancer or SCLC (very high incidence of brain metastasis)
- Hepatomegaly (liver failure is a very late complication and is more likely to be related to chemotherapy)
- Often metastasises to the adrenal and rarely can result in Addison's disease if metastases are bilateral (see page 629).

Paraneoplastic syndromes

NEUROLOGICAL

- Peripheral neuropathy (see page 312)
- Cerebellar signs (see page 347)
- Eaton–Lambert syndrome: proximal muscle weakness and fatigue. It is similar to myasthenia gravis, except that power is often improved after brief exercise and reflexes are restored soon after activity.

ENDOCRINE

- Ectopic ACTH (adrenocorticotrophic hormone) production: pigmentation resulting in Cushing syndrome, which occurs with small cell carcinoma.
- Hypercalcaemia: parathyroid hormone-related peptide production, usually by squamous cell carcinoma. Symptoms include confusion, polyuria, abdominal pain, lethargy, nausea and dehydration.
- SIADH (syndrome of inappropriate antidiuretic hormone production): confusion, nausea, vomiting.

DERMATOLOGICAL/RHEUMATOLOGICAL

- Dermatomyositis (see page 511)
- Clubbing
- Hypertrophic pulmonary osteoarthropathy: thickening of the distal end of the ulna and radius, most marked on radiograph with classic changes.

OTHER

- Recurrent venous thrombosis
- Pericarditis
- Marantic endocarditis.

Risk factors

- Cigarette smoking: pack-years are important
- Manufacturing: asbestos, beryllium, ether, polycyclic aromatic hydrocarbons, chromate, nickel, arsenic
- Radioactivity: uranium mining, radon.

Symptoms

- Cough, haemoptysis, breathlessness, hoarseness
- Weight loss, malaise
- Chest pain
- Lymphadenopathy
- Related to metastatic/paraneoplastic effects.

Initial investigations

- Chest radiograph: solitary pulmonary nodule or mass, pleural effusion, pulmonary collapse or area of consolidation, mediastinal lymphadenopathy.
- Sputum cytology: low sensitivity for peripheral masses, much higher for central lesions. Useful for patients who cannot tolerate bronchoscopy.
- Bronchoscopy or percutaneous transthoracic needle aspiration and/or biopsy: depending on location of mass (the latter for peripheral lesions).
- Pleural aspiration and biopsy – if effusion present.

Further investigations (staging)

- Ultrasonography of liver: liver metastases
- CT of the thorax with contrast (hilar lymphadenopathy), liver, adrenals: for diagnosis of lung cancer, to identify tumour morphology, evidence for local invasion and metastatic disease, and to determine the best means for biopsy – needle or bronchoscopy
- Liver function tests (LFTs), bone profile – metastases
- Pulmonary function tests
- Bone scan: bony metastases
- Positron emission tomography (PET)/CT: useful for solitary pulmonary nodules and solitary lesions, especially mediastinal disease; now approved by NICE guidelines
- Anterior median sternotomy: can be used for staging carcinoma of the left upper lobe.

Management

- Surgery: rarely suitable, as a result of frequent local spread. Only helpful in non-small cell lung cancer (NSCLC). Requires adequate lung function (FEV_1 > 1.2 l for lobectomy, > 1.5 l for pneumonectomy).
- Small cell cancer: the treatment is cisplatin-based chemotherapy with radiotherapy. Prognosis remains poor despite initial responses.
- Metastatic NSCLC: platinum-based agents are more effective as first-line therapy than non-platinum agents. Radiotherapy is useful for palliative relief of haemoptysis and bony pain.

- Endobronchial treatments: useful as palliative treatment of local bronchial obstruction. It can also be used in early NSCLC. Several types of endobronchial treatments exist:
  - photodynamic therapy: effective in managing small, superficial, squamous cell tumours
  - brachytherapy: delivery of local irradiation, limited evidence of its effects on symptoms and survival at present
  - laser ablation: direct thermal ablation; no evidence supporting its effectiveness in palliation or for cure.
- The TNM (tumour, node, metastasis) classification is commonly used for staging NSCLC whereas for SCLC the simple staging system introduced by VALC (Veterans' Administration Lung Cancer Study Group) has been found to suffice in most clinical situations. This separates patients into those with limited and extensive disease.

Question

1. What types of bronchial carcinoma are you aware of?

Small cell bronchial carcinoma

- Accounts for 20–30% of all lung cancer cases
- Arises from endocrine cells
- Commonly secretes polypeptide hormones that account for the neuroendocrine effects
- Most responsive to chemotherapy but chemoresistance occurs.

Non-small cell bronchial carcinoma

SQUAMOUS

- Accounts for 40% of lung cancer cases
- Commonly presents as obstructive lesions in bronchi/bronchioles, leading to infection (approximately 10% cavitate)
- Local invasion common – SVCO
- Metastasis late
- Usually well differentiated.

ADENOCARCINOMA

- Accounts for 10% of lung cancer cases
- Arises peripherally from mucous glands
- Commonly invades mediastinal lymph nodes and pleura
- Metastasises to bone and brain
- Often difficult to obtain tissue as a result of the peripheral nature of the lesion
- Common in women, with asbestos exposure, non-smokers, Far East origin

- EGFR (epidermal growth factor receptor) tyrosine kinase inhibitors work best in this tumour type.

LARGE CELL

- Accounts for 25% of lung cancer cases
- Poor differentiation
- Metastasises early.

SCENARIO 7. THORACOTOMY SCAR

Please examine this patient's respiratory system.

This case is similar to the unilateral pulmonary fibrosis case. However, here there is an obvious scar with dullness and reduced breath sounds unilaterally. There is no debate about infection as a cause.

Examination points

- A scar is visible on the chest wall.
- There is usually deviation of the trachea. If the surgery performed was a unilateral lower lobectomy, the trachea may remain central.
- Dullness to percussion and absent breath sounds over the area surgically removed. Coarse crackles can occur over this area.

A good candidate

- Will be able to identify the most likely reason for a thoracotomy
- Will identify associations with that cause.

Associated conditions

Lung malignancy

This can include either primary lung cancer or mesothelioma. Occasionally isolated metastasis from other sites can be removed, although there are few supportive data for this. This can result in bilateral scars.

SIGNS OF MALIGNANCY (LUNG CANCERS IN MOST CASES)

- Evidence of locally advanced disease (SVCO and lymphadenopathy).
- Look for evidence of metastasis hepatomegaly, cranial nerve lesions, bone metastasis or spinal cord compression
- Look for paraneoplastic signs such as finger clubbing, cachexia, cerebellar signs, skin lesions, hypercalcaemia and Cushing syndrome; it should be remembered that steroids are often used as treatment for these patients, which occurs more commonly than ectopic ACTH production
- Evidence of other treatment such as radiotherapy and chemotherapy. Remember that surgery is rarely performed on SCLC and adjuvant chemotherapy, after surgery, is given for NSCLC.

Bronchiectasis

Bronchiectasis associated with uncontrolled or recurrent haemoptysis can require surgery. This is most commonly associated with CF, but can be a result of childhood or adult infection and obstruction (such as a tumour).

SIGNS OF BRONCHIECTASIS

- Clubbing
- Central cyanosis
- Dyspnoeic: increased respiratory rate
- Cachexia and short stature
- Pleuritic chest pain: usually associated with infective exacerbations
- Cough with copious purulent sputum, intermittent haemoptysis and halitosis
- Coarse inspiratory crepitations, often over one or more areas of the lungs.

AETIOLOGY OF BRONCHIECTASIS

- Features associated with CF: young, cachectic, short stature
- Obstruction, ie malignancy: clubbing lymphadenopathy and cachectic
- TB: lymph nodes, cachexia, pyrexias and sputum.

Tuberculosis

TB was a common cause of thoracotomy in the past and is becoming increasingly common with MDRTB. Patients will often have no other clinical signs but you should consider sputum, pyrexia and lymphadenopathy, as well as the side effects of TB drug therapy. In reality patients with active TB will not appear in the exam. Factors to consider are:

- Skin rash
- Peripheral neuropathy
- Retrobulbar neuritis
- Arthralgia
- Hearing loss and vestibular problems
- Jaundice.

Investigations and treatment

A chest radiograph may be helpful, but investigations should be determined by the cause and may not be necessary.

STATION 2

The History-taking Examination

1. Chest pain
2. Abdominal pain
3. Chronic cough
4. Breathlessness
5. Acute-onset headache
6. New headache of recent onset
7. Chronic/intermitten headache
8. Back pain
9. Weak legs
10. Falls
11. Painful joints of the wrist and hand
12. Abnormal liver function tests
13. Alcohol dependence and abdominal pain
14. Diarrhoea
15. The HIV patient
16. Hypertension

HISTORY TAKING FOR PACES

Introduction

History taking is a special form of communication in which both parties study each other. It is one of the cornerstones of a doctor's skills. Although many candidates may already feel skilled in this discipline, the history-taking station in PACES is one that is commonly failed. This is usually because of poor technique, organisation or not covering all areas.

Key features of the station

Written instructions for the case, usually in the form of a letter from the patient's GP, are given to the candidate to read in the 5-minute interval before the station.

Then, 14 minutes are allowed for the history taking, 1 minute to collect your thoughts and then 5 minutes for discussion, during which the patient is asked to leave the room.

The examiners are present throughout and observe the history taking. Although they have guidelines as to the key areas on which they base their overall mark, you are not marked on the specific points.

General approach

Read the instructions carefully in the 5-minute interval before the station. Based on the symptoms given, consider the possible differential diagnoses to enquire about. If a medical condition is stated, consider its medical and social implications, associations with other conditions, complications and treatment.

It is essential to try to put the patient at ease and encourage him or her to talk freely. Common courtesy goes a long way towards this. Greet the patient, by name if possible, and tell him or her whom you are. The value of the patient's history and his or her confidence in you as a physician depend upon the rapport that is created.

When the patient is telling the story, watch for gestures and non-verbal clues, as it is as important to listen to what is not said as to what is said and how it is said. Make it clear from your posture, gestures and expression that the patient has your undivided attention. Do not sit there staring at the examiners, or out of the window, or spend the whole time furiously writing notes.

Remember to use a mixture of open and closed questions. Start the consultation with a series of open questions, ie ones that do not suggest a particular answer, eg 'Why have you come to see me today?' or 'Tell me what is wrong from your point of view'. Move towards more closed questions as you progress in the history, eg 'Any trouble with your water works?'. You may eventually need to use closed questions where the answer is suggested, eg 'When you wake at night, are you thirsty?'.

A good candidate: the marking sheet

History taking in PACES is marked in three sections:

1. Data gathering: this includes the well-established process of taking the history of the presenting complaint, past medical history, drug history, family history, social circumstances, smoking, alcohol, etc. It places particular emphasis on taking the history in a logical manner, good communication (responding to verbal and non-verbal cues) and a progression from open to closed questions. It specifically states that any leads on psychosocial factors should be pursued – this is best interpreted as making an assessment of the impact of the disease on the patient's life.
2. Identification and use of information: candidates are specifically marked on checking that the information given is correct, so (after introductions) candidates should always begin by reading out the information provided to the patient. Once information has been gathered, candidates are marked on their ability to process a problem list. This is not simply a numbered list of differential diagnoses; it summarises all the issues, both medical and non-medical, that need to be addressed. This is the cornerstone of the station.
3. Discussion related to the case: this assesses your interaction with the examiner rather than the patient. In particular, the ability succinctly to construct the problem list and then offer prioritised, pragmatic solutions is tested.

In general terms, examiners will be making a judgement about your ability to gather, interpret and present information in a manner that would make their ward rounds and clinics run smoothly.

Pitfalls

The actual gathering of data takes most of the time and accounts for only a small proportion of the available marks. Therefore, pursuing detailed information about any issue that is unlikely to appear in the problem list, for the sake of historical accuracy, must be avoided.

There is potentially a vast amount of information to be gathered in a history. Not all of it can be, or needs to be, collected in each case. The eight classic parts of a history must be included:

1. Age, marital status, occupation/social circumstances
2. Presenting complaints
3. History of presenting complaints
4. Past medical history including ongoing conditions

5. Treatment history
6. Social and occupational history
7. Family history
8. Review of systems, including menstrual history in women.

However, it is impossible to cover all these in detail in the time allowed. Detail should be extracted from those areas most relevant to the patient's problem; this is essentially the skill of passing the history station and distinguishes it from the real-life scenario when you have plenty of time to return and clarify aspects of the history that are unclear. Focusing in detail on only one specific problem is a common way in which candidates run out of time.

A large proportion of the marks is allocated to determining the interaction between social circumstances and disease. Squeezing a brief social history into the last minute for the sake of completeness is invariably fatal.

The construction of a holistic problem list rather than a simple differential diagnosis distinguishes the registrar from the senior house officer. This is why construction of the problem list is mentioned in two of the three sections of the marking sheet.

Strategy for history taking in PACES

Before launching into the history make sure that you:

● introduce yourself
● read out the details provided to the patient and confirm that these are correct.

Within PACES, limited time and the specific demands of the marking sheet mean that the strategy for history taking that should be adopted is very different from the one that you might find in a standard textbook on medical examination. The candidate who simply progresses through the usual stations of the history, eliciting facts under each heading, will usually fail, irrespective of whether the proffered differential diagnosis is reasonable.

The key point is to build a final problem list and plan of action as you go along. There is an important intermediary 'processing' stage in doing this and arranging the information elicited so far under the following subheadings can be useful.

Volunteered problems (and symptoms that the patient ignores): help you build a picture of his or her fears, expectations and beliefs about the condition. At least once during the history-taking process you should directly explore the patient's viewpoint, eg 'What are your own thoughts about this?' or 'Is there something worrying you in particular?'. Understanding the patient's belief system surrounding the condition gives you a clearer picture of which of the symptoms impact on day-to-day existence and also has important implications for the patient's future acceptance of investigations and treatment. Patients will focus on the most troublesome symptoms, not the most diagnostically useful ones. Failing to address these symptoms in your problem list – whether they are central to the condition or not – is invariably disastrous for the subsequent therapeutic alliance between doctor and patient and is thus marked negatively.

Alarm symptoms: are often elicited in the review of systems. The presence or absence of these has a major impact on the urgency of investigation and treatment. Some alarm symptoms are common to all conditions (eg weight loss) but it is imperative that, once you have a differential diagnosis in mind (which can usually be quickly divined from the provided vignette), you should prepare a mental list of the 'emergencies' associated with those disease categories. For example:

- The patient with cancer: symptoms of cord compression, hypercalcaemia, superior vena cava (SVC) obstruction, neutropenia.
- The patient with heart disease: chest pain at rest, syncope, family history of sudden death.
- The patient with liver disease: ascites, melaena, confusion, jaundice.
- The patient with abdominal pain: weight loss, jaundice, family history of intra-abdominal malignancy.
- The patient with back pain: loss of bladder or bowel control, leg weakness.

Disease interaction: multiple pathology is common in the PACES history case. Examiners will be specifically assessing your ability to recognise interactions between new conditions and established ones, eg the patient with ascending weakness after a bout of diarrhoea may well require admission to a ward and daily forced vital capacity (FVC) monitoring but a patient with the same symptoms and established chronic obstructive pulmonary disease (COPD) may require urgent admission to an intensive care unit (ICU) and plasma exchange to avert rapid respiratory failure.

Therapeutic success and failures: keep in mind the following questions once you have made a list of medications. Time does not necessarily allow asking each question for each drug – focus on the important ones relevant to the presenting problems:

- How effective is the drug at alleviating the problem for which it was prescribed?
- How often does the patient actually take it (general compliance rates are often estimated to be less than 50%)?
- What are the side effects?
- What symptoms does the patient rightly or wrongly attribute to the drug?
- Which drugs are being taken unnecessarily for conditions that have resolved?

Similar questions can be applied to any previous therapeutic procedures.

Risks to others: you have a responsibility for the health of others besides the patient in front of you, eg if you suspect a condition that is known to be hereditary it is crucial to identify which members of the family may be affected and need to undergo screening.

Daily life and disease: the social and occupational history is often the crux of the story. Demonstrating an appreciation of the impact of disease on daily life and vice versa is central to success in the history station. The following list of key areas is a useful aide memoire but it is not usually necessary to explore every area ("the six P's") in detail – the history so far should give you an idea which areas to focus on:

- **People**: marital status, other family members and their proximity, other dependants.
- **Place**: accommodation type, numbers of stairs, ownership.
- **Profession**: details of occupation, potential exposures/hazards, risk to themselves or others if their professional skills are impaired (eg taxi drivers).
- **Pocket**: financial status and if it is threatened by the current illness.
- **Public**: Social Services, Disability Allowance, unemployment benefits, home help, meals on wheels, district nurse, twilight nursing.
- **Pleasure**: smoking (how many pack-years, previous attempts to stop), alcohol (see below), risk factors for sexually transmitted infection (where appropriate), contacts who may need tracing, illicit drug use.

Concluding

Try to have a moment to summarise the history to the patient, thereby checking the details and jogging his or her memory for anything that may have been missed. Ask yourself why the examiners have chosen this case – there is likely to be at least one of the following:

1. Complex interaction of medical and social issues
2. Alarm symptoms that have not been addressed
3. Complex symptomatology that requires prioritised investigation
4. Additional iatrogenic disease burden
5. Implications beyond the patient (contact tracing, notifiable diseases, genetic testing for family members, etc).

If there are none of these it is likely that you have missed something. Identifying the likely diagnosis from a string of subtle cues is rarely the task at hand. If the history was not completed during the consultation do not panic; all you can do is take a structured history in a polite and competent manner and endeavour to use the time effectively.

Using this chapter

The history station is frequently neglected when candidates revise for PACES. One of the reasons for this is that many misguidedly feel that their history-taking skills are already sufficient (as supposedly evidenced by the successful clerking of several thousand patients to date). The other frequently cited reason is that finding patients with appropriately challenging problems is much more time-consuming than finding patients with interesting physical signs.

However, it is just as useful (if not more useful) to practise in pairs with a revision partner. The following sections are specifically designed to facilitate this. Using the 'key diagnostic features' and 'example problem lists', one revision partner can concoct an appropriately challenging scenario while the other has 14 minutes to take the history. Designing the history and acting as the patient gives you a useful insight into the viewpoint of the patient (increasingly an actor in the real exam) and the examiner. Most importantly, generic history-taking skills (eg responding to subtle cues, summarising information gathered so far, using open and closed questions) are best improved and polished by watching other people do them both well and badly.

There are a multitude of techniques and phrases that facilitate elicitation of all the important information in the given time in an empathic and sensitive fashion. Some of them you will have already acquired and some of them you won't. Reading a list of them will not make them stick in your mind – the best means of building up an effective armoury of skills is to practise with as many other candidates as possible and cherry-pick techniques and phrases that you feel are most effective.

1. Verify the information provided
Check the provided information with the patient and then ask: 'Tell me in your own words what the problem is ... .'

2. History of the presenting complaint (HPC)
Progress from open to closed questions keeping in mind the *differential diagnosis* There is usually more than one problem. For each, pursue specific symptom characteristics that limit the diagnostic possibilities

3. Previous investigations and treatments for the same problem

4. Systems review (SR)

5. Past medical history (PMH)
What are the current follow-up arrangements?

6. Drug history (DH) and allergies

7. Family history (FH)

8. Social and occupational history (SH)
Cover any points that have been missed so far (see the six 'Ps')

9. Summarise
'Is there anything else that we haven't discussed that you feel is important?'

10. Thank the patient

Volunteered problems – what does the patient's response to open questions reveal about his or her fears, expectations and beliefs surrounding the condition and how are these best addressed?

Alarm symptoms

Disease interaction: How do new problems interact with established conditions?

Therapeutic successes and failures

Risks to others

Daily life and disease: What is the impact of disease on daily life? How will treatment and investigation impact further? What is the impact of lifestyle/occupation on the disease?

Final problem list and plan of action

1. Address patient's fears, expectations and understanding of the condition. What are the key symptoms causing most misery and how can they be dealt with?

2. Triage the urgency of further investigation and treatment (eg does the patient require admission?) and determine which sources of expertise need to be called upon

3. Devise a feasible plan for therapy and investigations that is consistent with the limitations of established co-morbidities

4. Anticipate potential problems with compliance with the treatment or investigation regimen

5. May need to investigate and treat people other than the patient who might be at risk of disease

6. Outline the impact of the disease on the patient's life (and vice versa) and devise a strategy for improving the key areas

STATION 2

HISTORY-TAKING SCENARIOS

1. **Chest pain:**
- Unstable/stable angina
- Myocardial infarction
- Pulmonary embolism
- Pericarditis
- Pleurisy
- Oesophageal spasm
- GORD
- Costochondritis
- Anxiety

2. **Abdominal pain:**
- Gastro-oesophageal reflux disease (GORD)
- Peptic ulcer
- Gastric cancer
- Pancreatitis
- Functional dyspepsia

3. **Chronic cough:**
- Asthma
- Postnasal drip
- Sarcoid
- Drugs
- GORD
- Lung cancer
- TB
- Bronchiectasis

4. **Breathlessness:**
- Congestive cardiac failure (CCF)
- Chronic obstructive pulmonary disease
- Lung cancer and effusion
- Cryptogenic fibrosing alveolitis
- Recurrent pulmonary emboli
- Asthma

5. **Acute-onset headache:**
- Subarachnoid haemorrhage (SAH)
- Haemorrhagic stroke
- Viral meningitis/encephalitis
- Bacterial meningitis
- Cryptococcal meningitis

6. **New headache of recent onset:**
- Subdural haematoma
- Brain neoplasm, primary or secondary
- Brain abscess/toxoplasmosis
- TB meningitis
- Giant cell arteritis (GCA)

7. **Chronic/Intermittent headache:**
- Migraine
- Cluster headache
- Trigeminal neuralgia
- Analgesia overuse headache
- Sinusitis

8. **Back pain:**
- Spinal metastases
- Vertebral fracture (osteoporotic/pathological)
- Cord compression
- Mechanical lower back pain

9. **Weak legs:**
- Guillain–Barré syndrome
- Myopathy
- Multiple sclerosis/transverse myelitis
- Eaton–Lambert syndrome
- Cord compression
- Motor neuron disease
- Familial hypokalaemic periodic paralysis

10. **Falls:**
- Syncope
- Postural hypotension
- Epilepsy
- Vertebrobasilar ischaemia
- Parkinson's disease
- Myopathies

11. Painful joints of the wrist and hand:
- Rheumatoid arthritis
- Systemic lupus erythematosus (SLE)
- Osteoarthritis
- Crystal arthropathy

12. Abnormal liver function tests:
- Gallstones
- Acute viral hepatitis
- EBV
- PBC
- Autoimmune hepatitis
- Drug induced
- Non-alcoholic steatohepatitis (NASH)
- Haemochromatosis

13. Alcohol dependence and abdominal pain:
- Pancreatitis
- Peptic ulcer disease
- Spontaneous bacterial peritonitis
- Hepatocellular carcinoma
- Acute hepatitis

14. Diarrhoea:
- Irritable bowel syndrome
- Inflammatory bowel disease
- Infective diarrhoea/small bowel overgrowth
- Lactose intolerance
- Bile salt malabsorption
- Coeliac disease
- Chronic pancreatitis/insufficiency
- Diverticular disease
- Carcinoid
- Colorectal cancer

15. The HIV patient:
- Diarrhoea
- Weight loss
- Abdominal pain
- Headache
- Confusion
- Weak legs
- Jaundice

- Breathlessness
- Skin rash/lesion
- Chest pain
- Arthralgia/myalgia
- Visual disturbance

16. Hypertension:
- Essential hypertension
- Conn syndrome
- Cushing syndrome
- Phaeochromocytoma
- Renovascular hypertension
- Coarctation of the aorta

SCENARIO 1. CHEST PAIN

'Please would you see this 49-year-old man who has recently been complaining of chest pain when walking upstairs? His examination reveals a blood pressure of 140/96. Many thanks.'

'This 24-year-old, 30-week-pregnant woman has been experiencing sharp chest pains fro the last 48 hours. Please take a history.'

'I would be grateful for your opinion regarding the further investigation of this 28-year-old professional footballer. He has been complaining of severe chest pain after a recent match. He also describes a flu-like illness 2 days before.'

'This 62-year-old woman responded well to a course of antibiotics for a recent chest infection. However, she now complains of severe right-sided chest pains. Please take a history.'

'This 50-year-old man continues to suffer from angina despite a recent successful coronary bypass operation. This is usually postprandial and associated with low-grade nausea. Please take a history.'

'I would be grateful for your opinion about this 30-year-old woman who complains of palpitations and chest pains that are worse at night. A recent ECG, 24-hour tape and exercise tolerance test were reported as normal.'

1. Verify the information provided
'Tell me in your own words what the problem is ... .'

2. HPC:
Open to closed questions keeping in mind the *differential diagnosis*:
Unstable/stable angina
Myocardial infarction
Pulmonary embolism
Pericarditis
Pleurisy
Oesophageal spasm
GORD
Costochondritis
Anxiety

3. Previous investigations:
Chest radiograph? ECG?
Exercise tolerance test (ETT)?
Coronary angiogram?

4. SR:
Risk factors for coronary disease
Associated SOB, nausea, palpitations, headache

5. PMH
Known ischaemic heart disease (IHD), CVA, diabetes, dyslipidaemia, hypertension, autoimmune disease, DVT/PE

6. DH:
Contraindications to anti-platelet therapy/thrombolysis/β blockers/heparin/ACE inhibitors?
Current therapy for IHD, hypercholesterolaemia, hypertension

7. FH:
Premature IHD

8. SH:
Smoking history in pack-years, limitation of work by pain, recent travel (DVT/PE), Canadian Cardiovascular Society status, stress

9. Summarise
'Is there anything else that we haven't discussed that you feel is important?'

10. Thank the patient

Volunteered problems

Alarm symptoms:
Chest pain at rest/minimal exertion, crescendo symptoms

Disease interaction:
Is there more than one cause or more than one type of chest pain?

Therapeutic success and failures:
Has the condition improved with medications?
Did symptoms coincide with a change in medication?
Side effects (eg β blockers and impotence)

Risks to others:
Familial dyslipidaemia?

Daily life and disease:
What is the impact of symptoms on daily tasks and vice versa? Is stress and anxiety exacerbating symptoms or caused by them?

Final problem list and plan of action

1. Triage urgency of further investigation and treatment

2. Identify the best means of investigation (eg ETT or myocardial perfusion scan for suspected angina, endoscopy or pH manometry for suspected reflux disease)

3. Consider long-term secondary prevention and likely compliance, eg treatment of hypercholesterol-aemia, hypertension, smoking cessation, exercise, weight loss

4. Compliance with investigations and treatment (especially primary or secondary prevention)

5. 'Atypical' chest pain syndromes and abnormal disease behaviour may require clinical psychology input

Key diagnostic features	Example problem list and plan of action
Unstable angina	
Cardiac pain at rest or minimal exertion Typical or atypical (atypical more common in elderly people and women) Associated SOB/nausea Prevalence of other feature (GUARANTEE study 1996): • Hypertension about 60% • Previous angina about 60% • Hypercholesterolaemia about 40% • Family history of coronary artery disease (CAD) about 40% • Previous myocardial infarction (MI) about 40% • Previous angioplasty about 25% • Previous CABG (coronary artery bypass graft) about 25% • Diabetes mellitus about 25% • Current smoker about 25% • Previous CVA about 9%	Urgent risk stratification, eg ECG and troponin to collate a TIMI score (see p. 125) ETT or myocardial perfusion scan for further risk stratification Contraindications to ETT Anti-platelet drugs, antihypertensives, statins, β blockers and other secondary prevention medications DVLA rules and driving after an MI Debilitating chest pain may impair ability to work and impact on other areas of life
Stable angina	
Exercise tolerance before onset of pain Pain not affected by respiration or position Crescendo angina (falling exercise tolerance, increasing frequency of attacks) Pain abates with rest Risk factors for cardiac disease	Assess current anti-anginal therapy and potential for escalation Need for risk stratification if not done previously Impact on work and social life Side effects of medications (depression, impotence, etc) Anti-platelet drugs, antihypertensives, statins, β blockers and other secondary prevention medications
Pulmonary embolism	
PIOPED study: SOB (about 70%) Pleuritic chest pain (66%) Cough (about 33%) Haemoptysis (about 10%) Swollen calf/known DVT Risk factors for DVT (previous DVT/PE, hypercoagulable states, immobility, malignancy, smoking, oral contraceptive pill [OCP], pregnancy)	Wells' score to determine probability of PE (see below) Urgent investigation and therapy if needed Ventilation–perfusion scan vs CTPA Investigations and treatment in pregnancy (ventilation–perfusion scan > CTPA) Long-term anticoagulation and potential contraindications (eg falls) and risks

Key diagnostic features	Example problem list and plan of action
Pericarditis	
Chest pain: Severe ('devil's grip') Worse on lying flat, deep inspiration and swallowing Fever/flu-like prodrome SOB is common *PMH*: autoimmune disease, TB, renal failure, known malignancy	Exclusion of acute MI and other causes of pain Investigations to identify cause (see below) and implications for long-term treatment and risk of constrictive pericarditis
Pleurisy	
Chest pain on inspiration Fever SOB *PMH*: TB, recent/recurrent chest infection, known autoimmune disease, eg rheumatoid arthritis	Exclusion of PE Coxsackievirus B infection: are other family members affected? (Intrafamiliar spread of echoviruses and Coxsackievirus is common) NSAIDs unless contraindicated Need to provide adequate analgesia Time off work Postviral fatigue syndrome
Oesophageal spasm	
Chest pain (80%) Dysphagia (50%) Heartburn (20%) Globus and regurgitation are common	Need for pH manometry Diffuse oesophageal spasm (random contractions) vs nutcracker oesophagus (coordinated spasm of excessive amplitude) Treatment (eg Botox injection, PPI, calcium channel antagonists) Exclusion of cardiac pain
GORD	
See above	Exclusion of concomitant cardiac pain if cardiac risk factors are prominent
Costochondritis	
Insidious onset Movement related, deep inspiration Recent activity at unaccustomed level of exertion *PMH*: osteoarthritis elsewhere, inflammatory arthropathy, chest deformity (eg pectus excavatum)	Exclusion of PE/angina Address patient anxiety about heart/lung disease
Anxiety	
Palpitations, diaphoresis, sense of impending doom, SOB, dizziness, paraesthesiae History of depression/post-traumatic stress disorder/other anxiety disorder	Exclusion of underlying organic disorder Identification of precipitant factors Need for psychiatric review and likely compliance

Questions

1. What is the TIMI score?

The thrombolysis in myocardial infarction (TIMI) score predicts adverse outcomes in non-ST-elevation MI (NSTEMI) and correlates well with the degree of coronary artery stenosis. Each of the following scores 1 point:

- Aged ≥ 65 years
- Use of aspirin in the last 7 days
- Known coronary stenosis of ≥ 50%
- ST deviation on ECG > 0.5 mm
- Severe anginal symptoms (two or more or more anginal events in the last 24 hours)
- At least three risk factors for coronary disease
- Elevated serum cardiac markers (eg troponin I).

Score event	Risk of death from IHD (%)
0–1	4.7
2	8.3
3	13.2
4	19.9
5	26.2
6–7	40.9

2. How is the severity of angina assessed clinically?

The Canadian Cardiovascular Society grading scale for classification of angina:

Class I: angina only during strenuous or prolonged physical activity
Class II: slight limitation, with angina only during vigorous physical activity
Class III: symptoms with everyday living activities, ie moderate limitation
Class IV: inability to perform any activity without angina or angina at rest, ie severe limitation.

3. *What are the causes of pericarditis?*

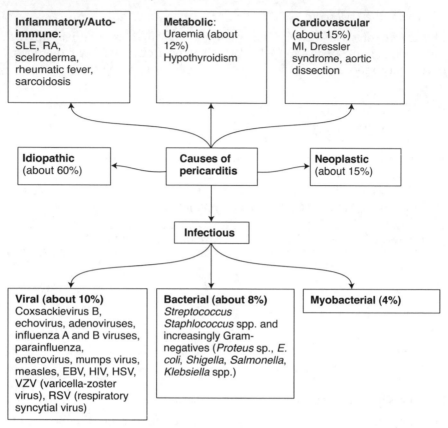

Figure 2.1 Causes of pericarditis.

4. *Are you aware of any scoring systems to assess clinical likelihood of a PE?*
Modified Wells' Score (Canadian score) for clinical probability of PE

Clinical feature	Score
Clinical signs of DVT	3
Alternative diagnosis less probable than PE	3
Heart rate > 100 beats/min	1.5
Recent immobilisation or surgery (4 weeks)	1.5
Previous DVT or PE	1.5
Haemoptysis	1
Cancer	1

Interpretation:

- Low probability: score < 2
- Moderate probability: score 2–6
- High probability: score > 6.

SCENARIO 2. ABDOMINAL PAIN

'This pleasant 55-year-old male car salesman has recently been made redundant. He has been suffering from epigastric pain for the last few months that has not responded to antacids. Please advise.'

'This 34-year-old woman has persistent heartburn despite using a PPI for many weeks. A recent endoscopy revealed mild oesophagitis. She is keen to explore surgical options for her problem but I thought referral to your clinic to ensure that we had maximised medical therapy would be prudent.'

'This 74-year-old man has just been diagnosed with a microcytic anaemia. He has also lost weight over the past 4 months. Please take a history.'

'This 40-year-old woman is now on Oromorph to control her recurrent abdominal pain. A recent upper GI endoscopy was normal. I would be grateful for your further advice.'

'This 18-year-old man has had a lot off time of work recently as a result of recurrent abdominal pain. This is only partially relieved by a PPI. He has noticed that his symptoms are much worse when at work. Please take a history.'

1. Verify the information provided:
'Tell me in your own words what the problem is … .'

2. HPC:
Progress from open to closed questions keeping in mind the *differential diagnosis*:
GORD
Peptic ulcer
Gastric cancer
Pancreatitis
Functional dyspepsia

3. Previous investigations:
Cardiac investigations?
Previous therapeutic trial of PPI/H$_2$-receptor antagonist?

4. SR:
Short of breath (SOB – anaemia)? Depression/anxiety?

5. PMH:
Cardiac disease, liver disease, pancreatitis
Functional (non-ulcer) dyspepsia has higher proportion of psychological co-morbidity

6. DH:
NSAIDs, bisphosphonates, aspirin, clopidogrel
Previous PPIs/H$_2$-receptor antagonists

7. FH:
Gastric cancer, peptic ulcer disease

8. SH:
Alcohol consumption in units, smoking in pack-years. Recent stress?

9. Summarise
'Is there anything else that we haven't discussed that you feel is important?'

10. Thank the patient

Volunteered problems

Alarm symptoms:
Weight loss, GI bleeding, jaundice, dysphagia

Disease interaction:
There may be an organic problem (eg gastritis) exacerbating a functional problem (eg postprandial distress syndrome)

Therapeutic success and failures
Is the pain relieved by PPI?
Side effects: gynaecomastia, diarrhoea, interactions (cytochrome P450 induction by some PPIs)
Is aspirin really needed or can an alternative anti-platelet be used?

Risks to others

Daily life and disease:
What is the impact of disease on daily life?
How will treatment and investigation impact further?
What is the impact of lifestyle/occupation on the disease?

Final problem list and plan of action:

1. Beware of over-investigation of patients with functional disorders.

2. Malnutrition and under-nutrition need to be corrected – a dietician's opinion is often very useful

3. Patient may be very reluctant to undergo invasive endoscopic investigations

4. Referral to a surgeon may be appropriate if there is gastric outlet obstruction/cancer/ treatment-resistant GORD, etc

5. Patients may not be willing to take a medication life long, even if effective

6. Diet and lifestyle factors often need to be addressed to prevent recurrent disease

Key diagnostic features	Example problem list and plan of action
Gastro-oesophageal reflux disease (GORD)	
Retrosternal burning pain Dysphagia Odynophagia Associated epigastric pain Waterbrash Regurgitation of food Acid in the back of throat Often worse at night lying flat Exacerbated by: large meals, tight belt, stooping over, fruit juice, spicy food, chocolate, caffeine, smoking *PMH*: diabetes (gastoparesis), co-morbidity precluding laparoscopic fundoplication *DH*: PPI (?working), motility agents (eg domperidone)	Need to establish the efficacy of current therapy and whether all basic advice is being followed (tilt bed towards feet slightly, eat evening meal early, avoid tight clothing, avoid alcohol, spicy food, etc) Those with symptoms despite a PPI (or with new unexplained symptoms and age of onset > 55) should have an upper GI endoscopy Use pH manometry to confirm reflux after a normal OGD (non-erosive reflux disease) and/or before referral for laparoscopic fundoplication Patients may have well-controlled symptoms with a PPI but do not like the idea of lifelong medication and would prefer to have surgery. They need to be aware of failure rate (15%) and complications (eg oesophageal stenosis and dysphagia in 5%) of surgery
Peptic ulcer disease	
Postprandial gnawing epigastric pain radiating through to back Duodenal ulcer: hunger pains before eating Nausea and vomiting (stricture and outlet obstruction) Anorexia, weight loss Melaena, haematemesis Recent alcohol binge *PMH*: established cirrhosis, previous ulcer disease *DH*: NSAIDS, steroids (recent alcoholic hepatitis?)	Identify and treat causative factors: NSAIDs, *H. pylori* infection, alcohol, steroids Triage urgency/necessity of upper GI endoscopy. Exclude perforation if unwell Need follow-up endoscopy to confirm healing of *gastric* ulcers only Non-healing ulcers need to be biopsied. Benign non-healing ulcers and pain despite a PPI raise the possibility of Zollinger–Ellison syndrome
Gastric cancer	
Constant abdominal pain Weight loss Nausea and vomiting (there may be gastric outlet obstruction) Anorexia Ethnic origin (very high incidence in Far East) *PMH*: previous gastric surgery (higher incidence of cancer). Known *H. pylori* infection *FH*: people with blood group A have higher incidence	Urgent endoscopy required if cancer suspected A multidisciplinary approach to staging and treatment. CT of chest/abdomen/pelvis, endoscopic ultrasonography Post-gastrectomy vitamin B_{12} replacement Consider co-morbidity and fitness for surgery Regular surveillance for recurrence

Key diagnostic features	Example problem list and plan of action
Chronic pancreatitis	
Relapsing/remitting severe central abdominal pain	Investigate and treat aetiology
Weight loss, fatty stools	Nutritional status and support (eg enzyme supplements)
Fat-soluble vitamin deficiency: vitamins A, D E and K	Malabsorption and vitamin deficiency screen
PMH: post-ERCP, known gallstones, recent mumps, EBV, pancreatic cancer, osteoporosis, fractures	Alcohol dependence and screening for other alcohol-related disease
DH: azathioprine, steroids, sulphonamides, methyldopa	Opiate dependence is common. In chronic severe pain, input from a chronic pain specialist is useful. Consider coeliac plexus ablation in resistant cases
SH: alcohol consumption	
Functional dyspepsia	
Rome III criteria for functional dyspepsia	Difficult to distinguish from functional abdominal pain syndrome (FAPS), which is not a primary dysmotility problem but an abnormal neuropsychological response to normal visceral stimuli
At least 3 months, with onset at least 6 months previously, of one or more of the following: Bothersome postprandial fullness Early satiation Epigastric pain Epigastric burning	
	Patients often require repeated reassurance that their symptoms do not result from serious pathology
No evidence of structural disease (including at upper endoscopy) that is likely to explain the symptoms	Spasmolytics, dietary modification, low-dose antidepressants and (increasingly) hypnotherapy are acknowledged treatment modalities
Exacerbation of symptoms with stress and anxiety is common	
PMH: depression and anxiety more common	

Question

1. *Which patients with dyspepsia should be referred for endoscopy?*

Clinical guideline (NICE 2006)

- Symptoms despite cessation of provoking factors (alcohol, NSAIDs, steroids, bisphosphonates, nitrates, calcium antagonists)
- Unintentional weight loss*
- GI bleeding*
- Iron deficiency anaemia*
- Dysphagia*
- Persistent vomiting*
- Epigastric mass*

- Suspicious barium meal result*
- Patients > 55 years with persistent symptoms and no obvious cause.*

*Warrants urgent endoscopy.

If endoscopy is not indicated, patients should be screened for *H. pylori* (a 2-week washout period off PPIs is required before breath tests) and treated if positive.

If *H. pylori* test is negative or treatment does not relieve symptoms, a therapeutic trial of a PPI can be tried, starting at the higher dose for 1 month then stepping down to the lowest dose that controls symptoms. Unsuccessful treatment or weaning off a PPI warrants referral to a gastroenterologist (who will almost always arrange an endoscopy).

SCENARIO 3. CHRONIC COUGH

'This 24-year-old woman is troubled by a persistent cough, worse at night. She says that it always seems to be a problem during the summer months. Please take a history.'

'This 30-year-old painter and decorator has been increasingly wheezy. His usual inhalers do not control his symptoms. I would be grateful for your further assessment.'

'This 60-year-old man is normally fit and well. He complains of paroxysmal coughing fits that can come on at any time. He is an ex-smoker and his past history is unremarkable apart from hypertension.'

'This 50-year-old woman with a 5-year history of asthma now complains of a chronic cough with occasional haemoptysis. Her asthma is becoming increasingly difficult to control. Please take a history.'

'I recently saw this 70-year-old man, a retired builder, when he attended my clinic with his wife (who was consulting for anxiety and insomnia). It emerged that he has had a nocturnal cough for the last 4 months that is keeping his wife awake at night. Furthermore, he has lost 4 kg in weight over that period which, although he seems unconcerned, is causing his wife considerable anxiety. I would be grateful for your further assessment of the man's problem.'

'This 35-year-old ex-IVD user works in a shelter for homeless people. Over the last 2 weeks he has been troubled by a persistent productive cough and night sweats. Please take a history.'

'The 40-year-old woman recently returned home after visiting relatives in Jamaica. She feels that she caught a chest infection abroad but a course of antibiotics has not improved her symptoms. She has a persistent cough and complains of general malaise and anorexia. In the last few days she has noticed a painful skin rash over her legs. Please take a history.'

1. Verify the information provided:
'Tell me in your own words what the problem is … .'

2. HPC:
Open to closed questions keeping in mind the *differential diagnosis*:
Asthma
Postnasal drip
Sarcoid
Drugs
GORD
Lung cancer
TB
Bronchiectasis

3. Previous investigations:
Chest radiograph?
Bronchoscopy?
Nasal endoscopy?

4. SR:
GORD symptoms

5. PMH:
Childhood asthma, atopy, nasal polyps, sinus problems, previous TB, recurrent pneumonias

6. DH:
NSAIDs (as precipitant of asthma)
ACE inhibitors (chronic cough)
Current inhaler regimen if known to have asthma
Any known allergies?

7. FH:
Asthma, atopy, lung cancer, TB exposure

8. SH:
Smoking history in pack-years, working conditions (recent dust/paint/solvent exposure), living conditions (damp, decorating work), pets, asbestos exposure, travel to TB endemic areas. Financial status. HIV risks (TB co-infection).

9. Summarise:
'Is there anything else that we haven't discussed that you feel is important?'

10. Thank the patient

Volunteered problems

Alarm symptoms:
Weight loss, haemoptysis, night sweats, progressive SOB, chest pain

Disease interaction:
eg GORD exacerbating asthma, steroid therapy in established osteoporosis

Therapeutic success and failures
Has condition improved with inhalers/steroids?
Did symptoms coincide with a change in medication?
How is their inhaler technique?

Risks to others:
TB exposure risk to close contacts

Daily life and disease:
Does the patient require a change in occupation or accommodation?
Are there legal/compensation issues?

Final problem list and plan of action

1. Patient anxiety regarding cancer is common irrespective of the most likely underlying diagnosis.

2. Need to triage urgency of further investigation and treatment

3. Exclude and treat non-respiratory conditions that may be exacerbating symptoms

4. Need to encourage compliance with maintenance therapy when well

5. Check inhaler technique

6. Infection control issues and their enforcement.

7. Help with smoking cessation

8. Occupational lung disease and employment/ financial/ compensation issues

Key diagnostic features	Example problem list and plan of action
Asthma	
Wheeze, cough and nasal congestion (polyps) are classic symptoms	Examination to assess severity (eg peak flow) and triage urgency of further investigation and management
Identify triggers: animal dander, dust, cold, exercise, pollutants, infection, emotion	Current inhaler technique adequate?
Duration, severity and frequency of attacks	Current inhaler regimen may be inadequate – need to step up therapy (see British Thoracic Society or BTS guidelines on page 139)
Green sputum?	
Reduced exercise tolerance?	
Previous skin testing?	Repeat courses of steroids – has bone density been checked?
PMH: previous ICU admission, atopy, nasal polyps	Working conditions may be exacerbating symptoms and a change of profession may be inevitable. What is the financial situation and what can the doctor do to assist (eg letters to employers for change of role at work)?
FH: atopy or asthma	
SH: smoking, occupational exposure to precipitants (eg sawdust, animal dander, solvents), living conditions and recent refurbishment, pets. Time off work/school	
	Compliance with treatment between attacks is a major issue. Specialist nurses have time to reinforce patient education
	Patients with brittle asthma should be included on an at-risk register to ensure rapid assessment and treatment in primary and secondary care
Postnasal drip	
Unpleasant taste in mouth	Need to exclude chronic sinusitis (CT of sinuses indicated?)
Nocturnal cough	
Nasal congestion	ENT referral may be necessary
Headache common (associated sinusitis)	May need to exclude a more sinister cause of cough
PMH: atopy, asthma	
DH: symptoms usually improve with topical steroids	
Sarcoid	
Fever, anorexia and arthralgias	Diagnosis: serum ACE, CT of chest, bronchoscopy and transbronchial biopsy
SOB on exertion	
Persistent cough	Assess severity: pulmonary function tests, transfer factor (D_{LCO})
Systems review (SR):	
Cardiac: cardiomyopathy, heart block	A multidisciplinary approach is frequently needed to identify and treat all involved systems
Neurological: lymphocytic meningitis, cranial nerve palsies	
Skin: erythema nodosum, lupus pernio	Patient may require simple monitoring or aggressive steroid therapy
Eye: uveitis	
FH: African–Caribbean origin or Scandinavian origin (Löfgren syndrome)	

Key diagnostic features	Example problem list and plan of action
Drug side effect	
ACE inhibitors	Angiotensin II antagonist may reduce cough, or choose alternative antihypertensive
GORD	
Retrosternal burning pain Dysphagia Odynophagia Associated epigastric pain Waterbrash Regurgitation of food Acid in the back of throat Cough worse at night or lying flat for extended periods Exacerbated by: large meals, tight belt, stooping over, fruit juice, spicy food, chocolate, caffeine, smoking *PMH*: diabetes (gastoparesis), co-morbidity precluding laparoscopic fundoplication *DH*: cough may improve with PPI	Poorly controlled asthma exacerbated by GORD may warrant laparoscopic fundoplication even if the oesophagitis or heartburn is minimal A normal OGD does not exclude asthma exacerbation by 'microdroplet' aspiration; pH manometry may be more useful Inhaled/oral steroid use for asthma may cause oesophageal candidiasis and symptoms of GORD
Lung cancer	
Local disease: cough, haemoptysis, non-resolving chest infection **Metastatic**: weight loss, anorexia, headache (most common cancer leading to brain metastases), behavioural change, SVC obstruction recurrent laryngeal nerve palsy **Paraneoplastic** (Eaton–Lambert syndrome) weakness, hypercalcaemia, DVT/PE *SH*: smoking history, occupational asbestos exposure	Multidisciplinary approach: oncology (clinical and medical), cardiothoracic surgeons, histopathology, respiratory physician, neurosurgeon Staging disease: staging CT of brain, chest, abdomen. PET (positron emission tomography) Bronchoscopy or CT-guided biopsy Endoscopic ultrasonography for hilar lymphadenopathy Does the patient qualify for compensation for asbestos exposure? Financial status and time off work for investigations/treatment Patient expectations may differ wildly from the likely prognosis

Key diagnostic features	Example problem list and plan of action
TB	
Symptoms often non-specific	Need to screen for HIV co-infection
Fever, anorexia, weight loss, haemoptysis, night sweats	Isolation and infection control.
Risks: potential exposure to TB, recent travel to TB endemic area, ethnic origin	Screening/prophylaxis of close contacts – implications for work and family life
PMH: HIV/AIDS	Stigma affects acceptance of diagnosis and compliance with investigations (often invasive) and long-term therapy. The patient's family may not always be supportive as a result of perceived risk of infection
DH: immunosuppressant therapy for other condition?	
	Screen for other organ involvement, eg abdominal TB, bone marrow infiltration, TB meningitis
	Monitor for adverse effects of anti-tuberculous medications (see questions below)
	Nutritional status may be poor and require correction
	Reduced efficacy of the oral contraceptive pill on rifampicin – recommend barrier contraception
Bronchiectasis	
Productive cough, SOB, wheeze, haemoptysis, weight loss	Diagnosis: chest radiograph and CT of chest
Causes (anything that obstructs mucociliary clearance):	Investigate and treat the underlying cause if treatable
Young syndrome (mild variant of cystic fibrosis presenting in middle-aged men)	Most causes are chronic progressive conditions that have vast implications for the patient's future
Cystic fibrosis	HIV and contact tracing, treatment, etc
Primary ciliary dyskinesia	
Allergic bronchopulmonary aspergillosis (asthmatic prodrome)	
HIV-related lung disease (chronic infection)	
Inhaled foreign objects	

Question

1. *Which patients with suspected TB should be isolated when admitted to hospital?*

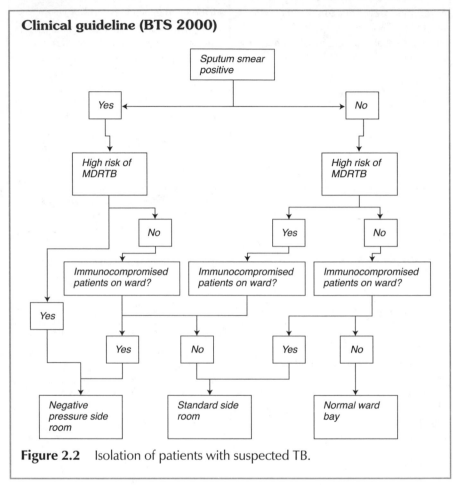

Figure 2.2   Isolation of patients with suspected TB.

2. *What are the common adverse reactions to anti-TB medications?*

- **Isoniazid**: raised liver enzymes (20%), acute hepatitis about 2%, peripheral neuritis, seizures, drug-induced lupus
- **Rifampicin**: hepatitis, reduced efficacy of cytochrome P450 (CYP450)-metabolised drugs, orange discoloration of body fluids
- **Ethambutol**: optic neuritis, gout, rash, peripheral neuritis
- **Pyrazinamide**: gout, hepatitis,
- **Streptomycin**: ototoxicity (audiovestibular disturbance), nephrotoxicity.

3. *What are the BTS guidelines on the use of inhaled and oral medication for asthma?*

Clinical guideline

Start therapy at the level most appropriate to the level of severity. Maintain control by stepping up therapy when control is poor and stepping down when control is good (Figure 2.3).

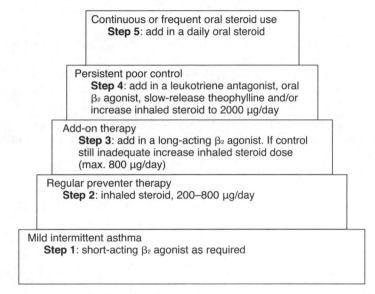

Figure 2.3   BTS guidelines for inhaled and oral medicine in asthma.

SCENARIO 4. BREATHLESSNESS

'Please see this 60-year-old man who has been complaining of nocturnal cough and breathlessness for the past 4 months. It is becoming increasingly debilitating these last few days such that he can no longer get about the house. Many thanks.'

'This 75-year-old man with a history of ischaemic heart disease (IHD) has been increasingly breathless over the last 2 weeks. Please take a history.'

'This 50-year-old woman complains of worsening shortness of breath on exertion. This seems to improve and then worsen again. Her past medical history is unremarkable apart from three miscarriages in her 20s. Please take a history.'

'This 45-year-old man has worsening shortness of breath. This is now impeding his ability to work as a postman. I would be grateful for your further advice.'

1. Verify the information provided
'Tell me in your own words what the problem is...'

2. HPC:
Open to closed questions keeping in mind the *differential diagnosis*:
Congestive cardiac failure (CCF)
Chronic obstructive pulmonary disease (COPD)
Lung cancer and effusion
Cryptogenic fibrosing alveolitis
Recurrent pulmonary emboli
Asthma (see above)

3. Previous investigations:
Echocardiography, coronary angiogram, lung function tests, CT of the chest

4. SR:
Reactive depression very common in CCF.

5. PMH:
Known heart or lung disease
Rheumatic fever
DVT/PE
Number of previous admissions to hospital with exacerbations

6. DH
ACE inhibitors, β blockers, diuretics
Drugs causing fibrosis, eg amiodarone, nitrofurantoin
Home oxygen

7. FH
α_1-Antitrypsin deficiency
Looking after a sick relative?

8. SH:
Occupational exposure to agents causing fibrotic lung disease, alcohol and dilated cardiomyopathy, smoking in pack-years, NYHA grade and specific limitations on hobbies, family life, ability to travel, etc

9. Summarise:
'Is there anything else that we haven't discussed that you feel is important?'

10. Thank the patient

Volunteered problems

Alarm symptoms:
Syncope or chest pain
Haemoptysis
Weight loss

Disease interaction:
eg COPD and CCF commonly occur together

Therapeutic success and failures:
Symptoms despite maximal medical therapy, treatment limited by side effects, compliance with secondary prevention (eg inhaled steroids)

Risks to others:
Oxygen at home and continued smoking

Daily life and disease:
What is the impact of symptoms on daily tasks and vice versa? Is stress and anxiety exacerbating symptoms or resulting from them?

Final problem list and plan of action

1. Triage urgency of further investigation and treatment

2. Assess likelihood of compliance with investigations and treatment

3. What is the degree of disability and need for additional help at home?

4. Optimise medical therapy and investigate potential complications (eg steroids and osteoporosis)

5. Ongoing smoker despite need for home oxygen?

6. Offer help with smoking cessation.

7. End-of-life decisions in patients with end-stage disease – set an appropriate ceiling of therapy

Key diagnostic features	Example problem list and plan
Congestive cardiac/heart failure (CCF/CHF)	
SOB at rest or on exertion Paroxysmal nocturnal dyspnoea (PND) Orthopnea Peripheral oedema Nocturia Confusion, lethargy Establish New York Heart Association (NYHA) status *PMH*: IHD, hypertension, alcohol, valvular disease *DH*: diuretics, β blockers, ACE inhibitors	Failing independence at home requiring additional support with activities of daily living (ADL) Inadequate/over-medication Medications that may exacerbate heart failure (eg β blockers, rosiglitazone) Possible reversible coronary insufficiency not investigated Reactive depression is common and often overlooked On maximal therapy but deteriorating – palliative care measures? Heart transplant candidate?
COPD	
SOB on minimal exertion Productive cough for more than 3 consecutive months for more than 3 years Wheeze Previous lung function tests? Consultation with a respiratory physician? *PMH*: previous hospitalisations and weight loss with anorexia imply a poorer prognosis *DH*: on home oxygen? Nebulisers? *SH*: usually > 20 pack-years smoking. Occupational lung disease	Further investigations to stage disease and identify cause Adequacy of current treatment Occupational lung disease and compensation Adequacy of current social support services Contraindications to home oxygen (eg ongoing smoker) Are the nebulisers helping? They may encourage patient to struggle on at home and present to hospital in a much worse state Exclude coexistent CHF or cor pulmonale
Lung cancer	
See above	See above
Cryptogenic fibrosing alveolitis (CFA)	
Insidious onset of SOB Flu-like symptoms and arthralgia common Wheeze and fever unusual Weight loss common *PMH*: chronic microaspiration from GORD may be implicated in some cases *SH*: smoking and occupational exposure to wood and metal dust slightly more common in CFA	Need to exclude other known causes of interstitial lung disease (eg drugs, occupational exposure) High-resolution CT (HRCT) of chest and transbronchial biopsy usually necessary Progressive condition – need to assess stage and plan long-term support

Key diagnostic features	Example problem list and plan
Recurrent pulmonary emboli	
May have no documented previous PEs (all subclinical)	May require cardiac catheterisation to determine pulmonary artery pressures if pulmonary hypertension suspected Risk of paradoxical embolism (history of stroke?)
Risk factors for DVT (previous DVT/PE, hypercoagulable states, immobility, malignancy, smoking, OCP, pregnancy)	
PMH: known prothrombotic disorder (antithrombin III deficiency, protein C/S deficiency, factor V Leiden mutation, antiphospholipid syndrome)	Anticoagulation and its contraindications Management of pulmonary hypertension (diuretics, prostaglandins, endothelin antagonists, home oxygen therapy)

Question

1. *What are the causes of lung fibrosis?*

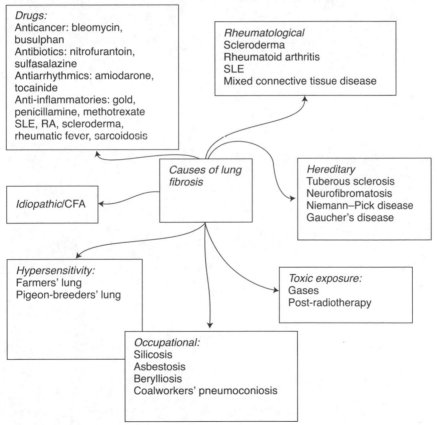

Figure 2.4 Causes of lung fibrosis.

SCENARIO 5. ACUTE-ONSET HEADACHE

'An HIV-positive man has referred himself to A&E with a headache. His partner thinks that he has recently been behaving slightly bizarrely. Please take a history.'

'A 34-year-old man presents to A&E with a headache that began earlier that day. It is now unbearable. Please take a history.'

'This 74-year-old man had a sudden-onset headache earlier today. He thinks that he may have lost consciousness for a moment and has been bedbound since. Please take a history.'

'This 18-year-old girl is suffering from a severe headache that woke her up in the early hours of the morning. Please take a history.'

1. Verify the information provided:
'Tell me in your own words what the problem is … .'

2. HPC:
Open to closed questions keeping in mind the *differential diagnosis*, eg
Subarachnoid haemorrhage (SAH)
Haemorrhagic stroke
Viral meningitis/ encephalitis
Bacterial/cryptococcal meningitis

3. Previous investigations:
Previous CT/MRI? HIV test? Renal imaging?

4. SR:
HIV risk factors. Symptoms of polycystic kidney/liver disease
Symptoms of AIDS-defining illnesses, meningism, photophobia, neck stiffness, non-blanching rash, fevers, rigors, seizures, cold sores (HSV)

5. PMH:
HIV and CD4 count
Polycystic kidney disease (PCKD)
Previous headaches
Previous splenectomy☐ prophylaxis (pneumococcal meningitis)
Base of skull fracture /trauma (pneumococcal meningitis)

6. DH:
Analgesia and efficacy
Anticoagulation and SAH
Immunosuppressants

7. FH:
SAH, renal cyst/renal failure

8. SH:
Risk factors for HIV (IVDU, high risk sex), contact with birds (cryptococci), contact with other case of meningitis

9. Summarise
'Is there anything else that we haven't discussed that you feel is important?'

10. Thank the patient

Volunteered problems

Alarm symptoms:
Impaired cognition/loss of consciousness
Neurological impairment
Meningism
HIV/high risk of HIV

Disease interaction:
eg recognition of sinister pathology on a background of frequent migraine

Therapeutic successes and failures:
Adequacy of current analgesia
Symptom control leading to prolonged delay in diagnosis
Opioids and drowsiness – jeopardises recognition of a fall in GCS (Glasgow Coma Scale)
New AIDS-defining disease and implications for possible resistance to HAART (highly active anti-retroviral therapy)

Risks to others:
Meningitis and treatment of close contacts
Contact tracing in HIV-related disease

Daily life and disease:
May need a long recovery period including rehabilitation. This may exacerbate existing financial/ social problems

Final problem list and plan of action

1. Such cases always require urgent investigation and treatment

2. Early involvement of neurosurgeon in appropriate cases

3. Screening for other organ disease/complications of sepsis/ AIDS-defining illnesses

4. Consent for investigation and treatment in the cognitively impaired patient

5. Medicolegal issues surrounding late presentations after missed diagnosis

6. HIV contact tracing

Key diagnostic features	Example problem list and plan of action
Subarachnoid haemorrhage	
Sudden-onset 'worse headache ever' like being hit over the head	Need for urgent investigation (CT of head 93–98% sensitive) and treatment
Nausea and vomiting	Early involvement of neurosurgeons in all cases
Neck stiffness, back pain	
Sudden loss of consciousness (about 40%)	Timing of lumbar puncture – greatest sensitivity 12 hours after headache onset
Sentinel bleeds (about 35%) – severe headaches that resolve quickly (usually around 2 weeks before a major bleed)	Close monitoring and surveillance for rising intracranial pressure (especially with blood in the fourth ventricle)
Neurological deficit evolving after headache onset	Prophylaxis for re-bleeding and vasospasm (fluids to keep hypervolaemic, nimodipine)
Mass effect symptoms – falling GCS score, nerve VI palsy	Also need to manage other complications:
PMH: renal cystic disease, hypertension, vasculitis, blood dyscrasias, fibromuscular dysplasia	• Seizures (25%) • Hydrocephalus (25%) • Neurogenic pulmonary oedema (up to 90%) • Arrhythmias
FH: intracranial aneurysm/early stroke/polycystic kidney disease	A quarter have residual neurological deficit and most have transient/permanent cognitive deficit – this has major implications for rehabilitation/career/support at home
DH: headache not responding to analgesia	Emotional lability and depression are common after recovery
	Secondary prevention of another event is crucial
Haemorrhagic stroke	
Sudden-onset headache	Complication of another treatment, eg thrombolysis for MI
Nausea and vomiting	
Seizures	Surgical intervention for cerebellar haematoma (high risk of brain-stem compression)
Focal neurological deficit	
Alarms: cerebellar or brain-stem symptoms (double vision, ataxia, slurred speech, vertigo)	Often decline rapidly – need early decision about resuscitation status support taking into account co-morbidities
Loss of consciousness common	Correction of anticoagulation
PMH: hypertension, known brain tumour, coagulopathies	Complex issues surrounding long-term support for survivors with neurological deficit – rehab potential (specialist centre or at home) and need to plan support at home
DH: anticoagulant	
SH: cocaine use in young patients	
	Secondary prevention of another event

Key diagnostic features	Example problem list and plan of action
Viral meningitis/encephalitis	
Swift onset of headache within the last 36 hours	CT needed before lumbar puncture (LP) (see below)?
Fever (> 90%)	Need for antibiotics until bacterial meningitis excluded
Prodromal coryzal symptoms and myalgia 48 hours before headache (50%)	Antiviral therapy (anti-HIV, ganciclovir for CMV, aciclovir for HSV) indicated if evidence of encephalitis (seizures, focal neurology, decreased GCS)
Nausea and vomiting	
Photophobia	
Cognitive impairment	Failure to improve after 24 hours? Investigate potential HIV, toxoplasmosis or tubercular meningitis which may give similar LP results
Neck stiffness	
Irritability	
Rash	
HIV risk factors (CMV, adenovirus, HIV, HSV encephalitis)	Long-term prognosis excellent unless concomitant encephalitis
Testicular pain – mumps	Barrier contraception for HSV-2-infected individuals
Diarrhoea – enterovirus	
PMH: immunosuppression/HIV Measles/mumps/immunisations	HIV contact tracing, etc if first presentation
Previous viral meningitis (HSV and EBV recur)	Beware neonatal death in pregnant women with Coxsackievirus B meningitis
DH: immunosuppressants (CMV, EBV)	
Analgesia	
SH: HIV risk factors, hamster/mouse/rat as pet: lymphocytic choriomeningitis virus	
Bacterial meningitis	
Classic triad of headache, neck stiffness and fever in 80%	Need for urgent treatment before further investigation
Onset in last 24 hours common (25%)	Need for CT before LP (see below)?
Cough/cold within last week (50%)	Vigorous resuscitation if septic
Vomiting (35%)	Aggressive control of seizures
Seizures (30%)	Prophylaxis for close contacts
Drowsiness	Close surveillance for immediate complications (50%): venous thrombosis, subdural/brain abscess, raised intracranial pressure (ICP) and hydrocephalus, SAH, infarcts
Indolent presentations in elderly and immunocompromised patients	
PMH: base of skull fracture (pneumococcal meningitis)	
Recent mastoiditis, sinusitis, otitis media	One-third of survivors have long-term neurological sequelae – need to plan rehabilitation and additional support
Splenectomy (pneumococcal meningitis)	
Ventriculoperitoneal shunt?	Surveillance for obstructive hydrocephalus within first month of episode
HIV/AIDS	
Immunised for meningococcus C or Hib (*Haemophilus influenzae* type b)?	
DH: may be partially treated by GP with course of antibiotics resulting in more indolent presentation	

continued on next page

Key diagnostic features	Example problem list and plan of action
Cryptococcal meningitis	
Known HIV-positive patient Similar presentation to bacterial meningitis but often less symptomatic in immunocompromised patients Contact with birds	May have a normal LP initially. India ink stain only 30% sensitive. CSF (cerebrospinal fluid) culture and latex agglutination test important Lifelong oral fluconazole after successful treatment with intravenous amphotericin

Questions

1. What are the guidelines for use of CT of the brain before LP?

Clinical guideline

The possibility of herniation after LP in the presence of raised ICP means that a CT of the head before LP is usually sensible. No national guidelines exist but most trusts have their own guidelines for out-of-hours CT in suspected meningitis. These are usually based around the findings of a 2001 paper in the *New England Journal of Medicine* (Hasbun et al. 01 Computed tomography of the head before lumbar puncture in adults with suspected meningitis. NEJM 2001, Dec. 13th 345(24): 1727–33), which prospectively studied 301 patients with suspected meningitis. The absence of any of the following features was associated with a normal CT of the head in 93 of 96 patients (all 96 of whom safely underwent an LP):

- Age > 60 years
- Immunocompromise
- Previous central nervous system (CNS) disease
- Seizure within the past week
- Abnormal GCS
- Inability to answer two consecutive questions or follow two consecutive commands
- Gaze palsy
- Abnormal visual fields
- Arm or leg drift
- Dysphasia/aphasia/dysarthria.

The presence of any of these features, or papilloedema, should prompt CT of the brain before LP.

2. *Outline the CSF profiles (protein, white cell count [WCC], glucose and opening pressure) associated with the different pathogens of meningitis*

Pathogen	Opening pressure (cmH$_2$O)	WCC (cells/mm^3)	Glucose	Protein	Further test
Bacterial	20–30	100–5000; > 80% PMNs	Low	High	Culture and Gram stain
Viral	10–20	10–300; lymphocytes	Normal	Slightly increased	PCR
TB	20–30	100–500; lymphocytes	Low	High	AFB stain, culture, PCR
Cryptococci	20–30	10–300; lymphocytes	Low	Increased	India ink, latex agglutination

AFB, acid-fast bacilli; PCR, polymerase chain reaction PMN, polymorpho-nucleocytes.

SCENARIO 6. NEW HEADACHE OF RECENT ONSET

'Please could you see this 70-year-old man who takes warfarin for atrial fibrillation. He has been increasingly frail and slow over the last year. Today he is confused and complaining of a headache.'

'This 24-year-old HIV-positive man is currently on highly active antiretroviral therapy (HAART). His latest viral load was undetectable. Today he presents with a 4-day history of worsening headache. He was having difficulty keeping up with a presentation at work today. Please take a history.'

'This 70-year-old Asian woman describes an intermittent worsening headache over the past 4 weeks. She speaks little English but her daughter tells me that she has lost weight and has been feeling generally unwell for some time. Please take a history.'

'Please could you assess this 56-year-old woman who has had a throbbing headache for the last 3 days. Today she was concerned to find herself unable to read the newspaper (she normally has perfect vision).'

'This 40-year-old woman has had a persistent cough for 2 months. She now complains of a constant headache (worse in the mornings), which is unbearable when she coughs. She has become increasingly anxious about the cause of her symptoms.'

1. Verify the information provided:
'Tell me in your own words what the problem is ... .'

2. HPC:
Open to closed questions keeping in mind the *differential diagnosis*, eg
Subdural haematoma
Brain neoplasm, primary or secondary
Brain abscess/Toxoplasmosis
TB meningitis
Giant cell arteritis (GCA)

3. Previous investigations:
Previous CT/MRI? HIV test?

4. SR:
Night sweats (lymphoma/TB), nausea and vomiting (raised ICP), weight loss, cough/haemoptysis (TB/bronchial carcinoma with cerebral metastases)
Myalgia (GCA)

5. PMH:
Known malignancy?
HIV/AIDS
Recent head injury/recurrent falls
Polymyalgia rheumatica

6. DH:
Analgesia and efficacy
Anticoagulation
Immunosuppressants

7. FH:
Primary brain tumours

8. SH:
Smoking history
TB exposure and recent travel
HIV exposure

9. Summarise
'Is there anything else that we haven't discussed that you feel is important?'

10. Thank the patient

Volunteered problems

Alarm symptoms:
Morning nausea and vomiting, weight loss, focal neurological deficit, altered mentation, haemoptysis, seizures

Disease interaction:
Implications of new illness for established disease (eg tumour progression, HAART resistance)
Co-morbidity and fitness for surgical intervention (subdural haematoma)

Therapeutic successes and failures:
Recent medications prolonging warfarin half-life resulting in over-anticoagulation
Non-compliance/adverse effects with anti-TB medications

Risks to others:
TB and HIV exposure

Daily life and disease:
May need a long recovery period including rehabilitation. This may exacerbate existing financial/social problems

Final problem list and plan of action

1. Urgent investigation and treatment

2. Compliance and consent for investigation and treatment in the confused patient

3. Patient anxiety regarding disease progression

4. Need to determine resuscitation status in metastatic disease through discussion with patient and family

5. Neurological impairment and rehabilitiation – implications for long-term self-care and independence

Key diagnostic features	Example problem list and plan of action
Subdural haematoma	
Acute (< 72 hours from injury) Subacute (3–20 days since injury) Chronic (> 20 days since injury) Insidious onset of symptoms: Headache (90%) – exacerbated by coughing or straining Cognitive dysfunction (50%) Irritability Asymmetrical motor weakness Aphasia Double vision on lateral gaze (nerve VI palsy indicating raised ICP) *PMH*: recurrent falls *DH*: warfarin or aspirin *SH*: possibility of non-accidental injury by carer	Urgent investigation (CT of head) and treatment (referral to neurosurgeon) May need a collateral history Aggressive control of seizures Chronicity of disease, neurological deficit and prognosis are crucial to determining whether neurosurgical intervention indicated Reversal of anticoagulation may not be straightforward, eg in context of metallic heart valve Exclude C-spine fracture Determine underlying cause of falls Non-accidental injury and possible elder abuse
Brain neoplasm (primary or secondary)	
Morning headache and/or vomiting Frontal tumours: depersonalisation, emotional lability, disinhibited behaviour Olfactory hallucinations/anosmia Parietotemporal tumours: seizures (often jacksonian), apraxia, memory loss, dysphasia, cognitive dysfunction, hemiparesis Pituitary fossa: bitemporal visual field loss, symptoms of panhypopituitarism/ prolactinaemia/diabetes insipidus Posterior fossa: ataxia, headache onset earlier in disease Brain stem: dysphagia, facial weakness, double vision Symptoms relating to primary tumour elsewhere, eg cough with haemoptysis (lung cancer most common site of primary in metastatic brain disease) *PMH*: HIV/immunocompromised – primary cerebral lymphoma Known malignancy *SH*: smoker	Multidisciplinary approach crucial (clinical and medical oncologist, radiologist, histopathologist, neurosurgeon, neurologist) Staging and treatment of extracerebral primary Control of seizures paramount to quality of life Patient's wishes are key – for metastatic lesions all treatment is palliative and may have profound side effects

Key diagnostic features	Example problem list and plan of action
Brain abscess	
Headache (about 70%)	Urgent treatment and investigation. Blood cultures before antibiotics
Altered mental state (about 65%)	
Focal neurological impairment (65%)	LP usually avoided
Fever (50%), seizures (33%)	Biopsy of lesion crucial
Nausea and vomiting (40%)	Surgical excision for single lesions, multiple decompressive aspirations for multiple lesions
Neck stiffness (25%)	
Headache may worsen suddenly if the abscess ruptures	Cover for *Toxoplasma gondii* infection if HIV suspected (treated with pyrimethamine and sulfadiazine)
Localised symptoms depending on location of abscess (see Brain neoplasm above)	
Symptoms from source of infection: sinusitis, otitis media, other chronic purulent focus	Good prognosis if onset of symptoms within a week. Otherwise residual deficit is likely and rehabilitation/additional support should be anticipated
PMH: immunocompromise (toxoplasmosis), congenital heart disease, endocarditis, recent dental surgery, penetrating trauma, transplantation	
DH: immunosuppressants	Treat underlying source of infection/immunocompromise
SH: HIV risks (toxoplasmosis, *Listeria*, *Mycobacterium*, *Nocardia* spp. and cryptococci), exposure to cats (toxoplasmosis)	
TB meningitis	
Immunocompetent: fever, headache, confusion, neck stiffness for several weeks	Requires urgent differentiation from other causes of meningitis
Immunocompromised: < 5% have meningism	Diagnostic difficulties, especially when CD4 count is low (acellular CSF)
Sudden-onset neurological impairment, including blindness	Screening of close contacts for TB
	Exclusion of other organ involvement
Fever, weight loss, anorexia, night sweats	HIV staging and treatment, including contact tracing
PMH: previous TB, known immunocompromise (HIV/AIDS), no BCG immunisation, positive test	
	Patient issues with stigma, relatives'/partners' fear of infection, compliance with long-term treatment
Ellispot/Quantiferon	
FH: contact with TB	Management of long-term neurological sequelae: rehabilitation, additional support

continued on next page

Key diagnostic features	Example problem list and plan of action
Temporal arteritis	
Unilateral temporal headache, often worse at night	Need to start steroid therapy urgently to protect against (further) visual loss
Jaw claudication (50%)	Non-urgent plan for temporal artery biopsy
Pain on combing hair/wearing hat or glasses	(but sensitivity decreases the longer steroid therapy continues)
Transient (amaurosis fugax in 10%) or complete visual loss	Maintenance therapy ± steroid-sparing agents, eg azathioprine
Proximal myalgia, low-grade fever, malaise	
PMH: known polymyalgia rheumatica. Recent deterioration in vision	Long-term consequences of steroids and need for bone protection agents (patients often elderly and at risk of osteoporosis)
DH: steroids (breakthrough vasculitis rare)	Monitoring for bone marrow suppression and hepatitis on azathioprine

Questions

1. *What other infections can mimic tuberculous meningitis in their clinical presentation?*

- Bacterial: partially treated bacterial meningitis, brain abscess, *Listeria* and *Neisseria* spp.
- Viral: herpes, mumps, HIV
- Fungal: cryptococci, *Histoplasma*, *Actinomyces*, *Nocardia* or *Candida* spp.
- Spirochaetes: *Borrelia burgdorferi* (Lyme disease), syphilis, leptospirosis
- Brucellosis
- Parasitic: toxoplasmosis, cysticercosis.

2. *What are the criteria for diagnosing GCA?*

Patients should have at least three of the following five criteria for a diagnosis of GCA:

1. Age > 50 years
2. New localised headache
3. Tenderness or decreased pulse of the temporal artery
4. Erythrocyte sedimentation rate (ESR) > 50 mm/h
5. Biopsy of artery characteristic of GCA.

3. *How does the CD4+ count relate to susceptibility to CNS infections in HIV?*

CD4 count < 50/mm³	CD4 count < 200/mm³	CD4 count > 200/mm³
Primary cerebral lymphoma	Toxoplasmosis	HSV
HIV encephalopathy/ progressive multifocal leukoencephalopathy (PML)	TB/bacterial meningitis	Bacterial meningitis
Cryptococcal meningitis	Non-Hodgkin's lymphoma	

SCENARIO 7. CHRONIC/INTERMITTENT HEADACHE

'This 28-year-old woman is known to suffer from migraines. Recently she has developed a tingling sensation in her right arm and difficulty word finding just before the headache begins. In light of these features I thought I should refer her for your opinion.'

'This 34-year-old woman has had a series of severe headaches over the last 3 weeks. She experienced a similar episode 2 years ago and a CT of the head was organised. I have been told that this was normal. She is currently unable to work because of the severity and frequency of her headaches. I would be grateful for your urgent investigation and further management of this problem.'

'I would be grateful if you could see this 33-year-old man who rarely attends my clinic except for a few exacerbations of asthma. He has had fevers and a severe frontal headache for the last week. He also describes some flu-like symptoms. Many thanks.'

'This 50-year-old woman has suffered from tension headaches for many years. She thinks that they are getting worse. Please advise.'

'This 40-year-old man has had a headache on and off for 2 years. He has noticed that it is associated with a bad taste in the back of his mouth. Please could you assess him.'

1. Verify the information provided:
'Tell me in your own words what the problem is ... .'

2. HPC:
Open to closed questions keeping in mind the *differential diagnosis*, eg
Migraine
Cluster headache
Trigeminal neuralgia
Analgesia overuse headache
Sinusitis

3. Previous investigations:
Previous CT/MRI?
Previous echocardiography?

4. SR:
Visual ticlopsia, lacrimation, nausea and vomiting, postnasal drip, nasal congestion

5. PMH:
Previous sinus surgery
Known structural heart disease/patent foramen ovale

6. DH:
Analgesia and efficacy
5HT$_1$ agonists

7. FH:
Migraine

8. SH:
Elicit any recent stress/bereavement
Time off work, financial problems

9. Summarise
'Is there anything else we haven't discussed that you feel is important?'

10. Thank the patient

Volunteered problems

Alarm symptoms:
Morning nausea and vomiting, weight loss, persistent focal neurological deficit, seizures

Disease interaction:
Co-morbidity: would the patient be fit for invasive interventional cardiac procedures (severe migraine) or trigeminal nerve decompression (trigeminal neuralgia)?

Therapeutic successes and failures:
Analgesics may be contributing to headache rather than attenuating it
Interaction between 5HT1 agonists and SSRIs (selective serotonin reuptake inhibitors)

Risks to others:

Daily life and disease:
Chronic pain and its impact on daily life – is there any secondary gain from symptoms?

Final problem list and plan of action

1. Patient acceptance of diagnosis/anxieties regarding more sinister pathology

2. Exclusion of sinister pathology, especially if focal neurological impairment

3. Involvement of ENT surgeon where appropriate

4. Referral for specialist management of chronic pain

5. Impact of debilitating pain on day-to-day life and how this can be assuaged

Key diagnostic features	Example problem list and plan of action
Migraine	
Preceding aura (1 in 5): • Scotoma • Zigzags (fortifications) • Scintilla (flashing lights) • Headache, usually unilateral • Nausea (80%) and vomiting (about 40%) • Photophobia (about 80%) • Aversion to loud noise (about 70%) • Migraine variants: • Hemiplegic migraine • Aura without headache • Basilar migraine (vertigo and ataxia) • Ophthalmoplegic migraine (double vision) • Cyclical vomiting syndrome (nausea without headache) • Precipitating food or alcohol *PMH*: previous episodes *FH*: migraine (80% have positive family history)	Rule out sinister pathology. CT indicated in atypical cases or where there is focal neurology Abortive therapy (eg $5HT_1$ agonists, high-flow oxygen) and prophylaxis (eg β blockers) Consider cardiology assessment for patent foramen ovale if migraine frequency severe/interferes with day-to-day life (MIST study)
Cluster headaches	
Short-duration severe periorbital headaches Episodes of frequent attacks, separated by at least 2 pain-free weeks Triggers: stress, extreme temperatures, sexual activity *SR*: autonomic periphenomena common (eg palpitations)	Psychosocial maladaption to this lifelong condition is common Abortive therapy similar to migraine therapy Neurosurgical ablation of cavernous sinus plexus in severe/resistant cases
Trigeminal neuralgia	
Hemifacial, lancinating pain Usually episodic with increasing frequency as the condition progresses Usually women aged > 40 Often triggered by sensory stimulation of trigeminal nerve territory *PMH*: ophthalmic zoster, trauma to trigeminal nerve	Referral for microvascular decompression (surgical correction of vascular compression of the trigeminal nerve) if medical therapy fails (carbamazepine) Management of chronic pain by specialists Other neurological symptoms/signs raises possibility of multiple sclerosis (MS) which should be investigated further Address associated depression. This is common – many cases of suicide are known

continued on next page

Key diagnostic features	Example problem list and plan of action
Analgesia overuse headache	
Headache present for more than 15 days each month (by definition) Headache reverts to less severe pattern when analgesics stopped	Persuading patient to reduce analgesia to attenuate pain often difficult
Sinusitis	
Nasal congestion, postnasal drip, anosmia, sore throat, chronic cough *PMH*: nasal polyps, septal deviation, allergic rhinitis, Wegener's granulomatosis *DH*: smoker	CT usually diagnostic and excludes other pathology Referral to ENT surgeon may be required for correction of osteomeatal obstruction

SCENARIO 8. BACK PAIN

'A 72-year-old man with known prostate cancer has been referred to the accident and emergency department with sudden-onset back pain when loading the washing machine. Current oral analgesia is no longer sufficient and the patient is now less mobile. Please take a history.'

'A 50-year-old woman with a previous history of breast cancer has been referred to the clinic with worsening back pain. She is otherwise completely well. Please take a history.'

'I would be grateful if you could see this 64-year-old man urgently. He has had back pain for many months but now complains of weakness in his left leg. He has also been unable to pass urine today.'

'This 36-year-old courier has recently been made redundant. He complains of lower back pain that began after lifting a heavy package. His pain is no longer controlled with NSAIDs or paracetamol. I have arranged radiographs of his spine and would be grateful for your further assessment.'

1. Verify the information provided:
'Tell me in your own words what the problem is … .'

2. HPC
Open to closed questions keeping in mind the *differential diagnosis*, eg
Spinal metastases
Vertebral fracture (osteoporotic/pathological)
Cord compression
Mechanical lower back pain

3. Previous investigations:
Previous bone scan? Bone densitometry? Spine radiograph/MRI? Mammogram?

4. SR:
Hypercalcaemia? (constipation, renal colic, depression, bone pain)
Bladder and bowel control
Leg weakness
Paraesthesiae/numbness

5. PMH:
Previous malignancy and stage when treated
Other conditions limiting mobility
Dates of the menopause

6. DH:
Calcium/Vitamin D supplements
Hormone replacement therapy
Bisphosphonates

7. FH:
Breast/prostate cancer, osteoporosis, coeliac disease.

8. SH:
Limitation of function in activities of daily life. Degree of improvement when pain controlled. Assistance from Social Services/family/friends. Smoking history

9. Summarise:
'Is there anything else that we haven't discussed that you feel is important?'

10. Thank the patient

Volunteered problems

Alarm symptoms:
Leg weakness, paraesthesiae, numbness, symptoms of hypercalcaemia, faecal/urinary incontinence

Disease interaction:
Fall in performance status and reduced fitness for further treatment or chemotherapy
Combined osteoporosis and metastatic disease

Therapeutic successes and failures:
Pain score and how it changes with activity/analgesia
Side effects (eg opiates and constipation, bisphosphonates and oesophagitis)

Risks to others:

Daily life and disease:
What is their performance status?
0 No symptoms
1 Ambulatory symptoms only
2 Symptoms requiring rest < ½ day
3 Symptoms requiring rest > ½ day
4 Bed bound
5 Moribund

Final problem list and plan of action

1. Potential oncological emergencies (hypercalcaemia, cord compression, SVC/IVC obstruction)

2. Identify patient's reservations about opiate analgesia (eg fear of addiction)

3. Does the patient require your help with arranging time off work (or even a lawsuit against employers) and is this appropriate?

4. Assess loss of independence and explore willingness to accept help from external agency

5. Do they require admission for pain control and/or occupational therapy or physiotherapy assessment?

Key diagnostic features	Example problem list and plan of action
Bony metastases (without cord compression)	
Severe pain, worse at night and after prolonged immobility/recumbent	Need for urgent radiotherapy and/or treatment of hypercalcaemia
Persistent pain after minimal injury/lifting	Implications for prognosis and further treatment
Multiple areas of pain, eg ribs and back	
Impairment of mobility	Associated depression and anxiety
Associated hypercalcaemia symptoms	Analgesia and the logistics of drug delivery at home (eg fentanyl patch, syringe driver) and follow-up (eg Macmillan service)
PMH: known breast, prostate, lung or renal cancer. Myeloma	
DH: side effects of analgesia especially NSAIDs (gastritis, peptic ulcer disease) and/or opiates (constipation, nausea)	Formal assessment of disability and need for help at home
Cord compression	
Gradually worsening back pain (90%)	Need for urgent investigation and treatment
Radicular pain	Availability of urgent MRI is a frequent problem
Worse lying flat	
Leg weakness or paraesthesiae	Urgent radiotherapy/decompressive surgery
Loss of bladder/bowel control	Implications for long-term care if neurological deficit permanent
PMH: known breast, prostate, lung or renal cancer	Litigious issues (if symptoms previously dismissed) are common
Pain often precedes neurological symptoms by many months	
Osteoporotic vertebral fracture	
History of minimal trauma suggests severe osteoporosis or pathological fracture	Need to minimise risk of further injury (eg hip protectors)
Date of menopause	Exclude cord injury/unstable fractures – refer to orthopaedic surgeons.
PMH: previous fractures to hip, pelvis, proximal humerus and distal forearm	Vitamin D and calcium supplementation (after assessment for deficiency)
Smokers, high alcohol consumption	
DH: previous steroid use, hormone replacement therapy	Exclude myeloma, malignancy, Pott's disease
SH: prolonged inactivity	Resulting immobility and acquisition of new problems during bedrest (pressure sores, pneumonia, DVT, PE)
Residence in TB endemic areas (Pott's disease)	Physiotherapy and occupational therapy assessment for discharge planning

Key diagnostic features	Example problem list and plan of action
Mechanical lower back pain	
Pain after twisting back while lifting a heavy object or after road traffic accident/operating vibrating machinery/a fall	Important to exclude sinister pathology but a thorough examination is usually adequate in the absence of alarm symptoms or trauma
Normal spinal imaging	Protracted symptoms may nevertheless require MRI to exclude herniated disc
Radicular pain, leg weakness, paraesthesiae, numbness – consider a possible associated disc herniation	Access and compliance with physiotherapy
PMH: previous back surgery/injury/ physiotherapy	Patient dissatisfaction without 'full scan'
Psychiatric co-morbidity	Opiate dependence
SH: if work-related injury, has there been time off work/poor job satisfaction/legal action against employer?	Poor prognosis when litigation against injurious party a factor

Questions

1. What is the definition of osteoporosis?

The WHO definition of osteoporosis is a bone mineral density (BMD) > 2.5 standard deviations (*T*-score) lower than mean BMD in a 25-year-old woman.

2. What are the guidelines for use of bisphosphonates in secondary prevention of fractures in osteoporosis?

Clinical guideline

Women should receive bisphosphonates under the following conditions:

- They are over 75 and have sustained an osteoporotic fracture (DEXA [dual X-ray absorptiometry] imaging unnecessary).
- They are aged between 65 and 74, have sustained an osteoporotic fracture and osteoporosis has been confirmed on DEXA densitometry.
- They are under 65, have sustained an osteoporotic fracture, and have a *T*-score < 3 on DEXA scanning, or if the *T*-score is < 2.5 and they have at least one of the following risk factors: low BMI (body mass index), family history of maternal hip fracture, chronic disease associated with bone loss (eg coeliac disease, Crohn's disease, rheumatoid arthritis) or prolonged immobility.

SCENARIO 9. WEAK LEGS

'This 40-year-old choreographer was recently treated by another practice doctor for a chest infection. She now re-presents with weak legs. She tells me that she has fallen twice at work when her legs seemed to just give way. I would be grateful for your urgent assessment and opinion.'

'Please could you assess this pleasant 60-year-old man who has a longstanding history of COPD. He is becoming increasingly weak and his daughter (his main carer) is having difficulty looking after him. He can no longer manage the stairs. Many thanks.'

'I would be grateful if you could see this 30-year-old artist. She had a seizure last year that was thoroughly investigated but no underlying cause could be found. Last week she developed shooting pains down her left arms and today, on getting out of the bath, she found that her legs were very wobbly. Many thanks for your further assessment of these worrying symptoms.'

'This 44-year-old man fell down the stairs last week. He feels increasingly weak in both legs and has also started to drop things. His wife tells me that she is concerned that he is more irritable than usual and recently nearly lost his job after an altercation with a senior colleague. I would be grateful for your opinion.'

'This 24-year-old Asian man describes being extremely weak on two occasions in the last month. On one of these episodes he was unable to get out of bed. The problem only lasted a few hours. Please take a history.'

'This 60-year-old man is avoiding a bronchoscopy to investigate a mass seen on CT in the right lung. He has recently had several falls which he described as his legs "giving way". Please take a history.'

'This 64-year-old woman with a history of breast cancer has had severe back pain for 2 weeks. She now feels that her legs are "wobbly". Please advise.'

1. Verify the information provided:
'Tell me in your own words what the problem is … .'

2. HPC:
Open to closed questions keeping in mind the *differential diagnosis*, eg
Guillain–Barré syndrome
Myopathy
Multiple sclerosis (MS)/
Transverse myelitis
Eaton–Lambert syndrome
Cord compression
Motor neuron disease (MND)
Familial hypokalaemic periodic paralysis

3. Previous investigations:
Previous CT/MRI?
Previous EMG/nerve conduction studies?

4. SR:
Visual disturbance, bladder dysfunction, emotional lability, cognitive impairment, myalgia, recent coryzal symptoms

5. PMH:
Known malignancy
Previous spinal surgery
Recent upper respiratory tract infection
Established COPD

6. DH:
Long-term steroids
Thyroxine

7. FH:
Periodic paralysis, thyroid disease

8. SH:
Alcohol consumption
Smoking history

9. Summarise:
'Is there anything else we haven't discussed that you feel is important?'

10. Thank the patient

Volunteered problems

Alarm symptoms:
Ascending weakness, weight loss, haemoptysis, back pain, loss of bowel/bladder control, visual disturbance

Disease interaction:
Implications of new episode on projected course of disease (eg primary progressive vs relapsing–remitting MS, progression of MND)
Interaction between new respiratory muscle weakness and established lung disease

Therapeutic successes and failures:
Drugs may well be causative/precipitant.
Is thyroxine therapy adequate?
Drug therapy available on the NHS (IFN-β1a)
Steroids can cause myopathy and treat it (eg polymositis)

Risks to others:
Care of other dependants may be jeopardised

Daily life and disease:
There are very few areas of one's life not affected by weak legs!

Final problem list and plan of action

1. Diagnosis of some of these conditions may take many months. Need to address patient's expectations and anxieties in the meantime

2. Many of these are devastating diseases affecting young individuals with young children

3. The socioeconomic impact must be anticipated and attenuated wherever possible (eg letters to employer, DSS for disability allowance, council for unpaid rent, etc)

Key points in the history	Example problem list
Guillain–Barré syndrome	
Symmetrical lower limb weakness spreading proximally	Investigations: LP may show raised protein and CT often performed to exclude other pathology. Neither is diagnostic
A benign respiratory or gastrointestinal illness some 2–4 weeks previously	Stool culture for *Clostridium jejuni* may support the diagnosis
Double vision (ophthalmoplegia – Miller–Fisher variant)	Alert ICU – one in three requires ventilatory support
Falls (impaired proprioception) and inability to walk	Cardiac monitoring if autonomic features/ heart block/arrhythmias present – the major cause of mortality after respiratory failure
SOB	
Paraesthesiae (also beginning distally and moving proximally)	Need to monitor forced vital capacity (FVC) at least twice a day (< 20 ml/kg is concerning)
Shooting pains	
Palpitation, dizziness on standing, facial flushing (autonomic dysfunction common)	DVT prophylaxis crucial because of immobility
PMH: recent immunisation for polio	Early referral for plasma exchange or intravenous immunoglobulin
DH: recent treatment for diarrhoea or chest infection	Most take months to recover – major implications for discharge planning and home support/financial status.
Note that no sensory loss/rising sensory level is found in Guillain–Barré syndrome	Residual neurological impairment in about 25%, often mild – need for careful occupational therapy and physiotherapy rehabilitation planning
Myopathy	
Difficulty standing from chairs or bath, difficulty climbing stairs, shaving, combing hair	Investigation and treatment of underlying cause with 'myopathy screen': thyroid function tests, 24-hour urinary cortisol, CK (creatine kinase), ESR, ANA, serum myoglobin
Distal muscle weakness: dropping objects, tripping over small obstacles, problems writing	EMG (electromyography) and nerve conduction studies sometimes useful
Falls	Muscle biopsy may be indicated
Timing of onset crucial:	Exclusion of acute rhabdomyolysis and its complications (renal failure, fulminant hepatic failure) is crucial in weakness of recent onset
• Over hours: toxic/periodic paralysis	
• Over a few days: dermatomyositis, rhabdomyolysis	
• Over weeks: endocrine myopathy (hypo-/hyperthyroidism, hyperparathyroidism, Cushing syndrome, Addison's disease), steroid myopathy, polymyositis, alcohol, infectious (HIV, cysticercosis)	Occupational therapy and physiotherapy to plan rehabilitation and support while recovering/on treatment
Malaise, fatigue	For alcohol dependence will need screen liver/pancreas/heart disease and encour self-referral to alcohol cessation group
PMH: endocrinopathy, renal failure, autoimmune disease, alcohol dependence	
DH: steroids, statins, colchicine, AZT (zidovudine)	(Alcoholics Anonymous, community and alcohol team)
SH: heroin/cocaine use	

continued

Key points in the history	Example problem list
MS/transverse myelitis	
Acute **partial** loss of motor, sensory, autonomic (bladder and bowel control) and reflex function beneath a particular vertebral level	Confirmation of MS as a diagnosis often requires prospective monitoring. There is no diagnostic test, although MRI is crucial to reveal demyelinating disease
Accompanying acute onset visual blurring and decreased acuity ('Devic syndrome' when occurring with a transverse myelitis)	CT is usually performed before LP to rule out mass lesions
Uthoff's phenomenon: symptoms worsen after a hot bath or exercise	Need to monitor over time for prognostic indicators:
Profound fatigue	● Primary progressive or relapsing/remitting?
Depression, mild cognitive impairment or low concentration span, sensory loss, psychiatric disturbance, ataxia, seizures (5%)	● Neurological recovery is rarely complete between attacks – a stepwise decline (secondary progressive MS) is common and has great implications for rehabilitation and social/medical support
Lhermitte's sign: neck movement results in shock-like pain radiating to extremities	While early assessment and ongoing management by a neurologist are obviously crucial, a multidisciplinary approach is often required (urologist, gastroenterologist, colorectal surgeon, stoma nurse, etc)
Symptoms distributed in space and time are the basis for a clinical diagnosis of MS	
A history of recent spinal injury suggests compressive spinal injury rather than MS	Identify and treat precipitants aggressively (eg early antibiotics for infections)
PMH: other causes of transverse myelitis: autoimmune (sarcoid, SLE [systemic lupus erythematosus], vasculitis), post-infectious (Lyme disease, *Mycoplasma pneumoniae*, syphilis, TB, viral – see Meningoencephalitis, above)	High-dose steroids often indicated for non-MS transverse myelitis (eg post-infectious). May require concomitant bone protection and surveillance for side effects
	Interferon (IFN-β1a) therapy – see below
Eaton–Lambert syndrome (ELS)	
Weakness of the proximal leg muscles is the most common complaint – difficulty rising from chairs, getting out of bath, climbing stairs, etc	Urgent investigation and treatment of the underlying malignancy (found in 75%)
More rarely:	Anti-acetylcholine (ACh) receptor antibodies, EMG and nerve conduction studies crucial to the diagnosis
● Oropharyngeal muscles: difficulty chewing, swallowing, dysarthria	Exclude ectopic ACTH as a cause of proximal myopathy if there are features of Cushing syndrome
⌐ular muscles: diplopia, ptosis	
┐ and symptoms of autonomic ┐potence) may be prominent	Avoid magnesium, calcium channel blockers, aminoglycosides
┐en progressing over	The prognosis is usually determined by the underlying disease, but ELS has major implications for day-to-day independence and end-of-life palliative support
┐rength	
⌐ant ent ⌐ies ⌐ater in ⌐ancy	

Key points in the history	Example problem list
Cord compression (see page 161)	
Familial hypokalaemic periodic paralysis	
This may present in adulthood (but usually before age 16) Attacks of symmetrical weakness, usually in the morning. Can develop complete paralysis Mild attacks may just affect a small group of muscles, often in the legs Weakness usually lasts a few hours but can last up to 3 days Precipitants: high carbohydrate meal, vigorous exercise the day before Permanent muscle weakness later on in the disease *DH*: may be precipitated by any drugs that cause hypokalaemia, eg salbutamol, steroids, insulin *FH*: usually hereditary	Exercise EMG and nerve conduction studies crucial in diagnosis. May require hypokalaemic provocation (with a glucose and insulin bolus) to induce the characteristic changes Avoidance of precipitating factors Carbonic anhydrase inhibitors for prophylaxis, oral potassium supplements to manage attacks Screening of family members is controversial: the genetic defect is heterogeneous with incomplete penetrance
Motor neuron disease	
Insidious onset, weakness, atrophy and fasciculation Symptoms often begin distally and progress proximally Common complaints include reduced manual dexterity, wrist drop, foot drop or cramps of the small muscles of the hand and/or foot Bulbar involvement leads to speech difficulties or difficulty swallowing. Tongue fasciculations are common Cognitive impairment, with frontal lobe symptoms, is sometimes reported	Diagnosis is usually arrived at after exclusion of other pathology over several months or years During this time clinicians will have to address patient's anxieties regarding a devastating progressive disease EMG (fibrillation and fasciculations) and nerve conduction studies more useful than imaging in diagnosis It is important to discuss end-of-life decisions with the patient, who may wish to instigate an advanced directive/living will. Advanced directives and the degree to which they should influence clinical decisions are controversial

Question

1. *What are the benefits of IFN-β1a therapy in MS and what are the guidelines regarding their use in the UK?*

Clinical guideline

IFN-β1a has been shown to:

- reduce the frequency of relapses in relapsing–remitting MS by around 30% (over the course of 2-year trials); the severity and duration of relapse are also significantly reduced
- delay the progression of disability by treatment.

Current NICE guidelines (2002) do not recommend the use of IFN-β1a on the basis of cost-effectiveness. Annual treatment costs approximately £7300. This decision was up for review in 2006–7.

SCENARIO 10. FALLS

'Please see this 69-year-old woman, who has had three falls. Apart from feeling a little more tired than normal over the last few months, she has been well. I could find no injury and her examination is normal except for a pulse of 46 beats/min.'

'You are referred a 28-year-old, right-handed woman by the accident and emergency SHO. She attended today having had an episode of loss of consciousness 2 days ago. The mother feels that she has not recovered completely as her daughter is not herself. She has a headache that has been present for the preceding 2 weeks.'

'This 78-year-old man is struggling to cope at home. His warden tells me that he is increasingly slow and hesitant on his feet and he has had two falls in the past month. I would be grateful for your further assessment.'

'This 66-year-old woman with rheumatoid arthritis had a blackout at the hair-dressers. An ambulance was called but she felt fine when it arrived and was not keen to go to hospital (she is the main carer for her husband).'

'This 60-year-old woman has been finding it increasingly difficult to get around the house. She had a fall when climbing the stairs 2 days ago. Please take a history.'

'This 50-year-old man with longstanding diabetes and hypertension (well controlled on medication) complains of periodic dizziness. Please take a history.'

1. Verify the information provided
'Tell me in your own words what the problem is ... .'

2. HPC:
Open to closed questions keeping in mind the *differential diagnosis*, eg
Loss of consciousness (LOC):
Syncope
Postural hypotension
Epilepsy
Vertebrobasilar ischaemia
No loss of consciousness:
Parkinson's disease
Myopathies

3. Previous investigations:
24-hour tape?
Carotid Doppler ultrasonography?
CT/MRI head?
EEG? Echocardiography?

4. SR:
Memory loss, ankle swelling, hypothyroid symptoms, tremor

5. PMH:
Hypertension, hyperlipidaemia/epilepsy
Rheumatic fever as a child.
Previous fractures
Known movement disorder

6. DH:
Sedatives, antiarrhythmic, β-blockers, antihypertensives, ACE inhibitors

7. FH
Cardiac risk factors?

8. SH:
Layout of house, support at home, support from outside immediate family, driving, alcohol, isolation, depression social responsibility (caring for others). Smoking. Driver?

9. Summarise
'Is there anything else that we haven't discussed that you feel is important?'

10. Thank the patient

Volunteered problems
Is the patient's insight intact?

Alarm symptoms:
LOC rather than loss of postural tone
Exertional syncope, family history of sudden death, serious injury following fall, socially isolated, injured, unclear/no collateral history (unable to triage risk)

Disease interaction:
eg osteoporosis and aortic valve stensosis
Is there adequate secondary prevention of hip fracture?

Therapeutic success and failures:
Iatrogenic hypotension/sedation/arrhythmias/long QT

Risks to others:
Continuing to drive after a syncopal event?

Daily life and disease:
Loss of confidence and independence very common after injurious falls

Final problem list and plan of action

1. Triage urgency of further investigations and treatment

2. Inpatient vs outpatient investigation depending on risk of injury

3. Early involvement of occupational therapist and physiotherapist

4. Preserved insight into dangers of further collapse?

5. Level of risk of injury given social/home/occupational circumstances

6. A spell in a rehabilitation centre may be warranted.

7. Need to improve social support – is the patient amenable to this?

8. Dependants may also need additional support while the patient is incapacitated

Key diagnostic features	Example problem list and plan
Loss of consciousness	
Syncope	
Dysrhythmias Palpitations before or after fall Previous pacemaker and recent checks Family history of sudden death Structural heart disease (eg aortic stenosis) Exertional syncope Rheumatic fever as child Previous valve disease Cardiomyopathy/CCF	Low pick-up rate of 24-hour tape – is the patient suitable for an implantable Holter loop recorder? Assess need for urgent pacing/pacemaker Are antiarrhythmics optimised? Risk assessment of further injury Get collateral history/witness Loss of confidence after the fall and rehabilitation Harbinger of poor prognosis and need for surgery in aortic valve disease. On ACE inhibitor with aortic valve disease?
Postural hypotension	
Fall after standing Altered vision before fall Recent change in medications (eg antihypertensives) Other autonomic disturbance, eg micturition syncope or associated diseases (eg diabetes, or Parkinson's or Alzheimer's disease) Cognitive impairment	Need for autonomic testing if a cause cannot be found and symptoms are severe Exclusion of metabolic causes (eg Addison's disease) Triage between inpatient and outpatient investigation and treatment (frequency of falls more important than severity of injury) Associated cognitive impairment and its further investigation and management
Epilepsy	
Pre-seizure 'aura' Postictal confusion or weakness (Todd's paresis) Injury (eg tongue biting) Incontinence Provoking factors Previous abnormal neuroimaging *PMH*: stroke, meningitis/encephalitis, alcohol excess *DH*: benzodiazepine/alcohol withdrawal? Side effects on anticonvulsants	Need to focus investigations on: 1. Is it true epilepsy? 2. What kind of epilepsy? 3. What is the cause? MRI is superior to CT of the head (CT misses half the lesions detected by MRI) but sometimes an urgent need to rule out serious pathology may make CT preferable EEG most sensitive within 24 hours of a seizure; sleep-deprived EEGs are more sensitive (50%) but should not be used to 'exclude' epilepsy as false positives are common DVLA rules (see below) and implications for the patient Address anxiety regarding recurrence: 'sword of Damocles' syndrome

Key diagnostic features	Example problem list and plan
Epilepsy (contd)	
	Assess need for anticonvulsant therapy. Risk of recurrent seizure higher if: night-time seizures, family history of epilepsy, prior seizures, Todd's paresis, known abnormal neuroimaging, abnormal EEG
Vertebrobasilar ischaemia	
Symptoms provoked by head position	MRI far superior to CT for posterior fossa imaging
Vertigo is the cardinal symptom	
Hemifacial numbness or paraesthesiae with contralateral symptoms in the extremities	Surgical options far more limited than in carotid stenosis but angioplasty and stenting may be of benefit (but high risk of stroke)
Dysphagia, dysarthria	Assessment of swallow reflex crucial
Previous strokes in posterior territory	Extra caution needed with new or changed antihypertensives – this may precipitate a hypoperfusion injury
Arm claudication suggests subclavian steal syndrome	
Risk factors: hypertension, smoking, etc	Anti-platelets (unless contraindicated) should be started
No loss of consciousness	
Parkinson's disease	
Asymmetrical resting tremor	Investigation by a specialist: MRI and CT are not diagnostic but can exclude multi-infarct disease, normal pressure hydrocephalus (ataxia, incontinence, dementia) and Wilson's disease
Clumsiness/reduced dexterity	
Stop–start symptoms	
Cognitive impairment	
Sleep disturbance	Single photon emission CT (SPECT) useful if available
Autonomic dysfunction: sexual dysfunction, constipation, sweating	Level of disability and implications for long-term care, especially if cognitive impairment is present (± Lewy body dementia)
Depression in up to 40%	
Drug induced: neuroleptics, antiemetics	
DH: Side effects of established L-dopa therapy, eg dyskinesias, hallucinations, impulse control disorders	Balancing effective control of rigidity vs peak dose-induced dyskinesias
Myopathy	
Proximal muscle weakness	Need to establish cause with appropriate investigations
Difficulty getting up stairs or out of the bath	
Fatigue	Supportive care while awaiting response to treatment
No sensory symptoms	
Dark urine (myositis)	If drug induced (eg steroids), can these be safely stopped?
Timing:	
Over hours: toxic/metabolic cause	Muscle biopsy crucial if polymyositis suspected
Over days: dermatomyositis, rhabdomyolysis	Crucial role of occupational therapist and physiotherapist
Over months: polymyositis, steroid induced, thyroid disease	
Drugs and rhadomyolysis (eg statins)	

Note that, with the exception of vertebrobasilar ischaemia, transient ischaemic attacks (TIAs) do NOT cause loss of consciousness; rather focal neurological impairment resolves within 24 hours.

Questions

1. What are the indications for an emergency temporary venous pacing wire?

Indications for a temporary pacing wire before the emergency setting differ according to whether or not the context is acute MI.

Acute MI likely	Bradycardia not associated with MI
Asystole	
Sinus bradycardia or Möbitz type I second-degree atrioventricular (AV) block leading to hypotension and unresponsive to atropine	Syncope at rest in association with any second- or third-degree block
Bilateral bundle-branch block (BBB): alternating BBB or right BBB (RBBB) with alternating left anterior hemiblock (LAHB)/left posterior hemiblock (LPHB)	Ventricular tachyarrrhythmias secondary to bradycardia
Bifascicular block with first-degree block	
Möbitz type II AV block	

2. What are the laws governing driving after a seizure?

One should consult specific advice from the Driver and Vehicle Licensing Agency (DVLA): *For medical practitioners: at a glance guide to the current medical standards of fitness to drive,* issued by the Drivers Medical Unit, DVLA, Swansea: www.dvla.gov.uk.

The following is a guide.

After a single loss of consciousness in which investigations have **not** revealed a cause, at least one year off is required before returning to driving as long as the driver has been free from such attacks during this period.

Epilepsy is defined as all events – major, minor and auras. For the purposes of the regulations, if more than one seizure occurs in a 24-hour period they are treated as a 'single event'.

- **Entitlement for cars and motorcycles**: a person who has suffered an epileptic attack while **awake** must refrain from driving for **1** year from the date of the attack before a driving licence may be reissued, or a person who has suffered an attack while asleep must also refrain from driving for **1** year from the attack, unless he or she had an attack while asleep more than 3 years ago and has not had an awake attack since that asleep attack, and, in any event, the driving of a vehicle by such a person should not be likely to cause danger to the public.

- If the seizure is related to alcohol withdrawal the licence will be revoked or refused for a minimum of 1 year from the event.
- **Entitlement for medium and large lorries, minibuses and buses**: for a licence to be issued or reissued the patient must be free of any attack for 10 years, and have not required any medication to treat epilepsy, and should not otherwise be a source of danger while driving.
- Taxi drivers fall under the jurisdiction of the Public Carriage Office or the local authority and will be subject to their medical standards

In all cases, it is the duty of the licence holder to notify the DVLA of the relevant details

SCENARIO 11. PAINFUL JOINTS OF THE HAND AND WRIST

'Please could you see this 50-year-old painter and decorator who complains of a swollen, painful index finger. This came on abruptly 5 days ago and is barely controlled with NSAIDs. He is overweight and drinks fairly heavily.'

'This 34-year-old architect complains of joint stiffness in her hands that is particularly troubling in the morning. She is concerned that she is not able to keep up with her workload. Radiographs of the hand were reported as normal. I would be grateful for your advice about further investigation.'

'This 30-year-old woman from Nigeria, who has previously attended my clinic for reactive depression after a miscarriage, now complains of painful wrists and knees. She is having trouble looking after her young daughter. She was very distressed and tearful about this when she attended my clinic today. Please advise about her further investigation and management.'

'The lawyer of this 50-year-old secretary recently contacted me requesting a medical report with regard to possible repetitive strain injury. She has attended once before complaining of painful wrists and joints while typing. Radiographs showed some small osteophyte formation, but were otherwise normal. I have informed her solicitor that a rheumatology opinion would be more appropriate.'

1. Verify the information provided:
'Tell me in your own words what the problem is ... .'

2. HPC:
Open to closed questions keeping in mind the *differential diagnosis*, eg
RA
SLE
Osteoarthritis
Crystal arthropathy

3. Previous investigations:
Previous radiographs?
Blood tests?
Seen by a rheumatologist?

4. SR:
Symptoms of serositis (pericarditis, pleuritis, scleritis) or vasculitis (eg neuropathies)
Recent gastroenteritis or sexually transmitted infections (STIs) (reactive arthritis)
Loin pain (urate renal stones)
Fatigue, weight loss, myalgia
Rash

5. PMH:
Cardiovascular disease, peptic ulcer disease (NSAIDs), previous TB (planned infliximab treatment?)
Previous DVT/PE (SLE)

6. DH:
NSAIDs and complications, DMARDs and side effects

7. FH:
RA, spondyloarthropathies

8. SH:
Occupational history and assessment of level of disability. Smoking. Sexual history may be important in reactive arthritis.

9. Summarise:
'Is there anything else we haven't discussed that you feel is important?'

10. Thank the patient

Volunteered problems

Alarm symptoms:
Leg/arm/hand weakness, sensory loss, anuria, chest pain

Disease interaction:
Impact of multisystem inflammatory disease on other organs or established disease (eg RA and high mortality from cardiac disease)
High mortality from non-arthritic disease (eg cardiac, pulmonary)

Therapeutic successes and failures:
Adverse events and monitoring after introduction of new immunomodulator (eg azathioprine and leukopenia)
Non-compliance with medication when well

Risks to others:
eg now unsafe in the workplace due to a new disability

Daily life and disease:
How do specific disbilities translate into limitations on daily life and work?

Final problem list and plan of action

1. Any features of RA should prompt urgent referral to a rheumatologist for early DMARD therapy to prevent deformity and disability

2. Exclusion of other organ involvement

3. Management of risk factors for associated disease (specially cardiac disease in RA)

4. Step-down approach to therapy in inflammatory arthropathies increasingly popular

5. Immunosuppresants and their side effects/risks

6. Steroids and bone protection/ osteoporosis risk assessment

7. Secondary prevention for cardiac risk factors (RA)

Key points in the history	Example problem list
Rheumatoid arthritis	
Establishing criteria for urgent rheumatology referral: • Morning joint stiffness lasting 30 min or more • Swelling of three or more joints • Involvement of the MCP joints or metatarsophalangeal (MTP) joints Constitutional symptoms: malaise, fatigue, symptoms of anaemia, weight loss, muscular aches and pains The minority have an abrupt onset of symptoms (about 15%) If the diagnosis is already established, look for symptoms suggestive of disease activity: • Worsening joint pain • Increased duration of morning joint stiffness • Increased fatigue • Worsening limitation of function SR: other system involvement – pleuritis, pericarditis, neurological deficit (mononeuritis multiplex), IHD, dry mouth/eyes (Sjögren syndrome) PMH: cardiovascular disease and risk factors (cholesterol, BP) DH: DMARDs (disease-modifying anti-rheumatoid drugs) and adverse effects Steroids – frequency and duration of use SH: level of disability, occupational impact, alcohol and DMARDs (eg methotrexate). Smoking (further risk of cardiac disease)	Need for immediate referral to rheumatologist for DMARD therapy to prevent joint disability Surgical intervention may be necessary, eg to improve joint function/stabilise joints/tendon repair/carpal tunnel release Exclusion of rheumatoid emergencies (renal failure, vasculitis, atlantoaxial subluxation) Management of long-term immunomodulators and their adverse effects (hepatotoxicity, nephrotoxicity, pneumonitis, infections) Assess for changes in level of ability and adjust social support accordingly Aggressive management of cardiac risk factors Management of other organ involvement (eg pulmonary fibrosis, pericarditis, pleurisy) and associated autoimmune disease (eg Sjögren syndrome, Raynaud's phenomenon) Steroid-sparing therapy, bone protection and monitoring for osteoporosis
SLE	
Joint pain is the most frequent presenting complaint Small joints of the hands commonly affected Disability is mostly the result of pain, which often migrates from joint to joint Other features: General: malaise, fever, lethargy Skin: malar rash, photosensitivity, discoid lupus, alopecia, Raynaud's phenomenon Renal disease (50%): nephritic/nephrotic syndromes Pericarditis/pleuritis Anaemia, thrombocytopenia (bleeding diatheses)	A multidisciplinary approach is crucial – several systems are frequently affected Exclusion of SLE-associated emergencies: vasculitis, glomerulonephritis, severe neurovasculitis, diffuse alveolar haemorrhage, profound thrombocytopenia Assessment of disease activity: C3 and C4 complement levels, CRP, ESR, dsDNA (double-stranded DNA) are all markers of activity Management of long-term immunomodulators and their adverse effects (hepatotoxicity, nephrotoxicity, pneumonitis, infections)

continued on next page

Key points in the history	Example problem list
SLE	
PMH: recurrent infection, neuropsychiatric disease, more than two recurrent miscarriages, previous DVT/PE (antiphospholipid syndrome) *DI l*: immunosuppressants – dose and duration important Note drug-induced lupus (procainamide, hydralazine, quinidine and 35 other drugs)	Monitor for renal disease with regular urinalysis Like rheumatoid arthritis, cardiac disease is more common and treatable risk factors should be attenuated aggressively (smoking cessation, cholesterol-lowering medications, BP control, etc) Steroid-sparing therapy, bone protection and monitoring for osteoporosis Anticoagulation for patients with previous DVT/PE and positive antiphospholipid antibodies
Osteoarthritis	
Pain and stiffness (< 1 hour) in any joint Distal interphalangeal (DIP) joint commonly affected Often asymmetrical History of excessive use/load bearing of affected joint *PMH*: previous orthopaedic operations *SH*: occupational history and limitation of work. Any legal action in process against employer (eg for repetitive strain injury)	Assessment of level of disability by occupational therapist and physiotherapist Referral to orthopaedic surgeon where appropriate Encourage weight loss, exercise, occupational adjustments Pain control with NSAIDs, paracetamol and steroid injection for analgesia-resistant joint disease
Crystal arthropathy	
Acute onset (often at night) of a hot, swollen, exquisitely tender joint, often the MTP joint of the great toe Pseudo-gout may have a more insidious onset than gout Fevers, rigors, malaise – common to both crystal arthropathies and septic arthritis *PMH*: renal calculi, haemoproliferative disorders, renal impairment *SH*: alcohol consumption	Always treat for septic arthritis until it is excluded (this may not be necessary in recurrent identical episodes of known gout or podagra) Establish adequate prophylaxis and lifestyle changes to prevent future attacks Low purine diet

Question

1. What are the diagnostic criteria for SLE?

The American College of Rheumatology require features of 4 of the following 11 criteria for a diagnosis of SLE (*mnemonic*: dam pain rush):

Discoid lupus
Arthritis
Malar rash
Photosensitivity rash
ANA positive
Imunological markers (dsDNA, anti-Sm, VDRL [Venereal Disease Reference Laboratory])
Neurological or psychiatric disorder
Renal disease (nephrotic/nephritic)
Ulcers (oral)
Serositis (pleuritis, pericarditis)
Haematological disorder (thrombocytopenia, leukopenia, anaemia).

These criteria have an 85% sensitivity and a 96% specificity when tested against control and SLE patient databases. They also constitute a useful mnemonic for recalling the main features of the disease.

SCENARIO 12. ABNORMAL LIVER FUNCTION TESTS (LFTS)

'A 40-year-old businesswoman, who only drinks alcohol occasionally, has been referred by the accident and emergency officer with abnormal LFTs. The woman was alert and orientated but did have some right upper quadrant (RUQ) tenderness. Her past medical history is unremarkable apart from an underactive thyroid. Please take a history.'

'This 50-year-old man has a strong family history of heart disease. He is obese and has a high LDL-cholesterol level. He also has hypertension. As he was first seen by his new GP 3 months ago his LFTs have deteriorated. Please take a history.'

'I would be grateful for your further input regarding this 44-year-old man. He gives a 4-month history of worsening shortness of breath (SOB) and palpitations. He also complains of profound lethargy but attributes this to stress after his recent divorce. I had previously treated him for sexual dysfunction before the separation. On routine tests I found that he had a mildly raised ALT (alanine transaminase) and slightly prolonged INR (international normalised ratio). Please advise.'

'A 50-year-old woman has been referred by her GP for pruritus. This seems to be resistance to standard treatment. Her bilirubin, ALP (alkaline phosphatase) and GGT (γ-glutamyltransferase) are slightly raised but the other LFTs are normal. Please take a history.'

'Please would you see this 24-year-old woman who developed RUQ pain suddenly 4 days ago. The pain has now reduced significantly but on routine testing I note raised ALP and GGT levels. She thinks that she may have had a similar episode 6 months ago.'

'I would be grateful for your opinion about this 18-year-old girl. She complains of extreme tiredness and low mood and is worried about her performance in an imminent exam. On routine testing I noticed her ALT and GGT were slightly raised.'

'This 40-year-old dentist has become jaundiced. She complains of general malaise only. She is concerned that this might be related to an extramarital affair that she had some 6 weeks ago. Please take a history.'

'I was about to start this 55-year-old obese man, who has a past history of ischaemic heart disease, on a statin. However, I note that his AST and GGT are slightly raised. I would be grateful for your advice.'

1. Verify the information provided: 'Tell me in your own words what the problem is … .'

2. HPC
Open → closed questions bearing in mind the following differential diagnoses:
· **Gallstones**
· **Acute viral hepatitis**
· **EBV**
· **PBC**
· **Autoimmune hepatitis**
· **Drug induced**
· **NASH**
· **Haemochromatosis**

3. Previous investigations: Liver ultrasonography? Blood tests? Upper GI endoscopy?

4. SR:
Liver failure screen – jaundice, encephalopathy (eg daytime somnolescence and night-time insomnia), bruising, melaena/haematemesis

5. PMH:
Autoimmune disease (PBC, PSC, AIH)
DVT/PE (Budd–Chiari syndrome/portal vein thrombosis)
Blood transfusions (viral hepatitis)
Obesity, high cholesterol, hypertension, diabetes (NASH)

6. DH:
Paracetamol (unintentional overdose?), herbal remedies, other common culprits (see below)

7. FH:
Autoimmune disease?
Gallstones?

8. SH:
Travel history (HAV), sexual history (HAV, HBV, HCV) background alcohol consumption (may compound other pathologies)

9. Summarise
'Is there anything else that we haven't discussed that you feel is important?'

10. Thank the patient

Volunteered problems

Alarm symptoms:
Weight loss, any decompensation symptoms, previous malignancy

Disease interaction:
Any ongoing illnesses that may interact unfavourably, eg HIV, established liver disease

Therapeutic successes and failures:
If drug induced can the offending drug be safely stopped? Potential contraindications to antiviral therapy with IFN (eg depression, renal failure)

Risks to others
Are there any contact tracing issues (explore these *sensitively*)?

Daily life and disease:
eg restrictions on health professionals with HBV or HCV

Final problem list and plan of action

1. Address patient's anxiety about cirrhosis or cancer (many patients interpret jaundice as a harbinger of inescapable doom)

2. Triage urgency of investigation or treatment depending on the likely underlying condition and clinical correlates of liver function

3. Monitor for complications of cirrhosis in patients with established chronic liver disease (eg hepatoma and varices surveillance)

4. Need to arrange regular surveillance after or during treatment to assess response and pick up complications of therapy

5. Identify transplant candidates in end-stage or fulminant disease and refer early to a transplant centre for assessment

6. Contact tracing issues/screening of family members for viral hepatitis or genetic disorders

Key diagnostic features	Example problem list
Gallstones	
History of present complaint (HPC) Often asymptomatic Postprandial (30 min–2 h) RUQ pain, rising to a crescendo then fading Transient dark stools and pale urine if stone passed through duct Ongoing epigastric or RUQ pain suggestive of pancreatitis or cholecystitis (Charcot's triad: RUQ pain, fever and jaundice) *Past medical history (PMH):* Saint's triad: peptic ulcer disease, diverticulitis and gallstones occur together commonly (this may just be a statistical phenomenon arising from three common conditions) Risks: obesity, hypercholesterolaemia, sickle cell disease (pigment stones), oral contraceptive pill, multiple pregnancies, rapid weight loss (eg after bariatric surgery) *Family history (FH):* 1 in 4 has a first-degree relative with gallstones	Management is determined by the presence or absence of stones in the duct and whether or not the LFTs are improving If there is no clear duct dilatation on transabdominal ultrasonography, leaping in with ERCP is increasingly unpopular even in the presence of obvious stones in the gallbladder (resulting from the approximately 4% risk of pancreatitis). Endoscopic ultrasonography and MRCP are the best means of visualising stones if transabdominal ultrasonography is normal while the LFTs remain obstructive If a stone in the duct is confirmed ERCP is usually indicated. Rarely, a cholecystectomy and on-table duct clearance are performed Arrangements need to be made for routine cholecystectomy (usually within 3 months) after a successful stone removal at ERCP and sphincterotomy Need to inform patient of risk of further pancreatitis/cholecystitis and to return if pain persists or if he or she develops fever
Hepatitis A	
RUQ discomfort/generalised abdominal pain (40%) Elderly or very young patient Flu-like prodrome and/or diarrhoea common Jaundice (80% – often noticed by partner rather than patient) Dark urine and pale stools Nausea, anorexia, vomiting, fever Rash affecting lower extremities Recent travel (2–6 weeks' incubation period) to an endemic area without immunisation *Social history (SH):* elderly patients in institutional care at greater risk, men who have sex with men (homosexual or bisexual), foreign travel, intravenous drug use (IVDU)	Confirm diagnosis with appropriate investigations (eg hepatitis A IgM) Requires notification to Centres for Disease Surveillance Can usually be managed as outpatient Must exclude other causes of an acute hepatitis Very elderly people often require considerable supportive medical care Fulminant hepatitis A is very rare but INR should be monitored in the unwell patient until the LFTs have repeatedly improved Symptoms and infection can relapse in very elderly people – close follow-up is necessary to pick this up

continued on next page

Key diagnostic features	Example problem list
Hepatitis B	
The patient may present during acute or chronic infection	Need to confirm stage of disease (acute versus chronic); 90% of acutely infected patients (positive anti-HBc IgM) will develop surface antibodies within a year and require no further treatment or surveillance
Acute infection:	
• Jaundice, fatigue, anorexia, nausea and vomiting	
• An arthritis–dermatitis prodrome is seen in a third of cases of acute infection	Follow-up to check for HBsAg-negative, HBsAb-positive status required
Fulminant acute infection is characterised by encephalopathy (night-time insomnia progressing to confusion and coma)	For chronic active hepatitis: refer to a hepatologist for treatment – the aim is to suppress viral replication and increase the year-on-year chances of seroconversion to 'e' antigen-negative status (see page 47)
Chronic active hepatitis (± cirrhosis): similar symptoms to the acute phase but less marked	
Screen for symptoms of decompensated liver disease or portal hypertension: encephalopathy, melaena, ascites	Resistance to lamivudine is common after 2 years of continuous therapy. A flare in hepatitis may indicate viral resistance and additional adefovir will improve viral suppression
Risk factors for hepatitis B: IVDU, homosexual or bisexual men, ethnic origin, occupational hazards	A flare in a chronic active hepatitis patient may also be a result of development of a pre-core mutant (see page 47)
Extrahepatic manifestations, eg symptoms of nephrotic syndrome, polyarteritis nodosa, cryoglobulinaemia.	Fulminant hepatitis needs to be managed in a specialist liver unit
These conditions often manifest as oedema, palpable purpura, weakness and arthralgias	A high level of suspicion is required to pick up extrahepatic syndromes
Drug history (DH): may have had previous IFN (interferon) therapy that failed to induce seroconversion	There may be contact tracing issues – family members (vertical transmission) and sexual contacts
On lamivudine more than 2 years?	Routine screening for HIV advisable
SH: ongoing risks of infecting others. Occupational history (eg doctor, dentist, nurse)	IFN therapy is fraught with adverse effects – need to exclude bone marrow suppression and depression

Key diagnostic features	Example problem list
Hepatitis C	
Acute infection is usually asymptomatic	Need to genotype virus (HCV) and refer to hepatology to determine optimal timing for treatment
May present with symptoms of chronic decompensated liver disease (pages 30–31)	
Risk factors are key (IVDU, high-risk sexual practice, first-degree relatives, tattoos, blood products pre-1985 or abroad)	Manage decompensated liver disease/ hepatocellular carcinoma (HCC) if present
Previous episodes of jaundice	Contact tracing of sexual contacts/screening of first-degree relatives
PMH: HIV co-infection?	Assess likely compliance with further investigation and treatment
DH: previous IFN therapy for known HCV	Exclude contraindications to antiviral therapy (depression, ongoing IVDU, renal impairment, established cirrhosis)
SH: sexual contacts and family members tested?	
Careful occupational history. Ongoing IVDU	Patients with HIV co-infection progress to cirrhosis more rapidly and often need input from tertiary HIV/hepatology centres
	Routine screening for HIV is recommended
	High rates of mood disorders and depression among HCV patients. These need to be treated and followed up
Epstein–Barr virus (EBV)	
Prolonged lethargy and malaise	IgM monospot to confirm acute infection
Sore throat	Monitor LFTs – these are disrupted in most cases to some degree and may take many months to resolve (especially GGT)
Raised lymph nodes	
Low-grade fever, anorexia	
SH: may recall close contact with person with pharyngitis	May need long period of time off work as a result of profound lethargy
	Beware rare complications: splenic rupture, meningoencephalitis, chronic fatigue syndrome
	Supportive management as an outpatient is usually sufficient

continued on next page

Key diagnostic features	Example problem list
Primary biliary cirrhosis (PBC)	
Long indolent history of lethargy (65%), pruritus (55%), RUQ pain (20%)	Need to confirm diagnosis (AMAs)
	Need to stage liver disease
Jaundice (often disproportionate to other indicators of chronic liver disease)	Exclude other autoimmune causes of symptoms (eg hypothyroidism)
PMH: hypercholesterolaemia, other autoimmune disease	Implications of profound lethargy for career, family and social life
	Treatment (ursodeoxycholate)
	Pruritus is often extreme and difficult to control. It also leads to insomnia and depression. There are documented cases of suicide attributed to this symptom alone
	Treat hypercholesterolaemia if present
	Regular follow-up and surveillance for HCC if cirrhosis established
Drug-induced liver injury	
See table on page 187	Stop offending agent and monitor LFTs. A rising INR requires immediate discussion with a liver transplant unit
May have used alternative/herbal remedies – does the patient still have them?	
	Exclude background liver disease of alternative aetiology
	Determine alternative treatments for original problem, eg anti-tuberculous therapy, immunosuppression for transplant
	There are frequently medicolegal issues surrounding iatrogenic injury
Autoimmune hepatitis	
Can present as an acute hepatitis (RUQ pain, anorexia, lethargy) or chronic decompensated liver disease (see above)	Confirm the diagnosis/exclude other causes Liver biopsy nearly always indicated when the ANA is positive and no other cause is obvious
PMH: Other autoimmune disease; especially Sjögren syndrome, SLE, autoimmune thyroid disease.	Refer to hepatology for treatment (steroids and azathioprine)
	AIH may interact unfavourably with other autoimmune disease (eg hypothyroidism)
	Consider bone protection for extended steroid therapy

Key diagnostic features	Example problem list
Haemochromatosis	
Patients may present with manifestations of arthritis, cardiomyopathy, diabetes and/or chronic liver disease	Diagnosis requires confirmation of *HFE* mutations after assessment of transferrin saturation
Most common symptoms are: • Profound lethargy • Arthralgia • Impotence/reduced sex drive/ amenorrhoea	A multidisciplinary approach is crucial (endocrinology, hepatology, rheumatology, cardiology)
Arthritis: painful second and third MCP joints are characteristic	Regular surveillance (ultrasonography and AFP every 6 months) is needed for HCC in patients with established cirrhosis
Cardiomyopathy: younger patients, palpitations, increasing SOB on exertion, ankle oedema, syncope	Compliance with twice-weekly venesection often problematic (especially in needle phobics)
Diabetes (50%): polyuria, polydipsia, weight loss, chance finding of glycosuria	All first-degree relatives must be screened Alcohol cessation advice and support may be necessary
Chronic liver disease (see above). Rates of HCC are high in haemochromatosis	
Non-alcoholic steatohepatitis (NASH)	
Abnormal LFTs are often a chance finding on routine blood tests	Need to exclude other causes of liver disease (may rarely require biopsy)
PMH: obesity, diabetes, hypertension, dyslipidaemia	The general strategy is aggressive treatment of causative co-morbidity while monitoring the LFT response
SH: concomitant alcohol excess is common	Dietician referral often useful
	10% progression to cirrhosis – those who do not improve with modification of risk factors or develop signs of chronic liver disease may require a staging biopsy

Question

1. *Which medications commonly cause abnormal LFTs?*

Acute necrosis	Chronic injury and fibrosis	Acute cholestasis	Chronic cholestasis	Veno-occlusive disease	Autoimmune hepatitis
Isoniazid		Contraceptives			Sulphonamides
Rifampicin					
Amiodarone		Co-amoxiclav (Augmentin)			Nitrofurantoin
Methotrexate		Macrolides	Co-trimoxazole		Methyldopa
Valproate		Cimetidine	Carbamazepine		
Halothane		Hydralazine			
Paracetamol		Allopurinol			
Ketoconazole		Quinolones			

Figure 2.5   Drug-induced hepatitis: common culprits

SCENARIO 13. ALCOHOL DEPENDENCE AND ABDOMINAL PAIN

'This 35-year-old man drinks half a bottle of whisky a day. He presented to my clinic with a 24-hour history of severe central abdominal pain. This is similar to an episode that he experienced 1 year ago. Since then he has lost at least 5 kg in weight. His pain is barely controlled with co-codamol and I am concerned that he may have an ulcer. I would be grateful if you would admit him for an endoscopy.'

'This 55-year-old woman with established alcoholic liver disease has been complaining of increased abdominal girth despite the diuretics that I prescribed recently. Over the last 24 hours she has had fevers and feels generally unwell. I would be grateful if you could see her and advise about further management.'

'This 40-year-old man was previously a heavy drinker but has been dry for 6 months. Despite that he now presents with increasing abdominal distension and right upper quadrant discomfort. He looks emaciated and says that he is off his food. Please take a history.'

'This 38-year-old lorry driver had an endoscopy last year which revealed a severe gastritis. His pain improved on a proton pump inhibitor (PPI) but has now returned. He also tells me that he passed black stools 1 week ago. I would be grateful for your advice about his further investigation.'

'This 35-year-old woman, recently divorced, visited my clinic 3 weeks ago feeling generally unwell. She complains of profound lethargy during the day and being unable to sleep at night. She also describes vague RUQ discomfort and today she appears jaundiced. Please take a history'.

1. Verify the information provided:
'Tell me in your own words what the problem is ... .'

2. HPC:
Open to closed questions keeping in mind the following *differential diagnosis*:
Pancreatitis
Peptic ulcer disease
Spontaneous bacterial peritonitis
Hepatocellular carcinoma
Acute hepatitis

3. Previous investigations:
Varices surveillance (OGD), HCC surveillance (ultrasonography), CT of the abdomen (pancreatitis)

4. SR:
Decompensation screen – ascites, encephalopathy (eg altered sleep–wake cycle), bruising, melaena/haematemesis, fever

5. PMH:
Withdrawal seizures/syndrome
Neurological sequelae (stroke, Wernicke's encephalopathy, etc)
Cardiomyopathy
Pancreatitis, peptic ulcer disease
Coping strategy for other chronic illness, eg depression

6. DH
Multivitamins
Acamprosate?
Propranolol for varices prophylaxis?

7. FH:
Children with fetal alcohol syndrome?

8. SH:
Impartial exploration of quantity of alcohol consumption. CAGE questionnaire for alcohol dependence. Impact of alcoholism on work/relationships/financial status

9. Summarise
'Is there anything else that we haven't discussed that you feel is important?'

10. Thank the patient

Volunteered problems

Alarm symptoms:
Weight loss, any symptoms of decompensation, previous malignancy

Disease interaction:
Impact of acute illness on other alcohol-related pathologies and further detriment to social circumstances and chances of cessation

Therapeutic successes and failures:
Interactions with alcohol, eg warfarin, antiepileptics, benzodiazepines
Compliance with prescribed therapy

Risks to others
Is the patient violent or continuing to drive?

Daily life and disease:
Is the patient drinking and driving? What are their occupational prospects? Sympathetic employer? Homeless? Vulnerable to abuse or risk to other dependants?

Final problem list and plan of action

1. Need to assess severity of disease and triage level of care (eg most complications of alcoholic liver disease are potentially life threatening)

2. Is the patient likely to comply with further investigation and treatment?

3. Need to screen for alcohol-related damage to other organs

4. Alcohol abuse has massive socioeconomic impact – are others at risk (eg does the DVLA need to be informed?)?

5. Encourage referral to alcohol cessation services (Alcoholics Anonymous, community drugs and alcohol team) after resolution of acute episode

Key diagnostic features	Example problem list and plan of action
Pancreatitis	
Severe central abdominal pain	CT is the best diagnostic modality
Nausea	Glasgow criteria staging for acute pancreatitis to triage level of care
Fever	
Loose, pale stools	Risk of opiate addiction in chronic pancreatitis
Recent alcohol binge	
PMH: alcoholic liver disease/ cardiomyopathy/neuropathy	Possible pancreatic insufficiency – diabetes? malabsorption? Fasting glucose and faecal elastase/faecal fat estimation are useful adjunctive tests
DH: opiate use for recurrent episodes of pancreatitis	
Note that may be non-alcohol related, eg gallstone pancreatitis	Chronic pain and alcoholism usually interact unfavourably
	Prophylactic treatment for alcohol withdrawal (reducing dose of chlordiazepoxide) unless encephalopathic
Peptic ulcer disease	
Postprandial, gnawing, epigastric pain radiating through to back	May have other risk factors besides alcohol that need to be addressed, eg NSAIDs/ *Helicobacter pylori*, recent stress or surgery
Duodenal ulcer: hunger pains before eating Nausea and vomiting (stricture and outlet obstruction)	In patients with alcohol problems presenting with a GI bleed for the first time, a variceal source must be suspected until proved otherwise
Anorexia, weight loss	
Melaena, haematemesis	Triage urgency/necessity of upper GI endoscopy. Exclude perforation
Recent alcohol binge	
PMH: established cirrhosis	Lifelong PPI may be necessary, especially if alcohol cessation is unlikely
DH: NSAIDS, steroids (recent alcoholic hepatitis?)	
	H. pylori infection rates higher among patients with alcohol problems so test and eradicate if positive
Spontaneous bacterial peritonitis	
One-third of cases asymptomatic	An urgent ascitic tap is needed in all patients with ascites and chronic liver disease.
Abdominal distension, generalised pain, fevers Worsening confusion/drowsiness	Antibiotic treatment while awaiting results
PMH: established chronic liver disease	Exclude and treat encephalopathy/ hepatorenal syndrome/varices
DH: diuretics	
	Nutritional status often poor and requires support
	Antibiotic prophylaxis on discharge
	Is the patient a liver transplant candidate?

continued on next page

Key diagnostic features	Example problem list and plan of action
Hepatocellular carcinoma	
Weight loss, malaise, RUQ pain, newly decompensated liver disease (abdominal distension, symptoms of encephalopathy, etc) Ascites often develops quickly as a result of portal vein thrombosis on top of cirrhosis *PMH*: higher rates of HCC	Need to stage disease to determine whether liver transplantation or resection feasible Multidisciplinary approach (hepatobiliary surgeon, interventional radiologist, oncologist, hepatologist) Tumour markers Avoid biopsy if candidate for transplant Exclude and treat encephalopathy/ hepatorenal syndrome/varices
Alcohol-induced hepatitis	
RUQ pain, recent binge or recent cessation (withdrawal hepatitis) Evidence of decompensation: jaundice, bruising, encephalopathy (eg nocturnal insomnia)	Exclude other concurrent causes of liver disease Exclude and treat encephalopathy/ hepatorenal syndrome/varices Long-term HCC and varices surveillance crucial Surveillance for varices with OGD once recovered Condition carries a high mortality rate (50% at 6 months) – should be managed by hepatology team. Steroids and pentoxifylline may be appropriate

For all diagnoses: consider financial status, ability to work/drive, likelihood of alcohol/IVDU cessation and encourage self-referral to AA or community drugs and alcohol team.

Questions

1. How is the severity and prognosis of acute pancreatitis assessed?

The modified Glasgow criteria for acute pancreatitis are easily remembered with the acronym PANCREAS:

	Score 1 point if	
P: Po_2 on arterial blood gas	< 60 mmHg (8 kPa)	
A: age	> 55 years	
N: neutrophil count	> 15 000/μl	
C: calcium	< 8 mg/dl	Severe pancreatitis likely with a score > 3
R: renal function (serum urea)	> 45 mg/dl	
E: enzymes – LDH (lactate de-hydrogenase)	> 600 U/l	
A: albumin	< 32 g/l	
S: sugar (blood glucose)	> 180 g/dl	

2. *What are the important features of an alcohol consumption history?*

An impartial approach is crucial, eg 'Lots of people drink more than the recommended amount without it affecting their day-to-day life. Do you drink more than is recommended? How much and what type (spirits, wine, beer)?'

If she or he is drinking much more than the recommended limit ask the following:

- Where, when and with whom?
- How does it affect your:
  - domestic life: relationship, friends, home and children?
  - work life: recent redundancies, drinking at work?
  - financial situation: jobs, mortgages, etc?

Other questions:

- Precipitating factors: relationship, work?
- Binge drinking?
- Has he or she sought help before?
- Violence or trouble with the police?

CAGE questionnaire

An affirmative reply to **two or more** of these four questions has a high sensitivity and specificity for alcohol dependence syndrome:

C: Have you tried to **cut down** the amount that you drink?
A: Do you get **angry** if people tell you that you drink too much?
G: Do you feel **guilty** about how much you drink?
E: Do you ever drink in the mornings (**eye-opener**)?

SCENARIO 14. DIARRHOEA

'Dear Colleague

This 39-year-old woman with a family history of colon cancer has suffered from intermittent diarrhoea over the last few months. Would you be kind enough to see her and advise on management?'

'Please assess this 25-year-old woman who has severe diarrhoea and some associated abdominal pain. She has noticed that this is worse during her periods. It is becoming increasingly difficult to continue her work as a shop-floor sales person. Many thanks.'

'This 30-year-old man has lost 2 stone (13 kg) over the past 3 months. He complains of loose stools with occasional blood mixed in. Please take a history.'

'This 50-year-old man has longstanding alcohol problems. He recently suffered from a fractured humerus after a fall. Today he presents with diarrhoea that has been troubling him for 6 months and is worsening. I would appreciate your advice regarding further investigation of this problem.'

'This 30-year-old woman presents with diarrhoea. She noticed that this worsened significantly on holiday in Italy, where she also developed an itchy rash. Please take a history.'

'This 28-year-old man had a small bowel resection 5 years ago after a gunshot wound. He now presents with weight loss and diarrhoea but a healthy appetite. Please could you assess him further.'

'This 70-year-old woman has had a recent change in bowel habit. She frequently has to rush off to the loo to open her bowels and on occasions has suffered from faecal incontinence. She is understandably very distressed about these symptoms. Please advise.'

1. Verify the information provided
'Tell me in your own words what the problem is … .'

2. HPC
Open to closed questions keeping in mind the *differential diagnosis*, eg
Irritable bowel syndrome (IBS)
Inflammatory bowel disease (IBD)
Infective diarrhoea/small bowel overgrowth
Lactose intolerance
Bile salt malabsorption
Coeliac disease
Chronic pancreatitis/insufficiency
Diverticular disease
Carcinoid
Colorectal cancer

3. Previous investigations:
Endoscopies? Stool collection?
CT abdomen? Blood tests?

4. SR:
Skin rash (eg erythema nodosum in IBD, dermatitis herpetiformis in coeliac disease)
Joint pains, eye inflammation
Fistulae: vaginal discharge, pneumaturia
IBS: symptoms worse with period, dyspareunia common
Infective: foreign travel, fever, HIV risks?

5. PMH:
Previous acute pancreatitis
Itchy skin rash (dermatitis herpetiformis)
Arthritis
Thyroid disease

6. DH:
A multitude of drugs cause diarrhoea.
Laxative abuse?

7. FH:
Colon cancer: which relatives and their age at diagnosis? IBD, coeliac disease

8. SH:
Does diarrhoea interfere with work (eg taxi driver) or social life? Smoking (exacerbates Crohn's disease), alcohol consumption and pancreatitis, other stressful events precipitating IBS symptoms

9. Summarise
'Is there anything else that we haven't discussed that you feel is important?'

10. Thank the patient

Volunteered problems
Is the patient's insight intact?

Alarm symptoms:
Weight loss
PR bleeding
Flushing/palpitations (thyroid disease or carcinoid)

Disease interaction:
Staggered presentation of multisystem disease, eg IBD-associated arthropathy?

Therapeutic successes and failures:
Inappropriate use of anti-diarrhoeals in infective or IBD
Non-compliance with therapy for established condition

Risks to others:
Infectious diarrhoea and need for isolation (eg *Clostridium difficile*)
Colorectal cancer and screening of relatives

Daily life and disease:
Is removing caffeine, alcohol and stress easily achieved given the daily demands on the individual?

Final problem list and plan of action

1. Identify and address any anxieties about cancer

2. Judge impact of symptoms and risk of sinister pathology and triage urgency of investigations accordingly

3. Assess willingness to have a colonoscopy if indicated

4. Determine if any relatives may require colonoscopic screening

5. Impact of diarrhoea on work and social life (eg long-distance lorry driver)

Key diagnostic features	Example problem list and plan of action
Irritable bowel syndrome (IBS)	
Abdominal pain	Set an appropriate limit of investigative depth when IBS suspected – if the patient is < 45 with normal examination and blood tests, endoscopic tests are not required
Usually relieved by defecation	
Mucus per rectum	
Bowels open several times in morning and not throughout rest of the day	Abnormal inflammatory markers or alarm symptoms in patient under 45° flexible sigmoidoscopy usually adequate
Rarely opens bowels at night	
No alarm symptoms	The patient may fulfil surveillance criteria for colonoscopy as a result of family history of colorectal cancer
Worse during periods	
Dyspareunia common	
Symptoms worse with anxiety	Avoid repeating previously normal invasive investigations
Episode of infective gastroenteritis within past year (post-infectious IBS)	High fat, high caffeine, high alcohol, spicy foods, low-fibre diet requires modification
Relapsing and remitting	
Intermittent constipation	Associated anxiety disorder or depression
	Poor response to previous medications (eg spasmolytics, Imodium)
Inflammatory bowel disease (IBD)	
Diarrhoea > 300 g day	If IBD suspected then colonoscopy superior to flexible sigmoidscopy
Bowels open at night	
Per rectum blood and mucus mixed in with stool	What is the extent of disease? May require small bowel imaging, eg MR enteroclysis, small bowel follow-through, capsule endoscopy, white cell scan
Abdominal pain	
Anaemia and fatigue	
Weight loss	Need for screening colonoscopy if total colitis for > 10 years
Malaise	
Triggering factor: stress, infection	Assessment for malabsorption if small bowel Crohn's disease suspected
Factors favouring Crohn's disease over ulcerative colitis (UC): intermittent bloating (partial obstruction), perianal fistulae and fissures (perianal pain worsened by defecation), vesicoureteric fistulae (pneumaturia, recurrent urinary tract infections or UTIs), anaemia (can also occur in UC but less common), less faecal urgency (rectal sparing), surgical intervention more common, less responsive to 5-ASAs (5-aminosalicylic acid derivatives)	Involvement of surgeons if unresponsive to medical therapy – planned surgery preferable to emergency
	Admission if symptoms severe (and/or undiagnosed)
	Need for steroid-sparing agents if recurrent flares on weaning steroids (eg azathioprine)
	Immunomodulators and their side effects
	Anti-TNF agents for poorly controlled disease and contraindications
SR: extra-articular manifestations, eg uveitis, arthropathy, erythema nodosum	Assessment of bone density if long-term malabsorption and/or if on steroids

Key diagnostic features	Example problem list and plan of action
Inflammatory bowel disease (IBD) (contd)	
PMH: previous operations, previous TB (contraindication to anti-TNF agents), heart failure (also a contraindication to anti-TNF agents), chronic renal failure (contraindication to ciclosporin) *DH*: 5-ASA maintenance therapy, azathioprine, 6-mercaptopurine, methotrexate (Crohn's disease), previous anti-TNF agents *SH*: symptoms began with smoking (Crohn's disease) or worsened on stopping (UC)	
Infectious diarrhoea/small bowel overgrowth	
Chronic infection: travel abroad (*Microsporum, Giardia, Cryptosporidium* spp., amoebiasis endemic areas), weight loss, depression HIV status: cryptosporidia, *Microsporum* sp., CMV (cytomegalovirus) colitis, HSV (herpes simplex virus) proctitis, lymphogranuloma venereum, colonic TB, drug side effect Small bowel overgrowth: vitamin B_{12}/folate deficiency (anaemia symptoms, neurological symptoms), previous bowel surgery/blind loop/jejunal diverticulum, weight loss	Need to obtain three stool samples – for *Giardia* sp. stool ELISA (enzyme-linked immunosorbent assay) OR therapeutic trial of metronidazole Replace vitamin deficiency, correct nutritional deficiencies and exclude other non-infective causes Dietician review – low-carbohydrate diet may be helpful in bacterial overgrowth Recurrent disease as a result of structural abnormality/jejunal diverticulum may require surgical correction HIV-related diarrhoea often requires colonoscopy and biopsy (with CMV and ZN [Ziehl–Neelsen] stains) as a result of wide differential diagnosis
Lactose intolerance	
Ethnic origin (80–90% of adults of Asian/African origin) Diarrhoea induced by dairy products/relieved by stopping dairy products Bloating, nausea, abdominal pain	Trial of dairy-free diet (lactose hydrogen breath test often positive but poorly predicts response to lactose restriction) Dietician consultation Need for supplemental calcium in patients at risk of osteoporosis (eg Asian women)
Bile salt malabsorption	
Diarrhoea, watery and nocturnal Previous small bowel surgery/known short bowel/terminal ileal disease, eg Crohn's disease Also associated with: small bowel overgrowth, irritable bowel of the diarrhoea type (33% have bile salt malabsorption), coeliac disease	Successful trial of cholestyramine usually sufficient to make the diagnosis SeHCAT test (Bile malabsorption study) useful for complex cases where diarrhoea may have multiple causes Need to identify any underlying small bowel pathology

continued on next page

Key diagnostic features	Example problem list and plan of action
Coeliac disease	
Oily light stools Weight loss Fatigue Abdominal pain Itchy papulovesicular rash (dermatitis herpetiformis) Bleeding diatheses (vitamin K deficiency) Treatment for iron deficiency anaemia in the past Bony pain, weakness, paraesthesiae (hypocalcaemia) Improves with cutting out gluten-containing products and worsens when gluten is re-introduced	If transglutaminase antibodies positive (see below) then proceed to duodenal biopsy to confirm the diagnosis Check total IgA levels (selective IgA deficiency may give a false-negative transglutaminase antibody result). Patients should be eating gluten-containing foods when tested May need repeat antibody testing while consuming wheat products if they stopped before previous test (patients often try wheat exclusion before consultation) Correct nutritional deficits Dietician support and problems with compliance (especially young women/girls who may use gluten to effect weight control) Exclude complications if deteriorating despite gluten-free diet (see below)
Diverticulitis	
Episodic diarrhoea associated with left iliac fossa (LIF) pain and bleeding per rectum Fever Longstanding constipation Fistulae: dysuria, pneumaturia, vaginal discharge	Need to involve surgeon if patient having recurrent bouts/fistulating disease/abscess/acute abdomen Usually resolve with conservative management (fluids, antibiotics) Need to exclude other causes of bleeding per rectum (usually occurs in patients > 50) High-fibre diet may reduce flares
Chronic pancreatitis	
Abdominal pain (unpredictable, sometimes severe) Steatorrhoea Weight loss Bleeding diatheses (vitamin K deficiency) *PMH*: alcohol excess, previous abdominal trauma, hyperlipidaemia, diabetes (endocrine insufficiency), osteoporosis (vitamin D deficiency) *DH*: opiate dependence for chronic pain	Need to exclude other end-organ damage from alcohol dependence if this is the likely cause Correct nutritional deficits Assess osteoporosis with bone densitometry Referral to alcohol cessation clinics Chronic pain team Enzyme replacement therapy may need increasing Diabetes management

Key diagnostic features	Example problem list and plan of action
Carcinoid	
Diarrhoea (80%) Weight loss Skin flushing (80%) if metastatic Abdominal pain Wheeze Palpitations	Logistics of diagnosis often tricky: 24-hour urine collection and avoidance of foods with high tryptophan beforehand Multidisciplinary approach to staging and treatment – radiology, oncology, surgery, gastroenterology and endocrinology input Adequacy of symptomatic control with octreotide/other medications
Colorectal cancer	
Abdominal pain (50%) Diarrhoea/constipation (about 33%) Anaemia/bleeding (about 33%) Weight loss Anorexia *PMH*: IBD, colonic polyps, other cancers, acromegaly *FH*: HNPCC, FAP (see below) Smoking and alcohol are powerful risk factors	May fulfil colonoscopic screening guidelines for patients with a positive family history Other diagnostic modalities may be preferable to the patient (eg CT of pneumocolon) Multidisciplinary approach to staging Address anxiety and investigate need for screening of other relatives Co-morbidity and fitness for potential surgery

Questions

1. What diagnostic serological tests are available for coeliac disease?

The sensitivities and specificities for coeliac disease antibodies

Antibody	Percentage sensitivity	Percentage specificity	Predictive value: percentage positive	Predictive value: percentage negative
A-EmA	97	98	97	98
ARA	65	100	100	72
IgG AGA	88	92	88	92
IgA AGA	52	94	87	74

A-EmA, anti-endomysial antibody; ARA, anti-reticulin antibody; AGA, anti-gliadin antibody.

Anti-tissue transglutaminase (tTG) antibodies are widely used but are also positive in IBD so may not be appropriate as an isolated diagnostic test.

2. What are the common causes of relapse in coeliac disease?

Common causes of recurrent symptoms include:

- **Non-compliance** with a gluten-free diet
- **Lymphoma**

- **Refractory disease**: some patients do not respond to a gluten-free diet; immunosuppression may be necessary
- **Collagenous sprue**: a thick band of collagen forms beneath the basement membrane of the mucosal epithelium impeding absorption. Parenteral nutrition is often required.

3. *How does having a relative with colorectal cancer affect an individual's lifetime risk?*

	Lifetime risk
Population average	1:50
Any family member	1:17
One affected first-degree relative < 45	1:10
Two affected first-degree relatives	1:6

4. *What are the criteria for screening colonoscopy where there is a family history of colorectal cancer?*

Patients who fulfil the following criteria should be offered colonoscopy at age 35 or at presentation, whichever is later:

- At least one affected first-degree relative < 45 years old
- Two affected first-degree relatives diagnosed at any age.

5. *What are the main inherited predispositions to colorectal cancer and how do they differ from each other and sporadic colorectal carcinoma?*

Hereditary non-polyposis colorectal carcinoma (HNPCC) and familial adenomatous polyposis (FAP) are the two of the most common hereditary colorectal cancer syndromes.

The adenoma–carcinoma sequence involves a common sequence of acquisition of genetic abnormalities ('loss of heterozygosity'), ultimately resulting in invasive and metastatic cells. This usually begins with *APC* (adenomatous polyposis coli), followed by *ras*, *p53* and *DCC* (deleted in colorectal cancer). In FAP, an abnormal *APC* gene is inherited. In HNPCC the DNA-repair genes (listed below) are defective, thus accelerating heterozygosity and malignant transformation.

The incidence of adenomas is similar in both conditions, but adenomas in HNPCC are more likely to undergo malignant transformation. In HNPCC, most tumours are proximal to the splenic flexure whereas in sporadic colorectal cancer (CRC) most are distal.

FAP syndrome is an autosomal dominant condition leading to multiple (often thousands of) polyps throughout the colon. Unless patients undergo prophylactic colectomy, CRC is inevitable. Children of FAP patients should begin colonoscopic screening in adolescence. If no significant polyps have developed by the age of 40 they have not inherited the syndrome.

	Sporadic CRC	HNPCC	FAP
Mean age (years)	69	44	39
Arise from adenomas	Yes	Yes	Yes (many hundreds)
Distribution	70% distal to splenic flexure	70% proximal to splenic flexure	Throughout colon and rectum
Genetic cause	Polygenic	HMSH2, hMSH1, hMSH6, hPMS1, hPMS2	APC
Malignancies at other sites	No	Yes	Yes

SCENARIO 15. THE HIV PATIENT

'This 35-year-old man was diagnosed with HIV 3 years ago. He has recently developed diarrhoea. Please advise.'

'This 28-year-old woman, who recently arrived from Zimbabwe and is HIV positive, has developed shortness of breath.'

'This 62-year-old man with longstanding HIV infection has symptoms of loss of appetite and weight loss. He has also developed a cough at night. I would be grateful for your opinion.'

1. Verify the information provided:
'Tell me in your own words what the problem is ... .'

2. HPC:
Establish the current problem (see list below)
- Establish mode of original presentation and likely mode of infection
- Establish disease history to date focusing on any AIDS-defining illnesses

3. Previous investigations:
What is the latest CD4+ count and viral load? Previous CD4 count viral load

4. SR:
Full screen of all systems to pre-empt emerging HIV-related problems (see table). Depression and anxiety common

5. PMH:
HIV-related disease (eg Kaposi's sarcoma) and previous screening for other STIs (eg HCV, HBV, *Chlamydia*, gonorrhoea)

6. DH:
Anti-retrovirals – focus on duration of therapy, recent changes (known viral resistance?), compliance and side effects. Other drugs that interfere with HAART metabolism?

7. FH:
Affected relatives/children? Plans for a family?

8. SH:
Current occupation and potential risk to others (eg health-care professional)

Sexual history: gender of partners, frequency and nature of sexual contact. Use of barrier contraceptives

Previous/ongoing intravenous drug use

9. Summarise:
'Is there anything else we haven't discussed that you feel is important?'

10. Thank the patient

Volunteered problems

Alarm symptoms:
Any new symptom should raise suspicion of HIV-related disease and disease progression

Disease interaction:
eg HIV and HCV/HBV co-infection (more rapid progression to cirrhosis)

Therapeutic successes and failures:
Many patients require at least one modification to their anti-retrovirals before the optimum regimen is found
Common side effects: lipoatrophy, dyslipidaemia, dyspepsia/GORD, rash, hypersensitivity reaction (see below)
Immune reconstitution disease (unmasking of pre-existing infections with immune recovery with HAART)

Risks to others:
What is the patient's perception of risk to self and others and is it accurate? Contact tracing issues must be elicited

Daily life and disease:
Assess impact of drug regimen, adverse effects and disease burden on life and relationships
How does the current problem further influence the situation?

Final problem list and plan of action

1. Need to establish stage of disease (CD4 count and viral load)

2. A lower CD4+ baseline (usually at presentation) limits the upper plateau of CD4+ count that can be achieved with therapy. The CD4+ count at presentation thus has prognostic significance

3. Triage urgency of further investigation of new symptoms (should this be done as an outpatient or inpatient?)

4. It is often difficult to disentangle medication side effects from new HIV-related disease – several consultations with changes in medications may be needed

5. New contact tracing issues may arise long after first diagnosis

Key diagnostic features	Example problem list and plan of action
Diarrhoea	
Consider all the causes of diarrhoea common in the non-HIV population and the following (in approximate order of decreasing prevalence): • HAART side effect: foscarnet – 30% • IFN-α – 29% • Nelfinavir – 25–30%, didanosine (ddI) 17–28% • Ritonavir – 12–18% • Zalcitabine (ddC) – 10% Cryptosporidia: cholera-like diarrhoea – severity inversely related to CD4 count. Often present with volume depletion *Cyclosporum* and *Microsporum* spp: waxing and waning watery diarrhoea, anorexia, fatigue, weight loss. May persist for several months in HIV CMV colitis: abdominal pain, fever, bloody diarrhoea, weight loss *Mycobacterium avium-intracellulare*: CD4 count usually < 150, fever, abdominal pain (often RUQ), anorexia, weight loss *Clostridium difficile*: bloody diarrhoea after a course of antibiotics for another infection. Lymphogranuloma venereum (LGV), *Chlamydia trachomatis*: can cause bloody diarrhoea in the tertiary phase in homosexual or bisexual men; painful inguinal lymphadenopathy is characteristic, fever, chills, malaise HSV proctitis: pain in sacral nerve root distribution, bloody mucus discharge, painful inguinal lymphadenopathy Intestinal TB: fever, weight loss, malaise, diarrhoea, abdominal pain *Escherichia coli*, *Campylobacter*, *Shigella*, *Entamoeba* and *Giardia* spp. are all more common in the HIV population IBD is also encountered and easily missed	Colitis: frequent small-volume bloody or mucopurulent stools, lower abdominal pain, tenesmus and faecal urgency Small intestine infection: watery diarrhoea, dehydration, weight loss, abdominal cramps Multiple stool samples for microscopy and culture are key. A high neutrophil count in the stool suggests bacterial infection, eg *Salmonella*, *Shigella*, *Listeria* or *Campylobacter* spp. or *E. coli*. Bloody diarrhoea without a high faecal neutrophil count suggests amoebiasis Specific tests that won't be done unless you ask: • Biopsy and staining: *Isospora belli*, CMV, TB, *Mycobacterium avium-intracellulare* • Stool culture (non-routine): *E. coli* O157 in McConkey sorbitol medium • Stool antigen test: *Giardia*, *Cryptosporidium* spp. Empirical therapy should be instituted immediately, eg a fluoroquinolone and metronidazole. Both drugs successfully treat the underlying bacterial infections most commonly associated with diarrhoea, ie *Shigella*, *Salmonella* and *Campylobacter* spp. Treat dehydration, electrolyte imbalance and any nutritional deficit Endoscopic investigation with biopsies is almost always appropriate, especially if diarrhoea fails to resolve or if the CD4 count < 200 (as multiple pathologies may be present) Changing medications may not be advisable even if the side effect of diarrhoea is severe. Loperamide may offer some relief The prevalence of diarrhoea in the HIV-positive population is approximately 40%, higher in developing countries. Rapid and thorough assessment is crucial to minimising the impact on day-to-day life

Key diagnostic features	Example problem list and plan of action
Weight loss	
HIV-associated wasting: involuntary loss of 10% of ideal body weight in the absence of another disease process that could account for it	Gaunt appearance can be stigmatising. This can have a major effect on compliance with HAART if the patient feels that this is the cause
Weakness, lethargy and fever are commonly associated. Can occur despite HAART therapy and a normal CD4 count	Degree of weight loss directly proportional to mortality in HIV-wasting syndromes
HAART-related fat redistribution: typically lipoatrophy occurs in the face and extremities with lipotrophy in the trunk and abdomen	Bioelectrical impedance analysis should be arranged: this is the cheapest and most accurate diagnostic test
HAART-related pancreatic insufficiency and malabsorption: bulky, pale, frequent stools. Weight loss despite adequate calorie intake. Nucleoside analogues and protease inhibitors are common culprits	Patients require careful systematic exclusion of underlying infection or malignancy as a cause of weight loss before diagnosing HIV-associated wasting
	Full dietician assessment: lean body mass is often lost before fat – high-protein and high-calorie diets are usually appropriate
	Thiazolidinediones ('glitazones') may be effective in reversing lipoatrophy
	Enzyme replacement with meals may counter pancreatic insufficiency
Abdominal pain	
HAART-related GORD and dyspepsia (see pages 130–131 for GORD and dyspepsia symptoms)	Always need to exclude infectious or malignant pathology before attributing symptoms to medications (the most common cause of GI upset in HIV)
HAART-related or pentamidine-related pancreatitis (see above for pancreatitis symptoms): combined didanosine and tenofovir therapy carries the highest risk of pancreatitis (about 13%)	Often the offending agent cannot be stopped – standard medical management of dyspepsia and GORD is appropriate
Cholecystitis (CMV, cryptosporidiosis), RUQ pain, jaundice, fever, pale stools, dark urine	Pancreatitis, cholecystitis and GI bleeding are emergencies that require immediate investigation and treatment
Gastrointestinal (GI) lymphoma: abdominal pain, weight loss, fever, pruritus, night sweats, alcohol-induced pain, diarrhoea, GI bleed	GI lymphoma and Kaposi's sarcoma are difficult to diagnose in the small intestine. Capsule endoscopy and MR enteroclysis are increasingly available and optimise pick-up rates in small bowel malignancy
GI Kaposi's sarcoma: abdominal pain, GI bleeding, symptoms of intermittent obstruction (bloating, vomiting and constipation)	

Key diagnostic features	Example problem list and plan of action
Headache	
CNS cryptococcosis: CD4 < 100. Indolent onset of headache (75%), fever (70%), neck stiffness (about 30%), altered mental state (20%), photophobia (about 20%) CNS toxoplasmosis: CD4 < 200. Constitutional symptoms followed by headache, drowsiness and confusion. Seizures and focal neurological deficits tend to develop later. Can progress to coma within days CNS lymphoma: CD4 < 100. Similar symptoms to toxoplasmosis but more indolent onset	Early CSF analysis and CT are key in all cases, eg EBV DNA in CSF (detected by PCR) is a useful corollary of CNS lymphoma Exclude extracranial disease Effective prophylaxis against further infection may be appropriate HAART-naïve patients usually benefit from immediate introduction of therapy. This especially improves the prognosis in CNS lymphoma
Confusion	
PML (demyelination caused by reactivation of endemic JC papovavirus): CD4 < 100. Usually presents with focal neurological symptoms, eg behavioural change, speech, cognitive dysfunction, motor weakness and visual impairment. Headaches are rare. It evolves over several weeks but progresses more rapidly than AIDS–dementia complex CMV encephalitis: may have other systemic disturbance caused by CMV (eg colitis, hepatitis, pneumonitis) plus three distinct presentations: 1. Ventriculoencephalitis characterised by abrupt onset and rapid-onset confusion and lethargy 2. Facial and oculomotor cranial nerve palsies 3. Slowly progressive cognitive impairment similar to AIDS–dementia complex HIV-1 encephalopathy and AIDS–dementia complex: CD4 < 200. Insidious onset of behavioural and/or mood change, apathy and/or loss of interest in social activities. Poor concentration and decreased libido are common. Progresses to global cognitive impairment especially affecting memory and language functions	Other causes of cognitive impairment must be excluded ('dementia screen', eg CT of head, thyroid function tests, vitamin B_{12}, syphilis serology) Depression and anxiety are commonly associated and need to be addressed Empirical initiation of intravenous ganciclovir may be appropriate until CMV encephalitis has been excluded Optimised HAART therapy must be achieved to slow progression of AIDS–dementia complex Beware an initial worsening of PML on commencing HAART as a result of immune reconstitution Often cognitive impairment is permanent, which has major implications for independence and working life. Multidisciplinary input is crucial

Key diagnostic features	Example problem list and plan of action
Weak legs	
HIV-1-associated vacuolar myelopathy: CD4 < 100. Gradual onset of lower limb leg weakness, numbness and loss of balance is common. Progresses to cognitive decline and sphincter dysfunction HTLV-1-associated myelopathy (tropical spastic paraparesis). This most commonly presents with insidious onset of leg weakness. Other symptoms include painful legs, paraesthesiae, back pain and bladder dysfunction. Neurological disability usually stabilises after a few years. An associated sicca syndrome, arthralgias and dermatitis are very common Elicit history of travel to (or originating from) endemic areas: southern Japan, the Caribbean, parts of Central Africa and South America	Early input from occupational therapist and physiotherapist may limit the impact of disability on day-to-day life HTLV-1-associated myelopathy requires long-term surveillance for development of T-cell leukaemias
Jaundice/abnormal liver function tests	
Non-nucleoside reverse transcriptase inhibitor (NNRTI)-induced hepatitis: concomitant administration of protease inhibitors increases the risk of liver toxicity. There is no clear evidence that prolonged HAART therapy is associated with liver fibrosis HBV and/or HCV co-infection: intravenous drug use is usually the mode of HIV transmission. Patients may present with features of decompensated liver disease (eg ascites, encephalopathy, jaundice) CMV hepatitis: CD4 usually < 100. CMV hepatitis frequently presents with isolated abnormal LFTs. Jaundice is unusual and progression to cirrhosis is rare Biliary tract disease: cryptosporidia, microsporidia, CMV and *Mycobacterium avium-intracellulare* can all cause biliary tract infection which may manifest as abnormal LFTs (GGT, bilirubin and ALP) rather than acute cholecystitis	Need to stage liver disease (Child–Pugh score, ultrasonography, varices surveillance if cirrhotic, etc) and exclude other causes of liver disease All patients with HIV should be screened for HBV and HCV infection Liver biopsy may be necessary to distinguish NNRTI-induced transaminitis from inflammation caused by viral hepatitis in HIV/HBV or HIV/HCV co-infection Patients with viral hepatitis co-infection tend to progress more rapidly to cirrhosis. This has a detrimental affect on HAART tolerance. Early, optimal control of both infections is therefore essential Liver transplantation is an increasingly successful option in HIV-positive individuals with chronic liver disease – survival rates at 1 year are similar to HIV-negative transplant recipients. Early assessment for transplantation is crucial (the HIV-positive pre-transplantation population have a higher mortality rate than HIV-negative individuals with a similar severity of liver disease) Treatment regimens for HBV and/or HCV co-infection are sometimes synergistic and sometimes antagonistic. Joint management by a hepatologist and HIV specialist is important

Key diagnostic features	Example problem list and plan of action
Breathlessness	
Pneumocystis jiroveci pneumonia (PJP; previously *Pneumocystis carinii* pneumonia or PCP): CD4 < 250. Progressive exertional dyspnoea, fever and a non-productive cough are almost universal presenting complaints Chest discomfort, weight loss, rigors and (more rarely) haemoptysis are also features Recent chest radiographs may have been normal *PMH*: recent oral thrush (susceptibility to other fungal infection is common) *DH*: not on co-trimoxazole prophylaxis *Mycobacterium avium-intracellulare* (MAI): CD4 < 50. Insidious onset of worsening cough, sputum production, weight loss, fever, lethargy and night sweats. Patients sometimes complain of RUQ pain. Haemoptysis is rare. Breathlessness is unusual unless there is an associated hypersensitivity pneumonitis. May have a history of exposure to MAI from using jacuzzis. Fever of unknown origin is a common presentation *PMH*: pulmonary MAI often associated with established chronic lung disease, eg COPD Lymphocytic interstitial pneumonia: dyspnoea with fever, cough and pleuritic chest pain. May follow an indolent course and present much later as fibrosis and/or bronchiectasis TB (see above): CD4 count variable (often normal) CMV pneumonitis: CD4 < 150. In addition to breathlessness the patient may have an associated mononucleosis syndrome (fever and lymphadenopathy) *Pseudomonas aeruginosa* infection: CD4 < 50. Recent inpatient stay and/or invasive ventilation, productive cough, anorexia, dyspnoea HIV myocarditis/cardiomyopathy. CD4 often < 100. Orthopnea, PND, exertional dyspnoea and ankle swelling HIV-related pulmonary hypertension (no clear relationship with CD4 count). Exertional dyspnoea, ankle swelling, lethargy, syncope (about 10%). Kaposi's sarcoma at other sites (human herpesvirus 8 appears to be the pathogenic organism)	Bronchoalveolar lavage (BAL) is often needed for definitive diagnosis of an opportunistic pulmonary infection An elevated LDH is a useful pointer towards PJP in an HIV-positive patient with an acute respiratory illness The severity of PJP needs to be determined by arterial blood gas (ABG) sampling. This affects management – only severe PJP seems to benefit from adjunctive steroid therapy Diagnostic criteria for MAI lung disease require specific numbers of acid-fast bacilli (AFB) stains of sputum or BAL, and positive mycobacterial culture Anti-mycobacterial therapy may adversely affect organs already impaired by HIV-related disease (eg ethambutol) and optic neuritis (eg rifampicin and hepatotoxicity). Close surveillance for complications is necessary Need to exclude extrapulmonary disease (eg disseminated CMV, MAI) Long-term infection with its associated anorexia and a catabolic state often results in undernutrition or malnutrition, which should be corrected For all opportunistic infections antimicrobial resistance is a growing problem. Sending repeat specimens for sensitivity testing is important especially if initial response to therapy is poor Prophylaxis against future infection is key, eg co-trimoxazole for PJP. It may be safe to stop prophylaxis if the CD4 count recovers above a certain number (eg CD4 > 200 in the cases of co-trimoxazole for PJP) Treatment for HIV cardiomyopathy is similar to non-ischaemic cardiomyopathy with β blockers and ACE inhibitors, while endothelin antagonists appear to be effective in HIV-associated pulmonary hypertension

Key diagnostic features	Example problem list and plan of action
Skin rash/lesion	
Kaposi's sarcoma: CD4 count variable, often normal. In the HAART era this usually manifests as subtle purple patches rather than large fixed plaques Molluscum contagiosum: CD4 < 50. Multiple small, round, shiny, wart-like lumps with a depression in the centre. Facial involvement is common Erythema nodosum (often associated with immune reconstitution and CD4 > 200): raised, large, red, painful nodules, typically over the shins Prurigo nodularis: itchy bumps over the arms and trunk. The itch is often maddening and unresponsive to antihistamines Photosensitivity: this is usually drug related and particularly affects those with a low CD4 count. Co-trimoxazole (PJP prophylaxis) is a common culprit	Skin biopsy is sometimes necessary to make the diagnosis (eg Kaposi's sarcoma, erythema nodosum) Most conditions associated with a low CD4 count will improve with HAART therapy and immune reconstitution Such visible stigmata of HIV/AIDS are rarely life threatening but have a profound effect on patient's level of social interaction and general well-being and should be treated aggressively Skin lesions are often indicative of advanced disease and should instigate a thorough screen for other AIDS-defining illnesses which may be initially asymptomatic (eg CMV retinitis, oral candidiasis)
Chest pain	
Stable/unstable angina: protease inhibitors, a main component of HAART, induce atherogenic metabolic effects such as dyslipidaemia and insulin resistance Premature IHD is an increasing problem in the HAART era	Ensure adequate primary and secondary prevention by early treatment of dyslipidaemia IHD may compound other HIV-related cardiac disease (eg cardiomyopathy)
Arthralgia/myalgia	
Myositis and/or rhabdomyolysis: painful muscles (often proximal groups) with associated weakness. Dark urine Causes: ● Zidovudine ● Infection (eg toxoplasmosis) ● HIV-related polymyositis HIV-associated arthritis: an oligoarticular, asymmetrical and peripheral arthritis predominantly affecting the knees and ankles. It is usually self-limiting (1–5 weeks) Septic arthritis: fever, pain and markedly reduced range of movement. Atypical organisms include *Staphyloccus aureus*, *Neisseria* gonorrhoeae, *Candida albicans* and *Mycobacterium tuberculosis*	Need to exclude emergencies (eg rhabdomyolysis or destructive arthritis) and triage investigation and treatment accordingly Cessation of a putative causative HAART agent should always be discussed with an HIV specialist

Key diagnostic features	Example problem list and plan of action
Visual disturbance	
CMV retinitis: CD4 < 100. Patients describe floaters, photopsias or visual loss, without a red or painful eye. On the whole, visual acuity is usually good at the time of diagnosis HIV retinopathy: insidious loss of visual acuity with loss of colour and/or peripheral vision Toxoplasma choroidoretinitis: insidious bilateral loss of visual acuity, which may occur many months or years after the initial infection	Need to exclude systemic manifestations of the causative organism Early treatment and regular monitoring are crucial to preserve vision

Question

1. *What does standard HAART therapy consist of and when should it be initiated?*

Clinical guideline: British HIV Association (BHIVA 2003)

Standard recommended initiation therapy consists of:

- two nucleoside reverse tanscriptase inhibitors (NRTIs)

plus either

- a protease inhibitor or
- a non-nucleoside reverse transcriptase inhibitor (NNRTI).

Changes in medication are then prompted by either viral rebound or intolerance to a particular drug. If the former is the cause, viral resistance testing is recommended to guide selection of a different agent.

Initiation of treatment is a balancing act between increasing risk of opportunistic infection as the CD4 count falls and risk of adverse effects and/or viral resistance once treatment is initiated. Treatment should be initiated when the CD4 count is between 200 and 350 cells/mm^3. A CD4 count of 200 cells/mm^3 is the minimum level at which treatment is advised.

SCENARIO 16. HYPERTENSION

'This previously healthy 38-year-old woman felt unwell at work today with a headache and attended my walk-in centre. I have found a blood pressure of 230/110 mmHg and would value your opinion.'

'This 40-year-old man complains of ankle oedema and facial swelling. I also noted that his blood pressure was high (for the second time in the last month) last week. Please advise.'

'This 60-year-old woman was recently diagnosed with hypertension that has been difficult to control. This seems to be associated with profound lethargy and she is struggling to get her day-to-day tasks done around the home. I would be grateful for your further assessment.'

'I would be grateful for your opinion regarding this 38-year-old man with inter-mittent headache associated with sweating and palpitations. I took his blood pressure today during an episode and it was 200/106. Please could you advise with regard to his further investigation and management?'

1. Verify the information provided:
'Tell me in your own words what the problem is ... .'

2. HPC:
Open to closed questions keeping in mind the *differential diagnosis*, eg
Essential hypertension
Conn syndrome
Cushing syndrome
Phaeochromocytoma
Renovascular hypertension
Coarctation of the aorta

3. Previous investigations:
Previous blood pressure recordings?

4. SR:
Visual symptoms (retinopathy), headache, heart failure (strain)
Paroxysmal headache or palpitations, panic attacks
Leg claudication
Lethargy/confusion

5. PMH:
Renal disease
Diabetes
Endocrine disease
Stroke/IHD

6. DH:
Current antihypertensives, steroids, sympathomimetics, OCP

7. FH:
Renal disease (eg cystic), multiple endocrine neopolasia (MEN) type 2

8. SH:
Smoking history (cessation ameliorates hypertension-associated mortality and morbidity more than antihypertensives)
Caffeine consumption
Alcohol raises BP in dose-dependent fashion
Regular cocaine use has a similar effect

9. Summarise
'Is there anything else that we haven't discussed that you feel is important?'

10. Thank the patient

Volunteered problems

Alarm symptoms:
Visual loss
Confusion
Severe headache

Disease interaction:
Hypertension perpetuating other diseases (eg renal function, IHD)

Therapeutic successes and failures:
Adequacy of current antihypertensives
Drug interactions?
Side effects?
Compliance?

Risks to others:
MEN syndromes will require family screening

Daily life and disease:
Is removing caffeine, alcohol, stress and smoking easily achieved given the daily demands on the individual?

Final problem list and plan of action

1. Triage between potential malignant hypertension and chronic non-malignant hypertension (note that a diagnosis of malignant hypertension requires retinopathy)

2. Assess compliance with therapy (compliance for an asymptomatic condition is often poor)

3. Screen for end-organ damage.

4. Assess willingness to adopt lifestyle changes

continued on next page

Key diagnostic features	Example problem list and plan of action
Essential hypertension	
Usually asymptomatic Symptoms resulting from end-organ damage (stroke, TIA, angina, cardiac failure, etc) Cardiovascular risk factors Alcohol intake Cocaine use Current medications for high BP Headache *less* common in essential hypertension than in general population	Need to document high BP on three separate occasions Screen/examine for end-organ damage The most important modifiable risk factor for IHD, stroke, CCF, end-stage renal failure (ESRF) and peripheral vascular disease Implement treatment (see below) with careful follow-up
Conn syndrome	
Alkalosis and hypokalaemia: weakness, myalgia, polyuria, fatigue, palpitations Symptoms resulting from end-organ damage	Need for high index of suspicion (up to 10% of people with hypertension may have Conn syndrome) Need to stop ACE inhibitors/diuretics before checking renin levels Need to differentiate bilateral adrenal hyperplasia from a solitary adenoma (CT) Referral to a surgeon if appropriate
Cushing syndrome	
Weight gain (in characteristic distribution) Striae, easy bruising, amenorrhea, depression, new diabetes, easy fractures Hirsutism in women, feminisation in men Symptoms resulting from end-organ damage Visual loss, polyuria, headaches, galactorrhoea (Cushing's disease) Difficult to control hypertension Exogenous Cushing syndrome – long-term steroid use	Differentiating Cushing syndrome from Cushing's disease (see below) Difficulty in diagnosis when other conditions disturb the hypothalamic–pituitary axis (see below) Associated depression/cognitive impairment and life impact Multisystem consequences of steroid excess
Phaeochromocytoma	
Diagnosis excluded if asymptomatic Episodic headaches, sweating and palpitations are classic triad Tremor, nausea, weakness, weight loss, flank pain, constipation Symptoms resulting from end-organ damage Resistant to antihypertensives *PMH*: MEN 2, neurofibromatosis, von Hippel–Lindau disease *FH*: MEN 2	Identification and treatment of hypertensive emergencies – encephalopathy, retinopathy, seizures, worsening renal function, aortic dissection Multidisciplinary approach to staging and treatment Logistics of 24-hour urine collection for creatinine, catecholamines, vanillylmandelic acid Rule out a familial syndrome, eg MEN 2 α Blockade and compensatory volume expansion with fluids and increased salt intake α and β blockade before surgery

Key diagnostic features	Example problem list and plan of action
Renovascular hypertension	
< 65 years with abrupt-onset hypertension	Exclude fibromuscular dysplasia rather than atherosclerosis as the cause
Resistant to antihypertensives	
Recurrent sudden-onset SOB (flash pulmonary oedema)	Established chronic renal failure (note hypertensive insult to unaffected contralateral kidney if unilateral) and risk of contrast-induced failure after renal artery angiography
PMH: stroke, IHD, peripheral vascular disease	
SH: smoker	Angioplasty versus surgical revascularisation
	Smoking cessation crucial
	Need aggressive BP control
Coarctation of the aorta	
Often asymptomatic	High index of suspicion required
Headache, palpitations, leg pain, cold feet, muscle cramps	Impact of claudication on day-to-day life
	Risks of surgery and associated co-morbidity
PMH: Turner syndrome. Known structural heart disease, eg ventricular septal defect (VSD). Previous subarachnoid haemorrhage	Women contemplating pregnancy will need surgical intervention beforehand
	Unfavourable interaction with aortic valve disease or poor ejection fraction

Questions

1. *Which common conditions alter the activity of the hypothalamic–pituitary–adrenal (HPA) axis?*

Increased HPA activity	Decreased HPA activity
Depression and other psychiatric disease	Hyperthyroidism
Alcoholism	Postpartum period
Obesity	Rheumatoid arthritis
Hypothyroidism	
Pregnancy	

2. *How is Cushing syndrome differentiated from Cushing's disease?*

Differentiation of ACTH-dependent and -independent hypercortisolaemia is usually straightforward; a plasma ACTH level < 10 pg/l suggests cortisol secretion by an autonomous site (Cushing syndrome) rather than a pituitary adenoma (Cushing's disease) or ectopic ACTH (EAS) production.

In cases of ACTH-dependent Cushing syndrome 85% are the result of Cushing's disease – pituitary adenomas. EAS, compared with Cushing's disease, is usually associated with higher ACTH levels, an obvious lung lesion, hypokalaemia and a rapid onset of symptoms. Small carcinoids (< 1 cm) may secrete ACTH ectopically and prove very difficult to identify. The cortisol-releasing hormone (CRH) test (which looks for a rise in ACTH after CRH administration) is a useful means of differentiating ectopic ACTH production (no change in ACTH) from a pituitary adenoma (further rise in ACTH levels) if combined with inferior petrosal sinus sampling (IPSS) for ACTH.

3. *What guidelines on blood pressure targets are you aware of?*

> ### Clinical guideline (British Society of Hypertension [BSH] 2004)
>
> Drug treatment should be started in all patients with:
>
> * sustained systolic blood pressures = 160 mmHg or sustained diastolic blood pressures = 100 mmHg irrespective of additional lifestyle measures
> * sustained systolic blood pressures 140–159 mmHg or diastolic blood pressures 90–99 mmHg if target organ damage is present, or in the context of established cardiovascular disease or diabetes, or if there is a 10-year cardiovascular disease risk > 20%.
>
> The target blood pressure should be 140 mmHg systolic and 85 mm/Hg diastolic. In the context of diabetes, renal impairment or established cardio-vascular disease, a lower target of 130/80 mmHg is recommended.

4. *How would you go about choosing an antihypertensive for a patient?*

An ABCD (A: ACE inhibitor or angiotensin II antagonist; B: β blocker; C: calcium channel blocker; D: diuretic) approach has recently been supplanted by an ACD approach. The increased risk of developing type 2 diabetes on β blockers has led to their removal from guidelines on the management of hypertension, unless there are specific indications (or as fourth-line therapy in resistant cases).

There are several 'compelling indications' for each class of drug and several clear contraindications depending on specific conditions accompanying hypertension.

In isolated hypertension, the best choice of antihypertensive is determined by ethnicity and age (modified from joint NICE and BHS guidelines 2006) (Figure 2.6).

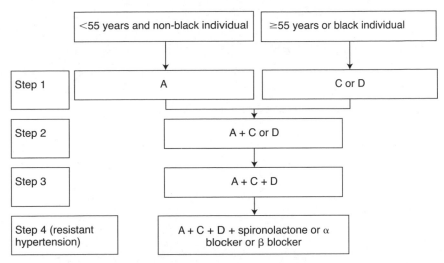

Figure 2.6   Choice of antihypertensive for patients.

Specific indications and contraindication to each class of antihypertensive (modified from BHS guidelines 2004)

Antihypertensive	Specific indications	Specific contraindications
A	Heart failure Post-MI/IHD Type 1 diabetic nephropathy (ACE inhibitor) Type 2 diabetic nephropathy (angiotensin II antagonist) Secondary stroke prevention	Renovascular disease Aortic stenosis: peripheral vascular disease worsening renal impairment Pregnancy
B	Post-MI Heart failure (chronic)	Heart failure (acute) Asthma COPD Patients with diabetes on insulin
C	Elderly patient Isolated systolic hypertension	
D	Elderly patient Isolated systolic hypertension Secondary stroke prevention	
α Blockers	Prostatic hypertrophy	Urinary incontinence, postural hypotension, heart failure

STATION 3

The Cardiovascular and Neurological Examinations

THE CARDIOVASCULAR EXAMINATION

The elucidation of the signs of disease in the cardiovascular system may follow a rather stereotyped pattern with the potential to reveal a wide range of signs and allow a broad differential diagnosis, including disease in many systems. Although it is inescapable that most cases will focus on valvular pathology, you must not focus too much on auscultation but look broadly at the totality of the case.

Introduce and expose

- Introduce yourself
- Ask 'Do you have pain anywhere?' or 'Are you comfortable?'
- Position the patient correctly, so that he or she is exposed from the waist up (a sheet can cover the chest initially if appropriate but will have to be completely removed) for a general inspection; the patient should be at 45° with the head resting on sufficient pillows to relax the sternomastoids
- Explain what you want to do briefly: 'I am just going to feel your pulse and listen to your heart; is that alright?' usually suffices.

Inspection

General

- Mitral facies: indicates pulmonary hypertension, classically from mitral stenosis
- Central cyanosis
- Differential cyanosis: suggests a patent ductus arteriosus (PDA) with pulmonary hypertension
- Pallor
- Dyspnoea
- Accessory muscles of respiration
- Down syndrome: look for a ventricular septal defect (VSD)
- Turner syndrome: look for coarctation, bicuspid aortic valve, aortic stenosis
- Noonan syndrome: look for pulmonary stenosis.

Hands

Consider the following:

- Dilated veins and palmar erythema in CO_2 retention
- Temperature: cool peripheries associated with poor flow; hyperdynamic circulation
- Peripheral cyanosis

- Clubbing: suggests cyanotic congenital heart disease, infective endocarditis, atrial myoxoma (very rare)
- Capillary pulsation: seen in aortic regurgitation (AR), PDA
- Osler's nodes, Janeway's lesions, splinter haemorrhages: suggest infective endocarditis
- Nailfold telangiectases: suggest collagen vascular disease
- Arachnodactyly: suggests Marfan syndrome, MEN 2 (multiple endocrine neoplasia type 2), homocysteinuria
- Xanthomas: suggest hyperlipidaemia.

Radial and brachial pulses

- Rate, rhythm and synchronicity
- Radiofemoral delay
- If the pulse is chaotic, it is usually atrial fibrillation (AF), although multiple premature ventricular beats can give the appearance of being chaotic; AF is a diagnosis made on an ECG
- Character: the only aspect of character that can be reliably assessed at these pulses is a collapsing or 'waterhammer' pulse
- Look over the brachial artery for scars from previous angiography
- Ask to measure the blood pressure and take the temperature.

Jugular venous pulse (JVP)

The JVP has three waves (a, c and v), and two descents (x and y).

By convention it is measured in the internal jugular vein, with the patient lying at 45°, when it is often visible just at the clavicle. The neck must be adequately supported by pillows so that the sternomastoids are fully relaxed; the head should be turned slightly to the side and a light shone obliquely across the neck to maximise the shadows of venous pulsations; it is measured in vertical height from the angel of Louis (sternal angle); the hydrostatic pressure of blood in the right atrium is a mean of 6–8 cm (of H_2O/blood); this is roughly at the sternal angle and hence just visible at the base of the neck, ie 0 cm. Alteration of the patient's position does not affect the *height* of the JVP but will alter its *position*; this helps to differentiate it from the carotid pulse, along with its:

- site
- double waveform
- ability to be compressed and obliterated
- presence of hepatojugular reflux.

If you cannot see the waveform, the vessel may be kinked and thus you cannot reliably use the JVP as a right atrium manometer; similarly if you can see pulsations in the external jugular vein and demonstrate the presence of hepatojugular reflux, it is perfectly acceptable to use this vein for the JVP.

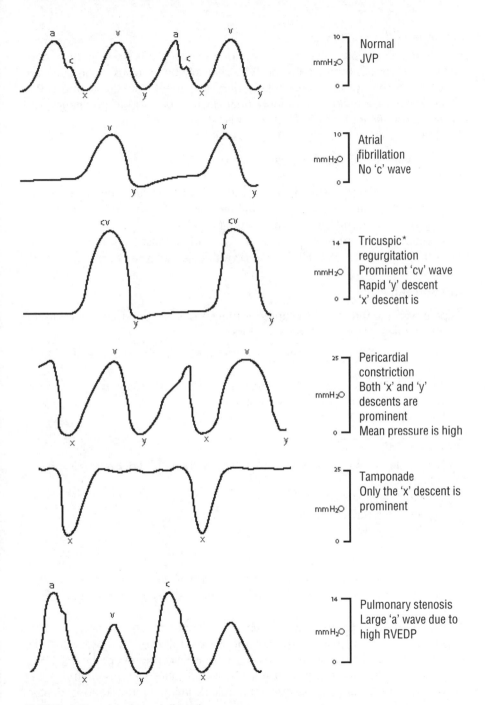

RVE DP, right ventricular end-diastotic pressure.

Figure 3.1   Jugular venous pulse.

Abnormal JVP

It is often under-appreciated that, alongside intravascular volume in the venous system, the venous tone affects the JVP; clinically this is of use when you are restoring volume to an intravascularly deplete patient. Practically, the JVP is raised in fluid overload – commonly heart failure, but also in pregnancy and over-enthusiastic intravenous fluid administration.

The following may be seen with their associations:

- Giant v waves: tricuspid regurgitation (TR)
- No a waves: AF
- Inspiratory filling (Kussmaul's sign): pericardial constriction (eg tuberculous pericarditis), tamponade (eg renal failure, post-myocardial infarction[MI], viral pericarditis, malignancy) and severe asthma
- Cannon waves: atrioventricular (AV) dissociation, most commonly complete heart block (CHB) and also ventricular tachycardia.

Carotid pulse

Palpate with the thumb on the anterior margin of sternomastoid alongside the thyroid cartilage; there are three components:

1. Percussion wave (P): the shock wave transmitted up the elastic wall of the artery
2. Tidal wave (T): the forward moving column of blood follows the percussion wave and might be palpable separately
3. Dicrotic notch (D): occurs with aortic valve closure.

Abnormal carotid pulse

- Large volume collapsing: very brisk upstroke then rapid diastolic run-off from the aorta:
    - aortic regurgitation (AR)
    - persistent ductus arteriosus
    - thyrotoxicosis
    - pregnancy
    - sepsis/fever.
- Anacrotic: slow rising with delayed percussion wave and sometimes a palpable judder (the anacrotic notch) on the upstroke found in aortic stenosis.
- Bisferiens: mixed aortic valve disease with significant regurgitation.
- Judder on the upstroke: the percussion wave is followed by a pronounced tidal wave, and thus a jerky pulse – hypertrophic cardiomyopathy (HCOM).
- Alternans: alternating large and small beats indicating very poor left ventricular (LV) function: severe ischaemic LV failure, aortic stenosis, dilated cardiomyopathy (DCM).

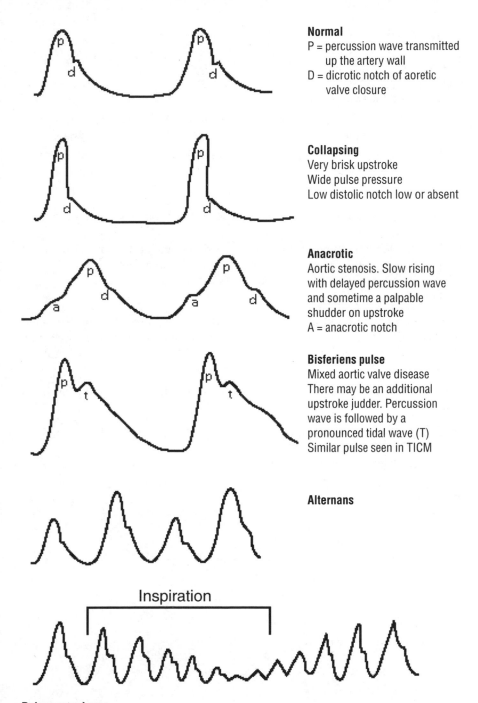

Normal
P = percussion wave transmitted
    up the artery wall
D = dicrotic notch of aoretic
    valve closure

Collapsing
Very brisk upstroke
Wide pulse pressure
Low distolic notch low or absent

Anacrotic
Aortic stenosis. Slow rising
with delayed percussion wave
and sometime a palpable
shudder on upstroke
A = anacrotic notch

Bisferiens pulse
Mixed aortic valve disease
There may be an additional
upstroke judder. Percussion
wave is followed by a
pronounced tidal wave (T)
Similar pulse seen in TICM

Alternans

Inspiration

Pulsus paradoxus
Excessive reduction in pulse pressure during inspiration (>10 mmHg) occurs in severe asthma

Figure 3.2   Carotid pulse.

Palpation

Palpate for the apex beat and over the whole precordium for any heaves, thrills or palpable sounds.

Consider the following features at the apex:

- Normally located at the fifth intercostal space in the midclavicular line; measure it from the angle of Louis. Palpable but does not lift the finger off the chest. It may be displaced but not necessarily signify an enlarged heart in pectus excavatum or scoliosis.

If abnormal decide whether it is:

- Volume loaded: mitral regurgitation (MR), AR or an atrial septal defect (ASD), hyperdynamic laterally displaced – 'thrusting'.
- Pressure loaded: aortic stenosis, hypertension or HCOM as long as the LV function is good – forceful minimally displaced – 'heaving'.
- Lateral and diffuse: LV failure, DCM.
- Double impulse (palpable atrial systole): HCOM.

Lay the flat of the hand along the left sternal edge to feel for the sustained pressure of a left parasternal heave, suggesting right ventricular hypertrophy (RVH) of any cause, eg pulmonary stenosis (PS), cor pulmonale or an ASD or VSD.

Palpate each valve area in turn with the flat of the fingers, for palpable heart sounds and thrills:

- Palpable in forceful closure:
  - S1: mitral stenosis
  - P2: pulmonary hypertension
  - S1 and S2: thin patients with tachycardia
- Thrills
- Systolic
- Aortic area: aortic stenosis
- Left sternal edge: VSD or HCOM
- Apex: MR (often caused by ruptured chordae)
- Pulmonary area: pulmonary stenosis
- Subclavicular area: subclavian artery stenosis
- Occasionally a diastolic thrill:
  - at the apex in mitral stenosis
  - left sternal edge in AR.

Auscultation

Listen to each valve area in turn and then the carotids. As already said, do not focus on auscultation to the exclusion of every other aspect of the case, but valvular pathology is common.

Heart sounds

- The valve sounds are all low frequency in health, best heard with the bell
- Any added sounds: murmurs, snaps, clicks or rubs
- Radiation from the valve areas
- M1 and A2 are louder than and precede T1 and P2; the split is wider in inspiration
- The split is reversed in aortic stenosis, left bundle-branch block (LBBB, eg ischaemic heart disease or IHD), RV pacing
- S2 is single in a large VSD, fixed and wide in an ASD
- S3: pathological over 30 years of age, when it is a result of rapid filling, eg MR or VSD or a dilated left ventricle with a high LV end-diastolic pressure (LVEDP), eg post-MI (when it is associated with a poor prognosis) or DCM
- S4: occurring at the end of diastole in hypertension, aortic stenosis, pulmonary stenosis, HCOM or after an MI. It disappears in AF.

Murmurs

Assess the murmur based on timing in the cardiac cycle, configuration, location and radiation, pitch, loudness and duration. Individual murmurs are discussed in their relevant section. Loudness *can* be graded as 1–4 for diastolic and 1–6 for systolic murmurs, but it is as helpful to grade as just audible, soft, moderate or loud.

Classification of murmurs

Systolic	Pansystolic
	Ejection systolic
	Early systolic
	Mid–late systolic
Diastolic	Early high pitched
	Mid-diastolic
	Presystolic
Continuous	

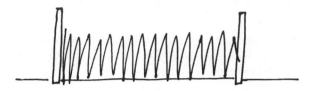

Pansystolic murmurs are generated when flow occurs between two areas with widely different pressures through systole, such that the gradient and jet begin early in contraction and last until relaxation is almost complete, eg from the left ventricle to either the left atrium or the right ventricle (see above).

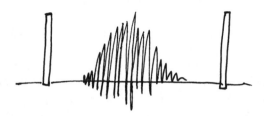

Ejection systolic murmurs, often crescendo–decrescendo in configuration, occur when blood is ejected across the aortic or pulmonary outflow tracts. The murmurs start shortly after S1, when ventricular pressure rises sufficiently to open the valve; as ejection increases the murmur gets louder and, as it declines, it gets quieter. With normal valves this murmur can represent an increased cardiac output, eg pregnancy, thyrotoxicosis, anaemia or arteriovenous fistula – ejection into a dilated vessel or normal transmission through a thin chest wall (see Innocent on page 228). Functional MR and more rarely TR can also produce this murmur.

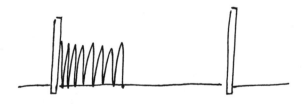

Early systolic murmurs are rarer. They begin with S1 and end in midsystole. They occur in TR without pulmonary hypertension or in acute MR. In a large VSD with pulmonary hypertension or small muscular VSD, the shunt towards the end of systole can be insignificant and thus the murmur may just be early systolic.

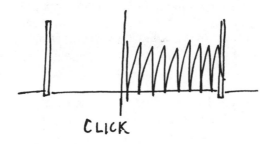

CLICK

Mid–late systolic murmurs are soft or moderate, and high pitched, heard at the apex; they start well after ejection and end before or at S2. They are often caused by mitral valve prolapse and can occur with or without a midsystolic click (see Mitral valve prolapse – page 238).

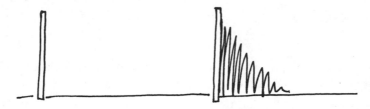

Early diastolic murmurs begin with or just after S2 when the pressure in the ventricle drops below that in the aorta or pulmonary artery, and are found in aortic and pulmonary regurgitation. They are usually decrescendo in quality

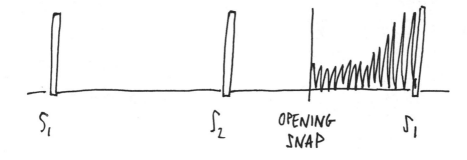

S_1 S_2 OPENING S_1
SNAP

Mid-diastolic murmurs originate from the tricuspid or mitral valves and occur early during ventricular filling and are caused by the relative disproportion between the valve orifice and the flow volume. They may also occur across the mitral valve (MV) and tricuspid valve (TV) in severe regurgitation, across the normal MV in a VSD or PDA or across the normal TV in an ASD where the flow volume is increased. The Austin–Flint murmur occurs in chronic AR and is often heard at the LV apex as a result of the regurgitant stream hitting the anterior MV cusp.

Presystolic murmurs occur during ventricular filling with atrial systole, ie at the end of ventricular diastole. They are usually caused by mitral stenosis (MS) or tricuspid stenosis (TS) in sinus rhythm (SR); an atrial myxoma may cause a similar mid-diastolic or presystolic murmur.

Innocent

Ejection systolic, between left sternal edge and the pulmonary valve and occasionally apical; no thrill, added sounds or cardiomegaly; normal ECG, chest radiograph and echocardiogram.

Pathological

- Organic: valvar, subvalvar, supravalvar
- Functional: dilated valve ring or increased flow.

Lung bases

Examine for oedema.

Abdomen

The examination of the cardiovascular system might stop at the lung bases; equally, however, it may be necessary to examine for the following:

- Hepatomegaly: if TR is suspected
- Splenomegaly: if infective endocarditis is a possibility
- Abdominal aortic aneurysm: elderly patient, smoker
- Renal bruits: if macrovascular disease suspected.

Periphery

- Palpate the peripheral pulses
- Examine for peripheral oedema (firm pressure for up to 30 seconds against the tibia 6 cm above the medial malleolus).

Dip the urine

The following references are useful for the cases: Swanton (1998), Brickner et al. (2000a, 2000b), Swash (2001) and Bonow et al. (2006).

Cardiovascular Scenarios

1. Mitral stenosis
2. Mitral regurgitation
3. Mitral valve prolapse
4. Aortic stenosis
5. Aortic incompetence
6. Irregular pulse/AF
7. Mixed valve diseases
8. Mitral stenosis and aortic regurgitation
9. Mitral stenosis and aortic stenosis
10. Aortic stenosis and mitral regurgitation
11. Ventricular septal defect
12. Eisenmenger syndrome
13. Atrial septal defect
14. Patent ductus arteriosus
15. Tricuspid regurgitation
16. Tricuspid stenosis
17. Hypertrophic cardiomyopathy
18. Prosthetic valve
19. Tetralogy of Fallot
20. Coarctation of the aorta
21. Pulmonary stenosis
22. Noonan syndrome

SCENARIO 1. MITRAL STENOSIS

The patient has a malar flush (mitral facies); the pulse is chaotic (completely irregular and irregularly irregular are alternative terms) (rate?) and of low volume. The JVP is of normal height. The apex is undisplaced and tapping. S1 is loud with an opening snap and a mid-to-late, rumbling, low-frequency diastolic murmur is best heard at the apex in the left lateral position, which radiates to the axilla and is accentuated by exertion.

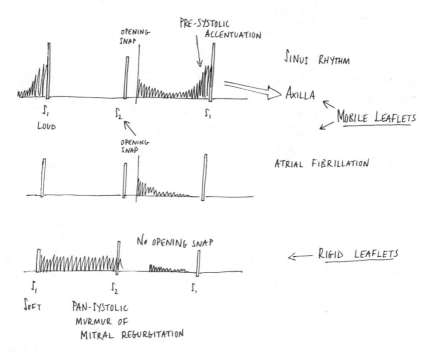

Figure 3.3 Mitral stenosis.

A good candidate

A good candidate will look for the following things that may be present:

- Left thoracotomy scar
- Prominent cv wave in the JVP: only if TR has occurred secondary to RVH
- Left parasternal heave: if there is RVH.

In severe disease there is:

- a short duration between S1 and opening snap
- longer duration of diastolic murmur
- worsening dyspnoea.

Questions

1. What is the aetiology?

Rheumatic valvular disease.

By far the most common cause is Lancefield group A streptococcal cell wall antigens which cross-react with the heart valve structural glycoproteins, causing inflammation and then commissural fusion.

Non-rheumatic disease causing mitral stenosis is very rare, eg

- Congenital: mucopolysaccharidoses
- Endomyocardial fibroelastosis
- Malignant: carcinoid.

2. What is the differential diagnosis?

- Inflow obstruction:
  - LA myxoma
  - ball-valve thrombus
  - Austin–Flint murmur: associated with AR with a collapsing pulse, volume-loaded ventricle and early diastolic murmur at the left sternal edge.

Symptoms

- Dyspnoea on exertion, orthopnoea and PND (paroxysmal nocturnal dyspnoea) as secondary pulmonary hypertension develops; pulmonary oedema may be precipitated by AF, pregnancy, exercise, a chest infection or anaesthesia
- Fatigue: because of the low cardiac output in moderate-to-severe stenosis
- Haemoptysis:
  - alveolar haemorrhage
  - bronchial vein rupture
  - pulmonary infarction because of the low cardiac output and immobility
  - bloody sputum, with chronic bronchitis caused by bronchial oedema
- Systemic emboli occur in 20–30%, eg cerebral, mesenteric, saddle or iliofemoral
- Chest pain: RVH with normal coronaries
- Palpitations and paroxysmal AF
- Right heart failure with TR and hepatic angina, ascites and oedema
- Dysphagia – from left atrial (LA) enlargement
- Infective endocarditis is unusual.

Investigations

- ECG: AF or if in SR p mitrale; RVH; low voltage in V1; progressive RAD (right axis deviation)

- Chest radiograph: splaying of the carina; double right heart border (enlarged left atrium); convex left heart border
- Echocardiography: necessary for differential diagnosis and to calculate the valve area
- Cardiac catheter: useful if non-invasive tests are inconclusive or if the clinical severity does not correlate with non-invasive tests, previous valvotomy, other valve disease, before surgery, angina or valve calcification on the chest radiograph.

Management (Bonow et al. 2006)

Infective endocarditis in isolated mitral stenosis (MS) is uncommon but appropriate endocarditis prophylaxis is recommended.

In those with more than a mild degree of MS, counselling the patient on avoidance of unusual physical stress is advised.

Tachycardia, by shortening the diastolic filling period, increases the pressure against the mitral valve (MV); in this situation, in patients in SR, where symptoms occur on exertion, β blockers or the negatively chronotropic calcium channel blockers may be of benefit.

Salt restriction and intermittent diuretics can be of benefit with small degrees of pulmonary vascular congestion.

Acute pulmonary oedema, especially from the development of AF, can be rapidly fatal, so patients must seek medical attention if they experience a sudden increase in dyspnoea.

Atrial fibrillation

Of patients with MS 30–40% develop AF. It occurs primarily in older patients with MS and is associated with a poorer prognosis – a 10-year survival rate of 25% compared with 46% in those who remain in SR.

Arterial embolisation, particularly stroke, occurs in 10–20% of patients with AF. The risk is related to age and the presence of AF. One-third of embolic events occur within 1 month of the onset of AF and two-thirds within 1 year.

In an acute episode of AF, anticoagulate with heparin and control the rate with digoxin, heart rate-regulating calcium channel blockers, β blockers or amiodarone.

If there is haemodynamic instability, DC cardioversion must be undertaken with heparin anticoagulation before, during and after the event.

Permanent AF can be controlled with β blockers, negatively chronotropic calcium channel blockers or digoxin – although the last is less effective at controlling the exercise-induced rate.

Elective cardioversion can be undertaken after either 3 weeks of warfarin or a transoesophageal echocardiogram excludes LA thrombus; heparin must be given before, during and after the event. Long-term anticoagulation will be necessary after any cardioversion.

Anticoagulation is indicated in patients with MS and:

- AF whether paroxysmal, persistent or permanent
- a prior embolic event, even if in SR
- LA thrombus.

Anticoagulation may be considered if the left atrium is $\geqslant 55$ mm or in severe MS, in an enlarged left atrium if there is spontaneous echo contrast.

The intervention of choice is percutaneous balloon valvotomy, which is the initial treatment of choice for symptomatic patients with moderate-to-severe MS who have a favourable valve morphology in the absence of significant MS or LA thrombus. If balloon valvotomy is unavailable or contraindicated, surgery should be contemplated with repair if possible or replacement. In the west, repair is performed as open commissurotomy but closed commissurotomy remains the treatment of choice in much of the developing world.

SCENARIO 2.   MITRAL REGURGITATION

The pulse is often chaotic and of small volume. The apex is laterally displaced and hyperdynamic. S1 is soft; A2–P2 may be wide; P2 is loud (if there is pulmonary hypertension); S3, if present, indicates rapid ventricular filling and thus negates any significant MS. There is an apical blowing pansystolic murmur, going through S2, radiating to the axilla.

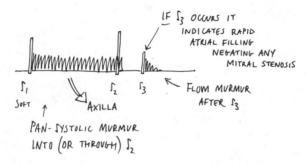

Figure 3.4   Mitral regurgitation.

The loudness of the murmur is of no significance.

In more severe disease:

- S1 is soft and an S3 is present.
- The apex is more laterally displaced
- Dyspnoea becomes progressively worse.

If the pressure is transmitted to the right ventricle a left parasternal heave may be present, indicating RVH.

The differential diagnosis in chronic MR is broad; consider the following:

- Aortic stenosis: regular slow rising pulse, pressure-loaded apex and ejection systolic murmur at the aortic area
- MV prolapse: midsystolic click: may have a late systolic murmur
- HCOM: jerky pulse – double, forceful pressure-loaded apex and ejection systolic murmur at left sternal edge (LSE)
- VSD: often a thrill and a pansystolic murmur, but both are maximal at the LSE
- TR: RV heave, murmur loudest at the left sternal edge in inspiration and giant 'cv' waves in the JVP
- ASD: right heart signs predominate, pulmonary ejection systolic murmur, but P2 does not move on inspiration (fixed splitting).

Questions

1. What symptoms will the patient have?

In chronic MR the regurgitation develops slowly, the left atrium enlarges and is fairly compliant, and thus the lesion can be well tolerated. The following occur:

- Chronic dyspnoea and fatigue
- Patient usually in AF
- Infective endocarditis is more common than in MS
- Haemoptysis is less common than in MS.

In acute MR the sudden volume overload imposed on the (left atrium and) left ventricle rapidly increases LV preload, which allows for a modest increase in the stroke volume (Starling's effect). There is no time for compensatory hypertrophy, however, and as such forward stroke volume and cardiac output are reduced. The unprepared left atrium and ventricle cannot accommodate the increased volume, causing large 'a' waves in the left atrium, which result in pulmonary congestion. Hence you may see both reduced forward output (even shock) and pulmonary congestion. The severe haemodynamic disturbance cannot be tolerated and emergency repair or replacement is necessary.

The following occur:

- The patient will almost always be severely symptomatic with sudden-onset dyspnoea and pulmonary oedema.
- As the left ventricle is normal size a hyperdynamic apex may be absent.
- The murmur may not be pansystolic and may even be absent.
- It is often ejection systolic.
- S3 or an early diastolic flow rumble may be the only finding.
- An apical thrill may be present because of chordal rupture.
- Patient is usually in SR.

2. What is the aetiology of MR?

This is varied and includes all structures involved in valvular function.

Functional

- Commonly secondary to dilatation of the MV annulus, either an ischaemic left ventricle or a DCM
- In elderly women more than men, you will see calcification of the annulus (lateral chest radiograph), which can extend to involve the cusps, causing MR, or it may be benign. It is associated with diabetes mellitus and Paget's disease, and doubles the relative risk of embolic stroke.

Structural

- Chronic:
  - rheumatic valve
  - floppy valve – one end of the spectrum of MV prolapse (see page 238)

- Acute:
  - chordal rupture: may be idiopathic or associated with the floppy valve because of myxomatous degeneration, or may be secondary to ischaemia
  - posterior papillary muscle dysfunction commonly occurs in an inferior MI, whereas anterior papillary muscle dysfunction, occurring in large anterior MIs with right coronary artery (RCA) involvement, is much rarer
  - infective endocarditis.

Investigations

- ECG: AF; SR with p mitrale; LVH ± RVH
- Echocardiography: shows the LA size and rapid filling; Doppler ultrasonography will show the size and site of the MR jet
- Chest radiograph: enlarged left ventricle; enlarged left atrium if chronic; MV calcification; Kerley B lines and pulmonary venous congestion
- Catheter: necessary only if valve repair is being considered, if non-invasive tests and symptoms do not correlate or are inconclusive, or the PA pressure is out of proportion to the severity of MR assessed by non-invasive testing. If necessary it will confirm the diagnosis, and assess the other valves and LV function. The LA/pulmonary wedge v wave can give a measure of severity.

In patients at risk of CAD coronary angiography should be performed.

Management (Bonow et al. 2006)

AF is best treated with rate-lowering calcium channel blockers, β blockers, digoxin or rarely amiodarone (see also NICE guidance on AF).

While the embolic risk of MR and AF is lower than in MS, treatment with warfarin is still recommended to maintain an international normalised ratio (INR) of 2–3.

In SR, warfarin is withheld unless there is a history of emboli, prosthetic MV regurgitation or coexistent MS with a low cardiac output.

Diuretics and nitrates decrease pulmonary venous congestion and LV preload in symptomatic MR.

In functional or ischaemic MR with systolic dysfunction, primary treatment with angiotensin-converting enzyme (ACE) inhibitors or β blockers (especially carvedilol) and biventricular pacing have all been shown to reduce the severity of functional MR.

In patients with MR who develop symptoms but have preserved LV function, surgery is the most appropriate therapy.

Acute MR is managed as cardiogenic shock – sodium nitroprusside reduces afterload and balloon pumping will both reduce afterload and improve coronary artery perfusion while surgery is arranged with all possible urgency.

SCENARIO 3. MITRAL VALVE PROLAPSE

There is a spectrum of disease and the following may be found:

- A midsystolic click or multiple clicks that move within systole with changes in LV dimensions, and/or a late-systolic or pansystolic murmur of MR heard best at the apex. The heart sounds are normal. There may be LA or LV dilatation.
- The condition is heterogeneous and can vary from benign with a normal life expectancy to adverse disease with significant morbidity and mortality.
- Involvement of other valves occurs; tricuspid valve prolapse occurs in 40%, pulmonary valve prolapse in 2% and aortic valve prolapse in 10% of those with MV prolapse.
- If there is a murmur, infective endocarditis prophylaxis is necessary. Reassurance is a major part of the management of MV prolapse. Those with mild or no symptoms and echocardiographic findings of milder forms of prolapse should be reassured of a benign prognosis, and a normal lifestyle and regular exercise are encouraged.

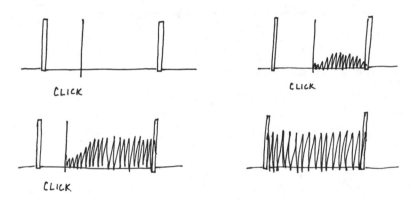

Figure 3.5   Mitral valve prolapse.

SCENARIO 4. AORTIC STENOSIS

The pulse is regular and anacrotic (slow rising with a judder – see page 222) with a narrow pulse pressure. The JVP is normal, and the apex minimally displaced and pressure loaded. In the aortic area there is a harsh ejection systolic (crescendo–decrescendo) murmur that radiates to the carotids.

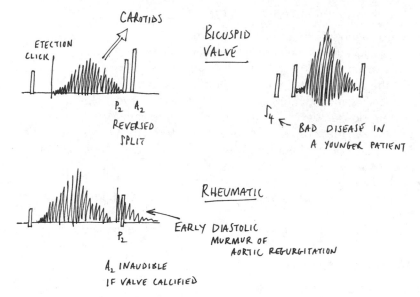

Figure 3.6   Aortic stenosis.

If the valve is bicuspid and mobile, S1 is soft, followed by an ejection click before the murmur.

If the valve is rheumatic and calcified, or the patient is old with a calcified valve, there is no ejection click, the murmur is harsh, but S2 is quiet, and there may follow an early diastolic murmur of aortic regurgitation.

In elderly people the carotid upstroke can be normal because of the effects of ageing on the vasculature, and the murmur may be soft or radiate to the apex. The only finding that is reliable in *excluding* the possibility of severe AS is a normally split S2.

Severe disease

- The carotids may be difficult to palpate
- S4 may be present in a young patient
- S2 may be reversed

- Pulsus alternans
- Aortic thrill
- Displaced apex: suggesting the development of cardiac failure.

Questions

1. What is the aetiology?

This is valvar, subvalvar or supravalvar:

- Valvar stenosis is *by far* the most common:
  - calcification of the normal tri-leaflet or congenital bicuspid valve
  - congenital in 70%, M:F 4:1: bicuspid aortic valves are present in 2% of the population (a third AS, a third mixed AV disease and a third normal). It is the most common cause of AS in 40 to 60 year olds
  - arteriosclerosis: in type IIa hypercholesterolaemia, gross atheroma can involve the aortic wall, major arteries, coronary arteries and aortic valve
  - inflammatory: rheumatic fever causing AS and AR, and invariably accompanied by MV disease (see page 249)
- Subvalvar: discrete fibromuscular ring; HCOM
- Supravalvar: a constricting ring of fibrous tissue at the upper margin of the sinus of Valsalva: associated with William syndrome – hypercalcaemia, giant 'a' wave in JVP, pulmonary valve stenosis – RVH, pulmonary thrill, elfin facies.

Differential diagnosis

- MV prolapse: see page 238
- VSD if very small: thrill and pansystolic murmur at LSE
- HCOM: see page 263
- Aortic sclerosis: there is no obstruction to outflow, so the pulse is normal in character and the apex is normal.

2. What symptoms might the patient have?

There is a long latent period during which the morbidity and mortality of AS are very low but eventually symptoms develop and the outlook changes dramatically. After the onset of symptoms, average survival is 2–3 years, and as such it is a watershed in the natural history. The symptoms are as follows:

- **Angina**: the increased muscle mass and increased pressure in the heart muscle in both systole and diastole increase oxygen demand while decreasing supply. Valvar calcification can extend to the coronary ostia.
- **Dyspnoea**: the increased pressure within the LV increases further with exercise.
- **PND and orthopnoea** supervene as the LV function deteriorates.
- **Giddiness and syncope**: on exertion the relatively fixed cardiac output cannot increase further.

- **Sudden death**.
- **Emboli**: from calcified valve.
- **Symptoms of infective endocarditis**.

Investigations

- Echocardiography: for diagnosis and assessment; indicated when there is a moderate (3/6) or louder murmur, single S2 or symptoms that might be caused by AS:
  - bicuspid valve
  - calcification
  - LV wall size and function
  - AR
  - gradient assessment
- ECG:
  - SR, but if in AF suspect MV disease or previous MI
  - P mitrale with a negative P in V1 because of the high LVEDP
  - LVH ± strain
  - LAD (left axis deviation), LAHB (left anterior hemiblock)
  - LBBB or CHB (with calcification of the valve ring in 5%)
- Exercise ECG: may be considered in asymptomatic patients with AS to elicit exercise-induced symptoms and abnormal blood pressure responses; should not be performed in symptomatic AS
- Chest radiograph:
  - LVH
  - calcification of the valve if > 40 years; on lateral views the calcification is above and lateral to the oblique fissure
  - poststenotic dilatation of the aorta
  - pulmonary oedema and LVF
- Catheter:
  - gradient assessment
  - LV function
  - coronary circulation
  - aortic root size.

Management (Bonow et al. 2006)

Antibiotic prophylaxis for prevention of infective endocarditis; in those with rheumatic AS it is indicated to prevent recurrence.

Medical

In those who are asymptomatic there is no specific therapy. Antihypertensives can be used cautiously in those with systemic hypertension.

Nitrates and ACE inhibitors should be avoided because they increase the gradient across the valve (reduce afterload).

Prospective trials of statin therapy in those with severe calcific AS have failed to show a benefit on progression. Trials in less severe AS are ongoing.

Attend to vascular risk factors.

Surgical

- Aortic valve replacement (AVR) is indicated for those with *severe* AS:
  - and symptoms
  - undergoing CABG (coronary artery bypass graft) or surgery on the aorta or other heart valves
  - and LV systolic dysfunction (ejection fraction < 0.5).
- AVR is reasonable for patients with *moderate* AS undergoing CABG or surgery on the aorta or other valves.
- AVR may be considered for:
  - asymptomatic patients with severe AS and an abnormal response to exercise – development of symptoms or asymptomatic hypotension
  - asymptomatic patients with AS if there is a high likelihood of severe disease progression – age, calcification and CAD
  - patients undergoing CABG who have mild AS where there is evidence, eg severe calcification, that progression may be rapid
  - asymptomatic patients with extremely severe AS (AV area < 0.6 cm², mean gradient > 50 mm/s) when the patient's expected operative mortality rate is ≤ 1%.
- AVR is not useful to prevent sudden death in asymptomatic patients with AS who have none of the above findings.
- Balloon valvotomy has little role in adults.
- The average survival (without surgery) once symptoms of angina/syncope occur is 2–3 years in angina/syncope, and 1–2 years in heart failure without surgery.
- The mortality rate of AV surgery is 3–4% for isolated AVR and 5.5–6.8% for AVR + CABG. If LVF is present it rises to 10–20%.

SCENARIO 5. AORTIC INCOMPETENCE

Several eponyms are associated with AR, mostly from the days of quaternary syphilitic aortic dilatation.

Observing the patient you may see the following:

- De Musset's sign: bobbing head
- Corrigan's sign: visible carotid pulsations
- Quincke's sign: visible nailbed capillary pulsations
- There is a regular, tachycardia (the regurgitant jet is reduced by shortening diastole) and full-volume collapsing ('waterhammer') pulse with a wide pulse pressure.

The carotid pulse has a rapid upstroke with no dicrotic notch (if the stroke volume is large there may be a judder); the apex is displaced inferolaterally and is hyperdynamic.

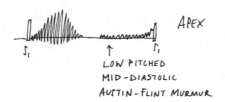

APEX

S_1 S_1

LOW PITCHED
MID-DIASTOLIC
AUSTIN-FLINT MURMUR

The heart sounds are normal and, at the LSE, there is a short, early diastolic, high-pitched, blowing (decrescendo) diastolic murmur, heard best with the patient sitting forwards and breath held in expiration.

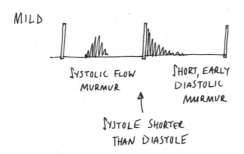

MILD

SYSTOLIC FLOW   SHORT, EARLY
MURMUR   DIASTOLIC
                     MURMUR

SYSTOLE SHORTER
THAN DIASTOLE

There is often a shorter systolic flow murmur across the aortic valve.

Duroziez's sign is present – an audible 'to-and-fro' murmur at the femoral artery – as is Traube's sign – 'pistol-shot' femorals.

In more severe disease the following findings may be apparent:

- As the regurgitation becomes more severe, the length of the murmur increases and, listening with the bell at the apex and with the patient in the left lateral position, you may find a rumbling, low-pitched, mid-diastolic murmur, as the regurgitant jet causes the fluttering of the anterior MV leaflet; this is the Austin–Flint murmur.

- As the regurgitation becomes more severe still and the LV diastolic pressure increases the MV closes prematurely (preventing forward flow and) thus S1 is soft, and the Austin–Flint murmur abolished. The diastolic murmur becomes full length and A2 is inaudible and P2 obscured (see below).
- If the ventricle is failing the waterhammer pulse may disappear.

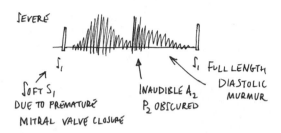

A good candidate will consider the rarer differential diagnoses.

- Pulmonary regurgitation: correction of tetralogy of Fallot or a postpulmonary valvotomy; Graham Steell murmur secondary to pulmonary hypertension of any cause.
- PDA: continuous machinery murmur usually loudest in second left intercostal space.

Aetiology (Bonow et al. 2006)

- Primary disease of the valve:
  - congenital valve lesions – most notably bicuspid valve
  - connective tissue laxity: Marfan or Hurler syndrome
- Aortic root disease with dilatation and stretching of the valve ring:
  - hypertensive root dilatation
  - dissection
- Secondary valve disease:
  - rheumatic fever
  - infective endocarditis
  - seropositive – rheumatoid arthritis
  - seronegative arthritides – ankylosing spondylitis, Reiter's disease
  - SLE (systemic lupus erythematosus)
  - syphilis – quaternary.

Investigations

Echocardiography is the main diagnostic technique, but if this is unhelpful radionuclide angiography or MRI (magnetic resonance imaging) may help.

Exercise stress testing is reasonable to assess functional capacity and symptomatic response where symptoms are equivocal or to guide participation in athletic activity.

Management

- Vasodilator therapy:
    - is indicated if surgery is not recommended in chronic severe AR, for short-term therapy to improve heart failure before AVR
    - is reasonable as a short-term measure to improve the haemodynamics of those with heart failure before proceeding to AVR
    - may be considered for long-term therapy in asymptomatic patients with severe AR who have LV dilatation but normal systolic function.
- Surgery/AVR is indicated if the patient:
    - has symptoms
    - is symptomatic on exercise stress testing
    - has an ejection fraction ≤ 50%
    - has chronic severe AR and is undergoing CABG, surgery on the aorta or other valves
    - is reasonable if the LV is enlarged.
- Consider AVR if:
    - enlarging heart on chest radiograph
    - pulse pressure > 100 mmHg
    - ECG deteriorating with lateral T-wave inversion: 65% of patients with all three will develop CCF or die within 3 years
    - postinfective endocarditis not responding to medical management.

SCENARIO 6. IRREGULAR PULSE/AF

The pulse is chaotic in both rhythm and volume ('irregularly irregular'); the radial rate is less than apical, 'pulse deficit'; there is no 'a' wave in the JVP. The apex is normal (unless other disease is present, eg MS). On auscultation S1 varies in intensity and S2 is normal.

A good candidate

A good candidate will consider the aetiology (eg features of MV disease or thyrotoxicosis) and either state the salient features or give the differential diagnosis and an investigation plan.

Aetiology

- IHD
- MV disease (especially stenosis)
- Hyperthyroidism
- Hypertension
- Pulmonary embolism
- Cardiomyopathies
- Alcohol
- Constrictive pericarditis
- Sick sinus syndrome
- Lung pathology, eg carcinoma, pneumonia.

Symptoms

- Usually none
- Palpitations, especially if paroxysmal
- Fatigue and dyspnoea
- Presyncope, dizziness
- Embolic symptoms, see Mitral stenosis, page 231
- Of the underlying cause.

Questions

1. *What is the differential diagnosis?*

- Ectopic beats: atrial or ventricular. Unifocal ectopics have a constant compensatory pause after the beat. Dropped beats are followed by a normal r–r interval. Multifocal ectopics can result in a truly chaotic pulse.
- Wenckebach's AV block has a progressively lengthening r–r interval, followed by a dropped beat; it is not chaotic.
- Sinus arrhythmia should present no difficulties.

2. *How will you investigate the patient?*

- ECG: chaotic baseline and absence of 'p' waves
- Chest radiograph: cardiac size and for the presence of lung disease
- Electrolytes: particularly potassium and calcium (high or low), hypomagnesaemia, acidosis (metabolic or respiratory)
- Arterial blood gases (ABGs): hypoxia and acidosis
- Free thyroxine (T_4) ± T_3 (triiodothyronine) and TSH (thyroid-stimulating hormone)
- Echocardiography: valve disease, cardiomyopathy, hypertrophy; indication for anticoagulation – chamber size or thrombus
- 24-hour tape or cardiac memo: may be necessary if paroxysmal
- ETT (exercise tolerance test) may be necessary rarely in the young patient with exercise-induced AF.

3. *What are the broad principles of management?*

- Accelerated tachycardia causing cardiorespiratory compromise may need treatment as a peri-arrest arrhythmia.
- Treat the underlying cause.
- Is the AF paroxysmal, persistent or permanent?
- Is the goal restoration of SR or control of the ventricular rate?

4. *Does the patient warrant anticoagulation?*

- In **paroxysmal AF**, the aim is cardioversion to, and then maintenance of, SR; if this is unattainable, aim to minimise the duration and frequency of AF.
- If **persistent AF**, there is a choice between rate and rhythm control; at least one attempt should be made to restore SR before opting for rate control. Many more attempts may be made (or none) to restore SR depending on, for example, age and presence of symptoms.
- If permanent AF, the aim is to control the ventricular rate:
  - β blockers or rate-limiting calcium antagonists should be the preferred initial monotherapy in all patients
  - digoxin should be considered as monotherapy only in predominantly sedentary patients (NICE 2006).

Atrial systole may contribute up to 25% of cardiac output by increasing the LV end-diastolic volume (LVEDV) and may be symptomatically critical in patients with a poor left ventricle. Cardioversion is either chemical or electrical.

Stroke risk

High	Previous ischaemic stroke/TIA or thromboembolic event Age > 75 with hypertension or vascular disease (CAD or PVD [peripheral vascular disease]) Clinical evidence of valve disease, heart failure or impaired left ventricle on echocardiography Anticoagulate with warfarin, target 2.5, range 2.0–3.0 Contraindication to warfarin – aspirin 75–300 mg/day if no complications
Moderate	Age ⩾ 65 with no high-risk factors Age < 75 with hypertension, diabetes or vascular disease Consider anticoagulation or aspirin
Low	Age < 65 with no moderate- or high-risk factors Aspirin 75–300 mg/day if no contraindications

The risks are not mutually exclusive and are additive to produce a composite risk; two or more moderate risk factors may favour warfarin use – echocardiography can help with risk stratification.

SCENARIO 7. MIXED VALVE DISEASES

In mixed aortic and mitral valve disease one lesion tends to predominate and the pathophysiology resembles that of the pure lesion.

Mixed mitral valve diseases

Predominant stenosis

The patient is comfortable at rest with a malar flush; the pulse is chaotic and small volume. The blood pressure is x/y mmHg (low). The JVP has no 'a' wave but is of a normal height.

The apex is tapping and minimally displaced or undisplaced and there may be a right parasternal heave.

On auscultation S1 is soft and of variable intensity. There is a moderate, blowing, pansystolic murmur heard at the apex, radiating to the axilla, and a long, low-pitched, quiet, rumbling diastolic murmur, also heard at the apex radiating to the axilla, heard best with the patient lying over to his or her left-hand side.

Predominant regurgitation

The patient is more likely to be in SR, and the pulse may be described as small volume collapsing. The JVP is normal unless there is significant pulmonary hypertension.

The apex is volume overloaded and very easily felt in the anterior axillary line; the whole left ventricle is hyperdynamic.

There may be a right parasternal heave. On auscultation S1 is soft and there is an LV S3, with a moderate, blowing, pansystolic murmur heard at the apex radiating to the axilla, and a short, low-pitched, quiet, rumbling diastolic murmur heard at the apex radiating to the axilla, heard only with the patient lying over to his or her left-hand side.

In either situation, if the pressure is transmitted to the right side, there may be RVH, a Graham Steell murmur and/or the signs of TR (see page 261).

If the patient remains in SR the JVP will contain 'a' waves and there will be presystolic accentuation at the end of diastole.

(see figure on next page)

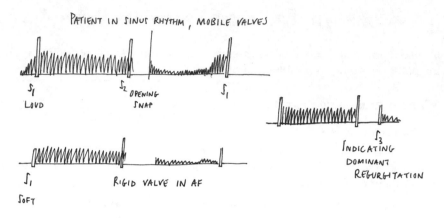

Figure 3.7   Mixed valve diseases.

Mixed aortic valve diseases

Stenosis dominant

The patient is comfortable at rest and on minor exertion. The pulse is regular, bisferiens in character and the rate is x. The blood pressure is y/z.

- *The pulse pressure is narrow.*
- The JVP is normal.
- There is a thrill over the aortic valve.
- The apex is minimally displaced to the anterior axillary line and pressure overloaded – heaving.
- S1 may be soft and S2 is reversed (ie P2 precedes A2).
- If the aortic valve is calcified A2 may be inaudible.

There is a *loud*, harsh, ejection systolic murmur heard best at the aortic area, radiating into the LV outflow tract (LVOT) and the subclavian and carotid arteries; there is also a quieter, *short*, decrescendo, diastolic murmur starting immediately after S2, heard best at the aortic area and down the LSE while the patient is leaning forwards with breath held in expiration.

The lung bases are clear.

Regurgitation dominant

The patient is comfortable at rest and on minor exertion. The pulse is regular, bisferiens in character and the rate is x (tends towards tachycardia). The blood pressure is y/z.

- *The pulse pressure is wide.*
- The JVP is normal.
- There might be a thrill over the aortic valve.

- *The apex is displaced to the anterior axillary line and is volume overloaded – hyperdynamic/thrusting and easily felt.*
- S1 may be soft and S2 might be reversed (ie P2 precedes A2).
- If the aortic valve is calcified A2 may be inaudible.
- There is a soft, long, decrescendo, diastolic murmur starting immediately after S2, heard best at the aortic area and down the LSE while the patient is leaning forwards with breath held in expiration; there is also a moderate, harsh, ejection systolic murmur heard best at the aortic area, radiating into the LVOT and carotid arteries.
- *The lung bases may have fine crackles indicative of pulmonary oedema.*

The eponymous signs associated with AR may be present.

A good candidate

A good candidate will consider the aetiology.

In severe bicuspid stenosis, where the patient has gone on to develop LVF with dilatation of the aortic valve ring, functional AR can occur.

S2 is of critical importance as to whether there is significant stenosis because in many cases of AR there may be a flow murmur across the aortic valve; the pulse character is also useful with the proviso that, as the patient gets older, the pulse can be normal in AS (see page 239).

In cases of doubt you must make note of these difficulties and mention the utility of the appropriate investigations to make a more precise diagnosis.

SCENARIO 8. MITRAL STENOSIS AND AORTIC REGURGITATION

The most common situation when these two lesions are present is for severe MS to coexist with mild AR with pathophysiology of isolated MS. However, the coexistent AR is occasionally severe; severe AR and severe MS can be confusing and lead to misdiagnosis.

MS restricts LV filling, blunting the impact of AR on the LV volume. Therefore even severe AR may fail to produce a hyperdynamic circulation with a consequent lack of some, or all, of the traditional signs of AR.

SCENARIO 9. MITRAL STENOSIS AND AORTIC STENOSIS

The physical findings of AS generally dominate and the signs of MS can easily be overlooked. However, the patient's symptoms are usually much more suggestive of MS. It is almost always secondary to rheumatic heart disease.

SCENARIO 10. AORTIC STENOSIS AND MITRAL REGURGITATION

Severe AS will worsen the degree of MR. The degree of MR may make it difficult to assess the degree of AS because it tends to reduce forward flow across the aortic valve; it will, however, tend to improve the LV ejection performance, thereby masking early LV systolic dysfunction caused by AS.

The development of AF with the loss of atrial systolic may further reduce forward output because of impaired filling of the hypertrophied left ventricle. It is often secondary to rheumatic heart disease but congenital AS and MV prolapse may occur in younger patients as may degenerative AS and MR in elderly people.

SCENARIO 11. VENTRICULAR SEPTAL DEFECT

Very small

The pulse is x beats/min and has a normal character and rhythm; the blood pressure is y/z mmHg; the apex is normal and there are no thrills; the heart sounds are normal (A2 is easily heard); at the LSE there is a loud, early, ejection systolic murmur. These signs indicate a very small, clinically insignificant VSD – 'maladie de Roger'.

The differential diagnosis includes mild AS and PS.

Small

The apex may be normal or reflect slight LVH. There is a thrill at the LSE. S2 splits on inspiration but A2 is obscured by a loud pansystolic murmur at the LSE radiating to the apex and the PA.

The differential diagnosis includes MR, TR, HCOM and PS.

Moderate VSD

There is slight RVH and LVH and a thrill at the LSE. There is a loud pansystolic murmur at the LSE obscuring S2 with an additional mitral diastolic murmur heard at the apex.

The differential diagnosis is of MR, TR and PS.

Large VSD

There is RVH and LVH and a thrill at the LSE. A2 is obscured but P2 may be loud. There is a pansystolic decrescendo murmur right up to S2, with a pulmonary ejection systolic murmur and click; occasionally PR may be heard. The differential is severe MR or mixed aortic valve disease.

Eisenmenger syndrome (see page 255)

There is RVH with palpable pulmonary arteries; there is no thrill. S2 is loud, single and palpable. There is no murmur at the LSE, but a soft ejection systolic murmur may be heard into the PAs with regurgitation over the pulmonary valve.

Aetiology

Congenital	
VSD as integral part of syndrome	VSD associated with syndrome
Tetralogy of Fallot	Tricuspid atresia
Double-outlet right ventricle	Pulmonary atresia
Truncus arteriosus	Transposition of great arteries
	Coarctation

Post-MI	

Symptoms

Small VSDs are common and asymptomatic

As pulmonary hypertension develops, fatigue, dyspnoea and symptoms of RV failure occur (see cor pulmonale).

Pathological considerations

An isolated VSD is the most common congenital heart lesion occurring in 2 per 1000 births with an equal sex incidence. Small VSDs are common and asymptomatic; about 50% close spontaneously in infancy.

At birth, when pulmonary vascular resistance (PVR) falls, blood starts to be shunted from left to right. Consequent upon this increased flow, irreversible pulmonary changes start in early childhood with initial hypertrophy and secondary thrombotic occlusion of the pulmonary arterioles, leading to pulmonary hypertension and eventual shunt reversal.

All grades need endocarditis prophylaxis.

Of VSDs 30–50% close spontaneously, commonly in muscular defects and defects in the membranous septum; this does not occur in lesions adjacent to valves or if there is septal malalignment, eg

- VSD + shift of septum to right: tetralogy of Fallot
- VSD + shift of septum to left: double-outlet left ventricle with subaortic stenosis.

Once significant pulmonary resistance has developed, closure of the VSD will be of no benefit.

Post-MI VSDs require urgent surgery.

SCENARIO 12. EISENMENGER SYNDROME

The patient is centrally cyanosed and plethoric, but comfortable if he or she remains at rest. There is digital clubbing and the pulse is regular and small volume. The venous pressure is normal (it might be raised if RV *failure* has developed) with a prominent 'a' wave (the atria are contracting against a raised RV pressure); there may be a prominent 'v' wave (if TR is present).

On palpation a left parasternal heave indicates RVH and the PAs and P2 are palpable. The absence of a thrill is worthy of note (consider the thrill present in tetralogy of Fallot – see page 267).

S2 is loud (pulmonary hypertension has developed, so P2 is loud). There is usually an (RV) S4.

You may find a pansystolic murmur over the tricuspid area (indicating TR because the valve cusp dilates consequent upon RVF), as well as an early diastolic murmur over the pulmonary valve (similarly PA dilatation causing PR – the Graham Steell murmur).

A good candidate

A good candidate will take a reasoned approach to a precise diagnosis based on the following:

- Cyanotic heart disease in the adult usually occurs in the context of a congenital VSD, an ASD or PDA.
- As a consequence of the increased pulmonary blood flow, the PVR rises.
- When the pulmonary pressure exceeds the systemic pressure, the left-to-right shunt reverses to become right to left, and Eisenmenger syndrome develops.

The differentiating features of the underlying pathologies are:

- VSDs have a single S2: the ventricular pressures are equal.
- ASDs: S2 is widely split and this does not vary with breathing (A2 precedes P2; P2 does not move, as the increased RV stroke volume does not vary with breathing).
- PDA: S2 is normal, ie A2 precedes P2 and P2 moves with breathing. There may be differential cyanosis, pink fingers and blue, clubbed toes (preferential passage of deoxygenated blood into the descending aorta, because the PDA is distal to the origin of the left subclavian artery).

Investigations

- FBC: polycythaemia
- ECG:
  - p pulmonale
  - RAD
  - tall r waves
  - inverted T waves in the right precordial leads (the RV strain pattern), atrial arrhythmias
- Chest radiograph:
  - PA dilatation
  - pruning of the peripheral vessels
- Echocardiography:
  - underlying anatomical defect will be localised, flow seen with Doppler ultrasonography
  - catheter
  - PA pressures with evidence of shunting on saturation run through the heart.

Management

Endocarditis prophylaxis; avoid pregnancy, venesect to keep the haematocrit < 0.45. The development of Eisenmenger syndrome negates any benefit from heart transplantation, but heart–lung transplantation does offer the potential for cure in a few selected young patients.

SCENARIO 13. ATRIAL SEPTAL DEFECT

Ostium secundum ASD

More common in females; may occur as part of Holt–Oram syndrome – triphalangeal thumbs, ASD or VSD.

Right heart signs dominate the picture:

- The patient is usually in SR. The JVP is raised with equal 'a' and 'v' waves. There may be a systolic thrill over the pulmonary outflow tract representing high flow and does not necessarily indicate PS. There is fixed splitting of S2–A2 precedes P2, with a tricuspid diastolic flow murmur and a pulmonary ejection systolic flow murmur that is so soft that it is often mistaken for a physiological flow murmur.
- AF often occurs with signs of TR.
- As pulmonary hypertension develops (it is often diagnosed later in life than primum defects) the ejection systolic murmur becomes softer, perhaps with an ejection click. The tricuspid murmur disappears and P2 becomes loud.
- Pulmonary regurgitation may occur – the Graham Steell murmur.

Eisenmenger syndrome may occur as pulmonary hypertension approached systemic pressures.

The ECG shows (incomplete) RBBB and RAD.

Secundum defects make up 75% of all ASDs.

Differential diagnosis

Mild pulmonary stenosis – P2 is delayed, softer and moves with ventilation.

As pulmonary hypertension, with cardiac failure, develops, the following may be confused with a secundum ASD:

- Mixed mitral valve disease (see above)
- Pulmonary hypertension and/or cor pulmonale.

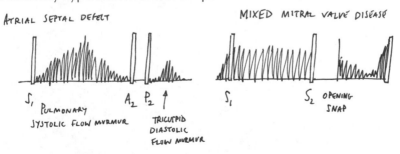

Figure 3.8 Atrial septal defect.

If AF develops with lower cardiac output, the right heart sounds do not dominate the picture as much and this can lead to difficulty. Listen for fixed splitting.

Primum ASD

This is a rarer, more severe lesion that usually presents in childhood or infancy. The signs are as a secundum defect but MR is often present and can be severe.

The ECG shows RBBB and LAD.

Primum defects make up 15% of all ASDs.

If there is a VSD component consider the presence of Down (common), Klinefelter or Noonan syndrome.

Endocarditis prophylaxis is not recommended for ASDs unless there is concomitant valvular abnormality.

SCENARIO 14. PATENT DUCTUS ARTERIOSUS

Very small

This may show no signs except a continuous machinery murmur heard in the second left interspace. Although there is always a pressure gradient between the aorta and the PA, it is greatest towards the end of systole. Thus, although there may be a continuous machinery murmur, it is accentuated at about the time of S2 (which gives the murmur its particular character).

There may be only a late systolic, or also an early diastolic, murmur, heard best in expiration at that site, or towards the left clavicle.

Moderate

The pulse is regular, bounding/full volume and collapsing with a normal rate, the pulse pressure is wide and the JVP is normal. The apex is displaced inferolaterally and is hyperdynamic (the left ventricle is chronically volume overloaded) and there is a thrill in the second left intercostal space in systole and/or diastole. S1 is normal; there is a continuous machinery murmur in the left second intercostal space, heard best at the end of systole, in expiration, which may obscure S2. It radiates towards the left clavicle and may be heard posteriorly.

With a large shunt, mid-diastolic and systolic murmurs from increased flow through the mitral and aortic valves may be noted.

If pulmonary hypertension develops a Graham Steell murmur may be heard.

If pulmonary pressure approaches systemic, shunt reversal and Eisenmenger syndrome will occur.

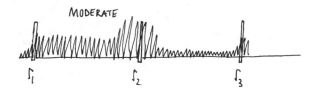

Figure 3.9   Patent ductus arteriosus.

Differential diagnosis of a continuous murmur

- Pulmonary AV fistulae, coronary AV fistulae or communications between the ascending aorta and PA.
- Venous hum: particular care must be taken not to confuse this with the murmur of PDA. It occurs in young children because of kinking or partial obstruction of one of the larger veins in the neck, thus preventing

continuous flow through the vein. It should be suspected because of its loudness in the neck and the youth of the patient! It can be obliterated by pressure on the neck, which completely compresses the offending vein, or merely by altering the position of the neck, or lying flat.

- Mammary soufflé
- MR and AR.
- VSD with AR.

Question

1. *What do you know about the aetiology of PDA?*

It is more common in:

- children born prematurely (up to 50%)
- females
- births at high altitude
- maternal rubellar infection in the first trimester – PDA is the most common congenital heart lesion following maternal rubella.

SCENARIO 15. TRICUSPID REGURGITATION

The pulse is chaotic and of low volume (rarely the patient might be in SR). The venous pressure is raised and there are giant systolic 'cv' waves with a rapid 'y' descent, (with prominent 'a' waves only if in SR). A left parasternal heave and a soft pansystolic (or late systolic) murmur at the LSE are present, accentuated on inspiration (Carvallo's sign) or Müller's manoeuvre (which causes increased venous return to the right side of the heart).

S3 may be heard at the LSE, ie an RV S3.

A good candidate

A good candidate will immediately proceed to examine the abdomen for the other signs of TR:

- Tender pulsatile hepatomegaly
- Ascites and other signs of chronic liver disease
- Peripheral and central cyanosis
- Peripheral oedema.

Then go on to examine the lungs for a cause of pulmonary hypertension.

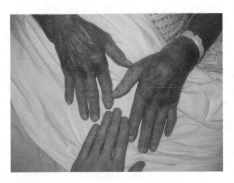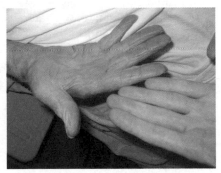

Figure 3.10

Note that, in establishing the diagnosis of TR, the presence of a systolic murmur is of less importance than the observation of a giant systolic 'cv' wave followed by a rapid 'y' descent in the JVP.

Rarer signs of severe TR are systolic propulsion of the eyeballs, pulsatile varicose veins, a venous systolic thrill and murmur in the neck.

Aetiology

- Functional: most common:
  RV systolic dysfunction:
  - secondary to pulmonary hypertension
  - MS
  - PS
  RV diastolic dysfunction:
  - DCM
  - RV infarction
  - RV failure of any cause
  Pacemaker-induced TR (rare)
- Organic: uncommon:
  Infective endocarditis: intravenous drug abusers
  Floppy TV may be associated with the floppy MV:
  - Marfan syndrome
  - TV prolapse
  Associated with congenital heart disease:
  - as a primary phenomenon, eg tricuspid atresia/hypoplasia and Ebstein's anomaly
  - secondary to right heart enlargement, eg ASD
  Rheumatic tricuspid valve disease; invariably occurs in association with aortic and mitral disease – rarer causes are:
  - tricuspid endocarditis as part of the carcinoid syndrome
  - secondary to the centrally acting appetite suppressants phentermine, fenfluramine and dexfenfluramine (all unavailable in the UK as a result of concerns about causing pulmonary hypertension)
  - radiation therapy.

Symptoms

- Abdominal distension and discomfort
- Hepatic angina
- Jaundice
- Peripheral oedema
- Fatigue and dyspnoea.

SCENARIO 16. TRICUSPID STENOSIS

The JVP has a slow 'y' descent and, if the patient is in SR, a giant 'a' wave; there is no RV heave. At the LSE there is an opening snap and a diastolic murmur with presystolic accentuation heard best on inspiration or after effort.

It is rare, almost always rheumatic and associated with additional MV or AV disease. The symptoms are those of TR.

SCENARIO 17. HYPERTROPHIC CARDIOMYOPATHY

The pulse is normal volume but may be jerky in character with a large tidal wave: The apex is prominent and minimally displaced, pressure loaded with a characteristic lift. The atrial impulse can (often) be felt – the double apex; the LV can be described as muscular. A systolic thrill is present at the lower LSE. On auscultation there is an apical S4 and a harsh ejection systolic murmur starts well after S1 and radiates from the apex to the LSE and towards the axilla.

The murmur is accentuated by forced expiration or Valsalva's manoeuvre (raising the intrathoracic pressure), and is diminished by deep inspiration or Müller's manoeuvre.

You may hear a mid-diastolic rumble in inflow obstruction.

The systolic murmur of HCOM not only can radiate to the apex and axilla but also can merge with the MR caused by the systolic anterior motion (SAM) of the anterior MV leaflet.

In severe HCOM S2 might be reversed.

Differential diagnosis

- Aortic stenosis: the pulse in AS is slow, rising but not jerky, the thrill is at the base, there is often an ejection sound and manoeuvres to vary obstruction do not change the murmur
- Subvalvar mitral regurgitation, eg chordal rupture
- VSD: in an VSD or subvalvar MR the pulse *can* be jerky and the thrill anterior or at the LSE with a late or ejection systolic murmur. Therefore the key feature to look for is the lack of variability with manoeuvres to vary the obstruction, eg Müller's and Valsalva's manoeuvres.

Questions

1. What do you know about the aetiology?

Up to 70% are inherited as autosomal dominant with variable penetrance and an equal sex distribution. Spontaneous mutations occur and account for the rest. There is a degree of genetic heterogeneity that affects prognosis within kindreds. The identification of the gene in an individual or family may enable an earlier and more precise diagnosis, and more useful prognostic information to be given.

The pathogenesis is unknown but the microscopic features of thickened and haphazardly arranged muscle fibres may be the result of excessive catecholamine stimulation caused by a genetic abnormality of neural crest tissue (note an association of HCOM, hypertension, lentiginosis and phaeochromo-cytoma).

2. What symptoms might the patient have?

Often asymptomatic, although a patient can present at any age with palpitations (associated with Wolff–Parkinson–White syndrome), syncope or sudden death (as in AS). Angina occurs even with normal coronary arteries. Dyspnoea can be caused by a stiff left ventricle in diastole, reducing atrial transport.

Symptoms may become rapidly worse if AF develops. MR often coexists.

3. What might you find on echocardiography?

Several features in association are diagnostic:

- Midsystolic aortic valve closure
- Asymmetrical septal hypertrophy
- Small LV cavity with a hypercontractile posterior wall
- SAM of the MV.

Management

- Avoid nitrates for angina because they increase the outflow obstruction (so using amyl nitrate is a useful diagnostic test).
- β Blockers are the mainstay of treatment for giddiness, syncope, angina and dyspnoea.
- Infective endocarditis may occur.
- It is well tolerated in pregnancy but there is a strong possibility that the child will be affected.
- Genetic testing, but the genotype–phenotype correlation is uncertain.
- Dual chamber pacing with depolarisation from the RV apex alters septal motion and is a promising alternative to surgery. Dual chamber pacing is required because atrial transport is so important in HCOM.
- Surgical myotomy or myomectomy through the aortic valve effectively reduces the LVOT gradient more than pacing but with higher risk.

SCENARIO 18. PROSTHETIC VALVE

The abnormal heart sound is the prosthetic valve and there should be no excuse for getting it wrong; however, it can be more complicated than that:

- Expect an opening sound and a closing sound
- There may be flow across the valve.

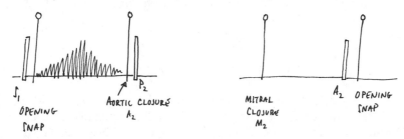

Prosthetic sounds: aortic Starr–Edwards valve – normal S1 followed by a prosthetic opening sound, then a soft murmur across the valve; S2 is the ball valve closing and P2 will be heard only if the split is wide. Mitral Starr–Edwards: S1 is the mitral ball valve closing. There should not be a systolic murmur in this situation. A2 should be heard distinct from the ball opening sound that follows. Diastole should be silent.

Figure 3.11   Prosthetic valve.

Look for the distal stigmata of infective endocarditis, particularly fever, splenomegaly, haematuria and splinter haemorrhages.

A forward flow murmur, eg ejection systolic murmur across an aortic valve or diastolic murmur over an MV, is normal. They are particularly prominent with mechanical valves.

A regurgitant murmur, eg a systolic murmur across an MV, should always be regarded as pathological and indicative of valve failure.

Look for evidence of valve failure: regurgitation and heart failure.

Inspect the teeth – meticulous dental care is vital.

The opening and closing sounds of either ball or disc should be clear and sharp and not muffled. Vegetations may muffle the sounds and restrict movement.

Are there stigmata of anticoagulation or embolic disease?

Question

1. *If you are seeing a patient with a prosthetic valve what symptoms might you look for?*

- Prosthetic valve endocarditis
- Any unexplained malaise, fever, weight loss, dyspnoea, etc; they will be told to avoid antibiotics until seen by a cardiologist
- Any dental treatment in the last 6 months with no antibiotics
- Change in valve sounds
- New symptoms, however vague
- Systemic embolisation:
    - most common with mechanical valves, approximately 1% per year even with ideal anticoagulation
    - dyspnoea, associated with failing valve – this is a predictable feature of biological valves, which fail more rapidly than mechanical valves
    - haemolysis, valve thrombosis, valve dehiscence, myocardial failure and arrhythmias occur.

If endocarditis occurs on a prosthetic valve it has a mortality rate of up to 60%. The patient requires urgent referral to a cardiothoracic centre. Most cases require a valve replacement, after prolonged systemic antibiotics.

If systemic embolisation occurs check for endocarditis

SCENARIO 19. TETRALOGY OF FALLOT

This young patient has central cyanosis and digital clubbing. The peripheral pulses are normal. The JVP does not have a large 'a' wave (contrast with PS with an intact septum).

An RV heave is palpable and (in some patients) a systolic thrill – caused by turbulent flow across the RVOT – is palpable. S1 is normal, but S2 is single (there is no P2) and often palpable.

After an aortic ejection click (occasionally present) there is an ejection systolic murmur, audible along the left sternal border, radiating up to the pulmonary area; this is caused by the obstruction to the RV outflow rather than the VSD.

The intensity and duration of the murmur are inversely related to the severity of the obstruction of RV outflow; a soft, short murmur suggests that severe obstruction is present.

A diastolic murmur of AR may be heard because of the very large aortic root.

A continuous murmur is the result of large aortopulmonary collaterals.

Polycythaemia is to be expected and the patient should be receiving regular venesection. Consider the clinical features of polycythaemia:

- Arterial or venous thromboses, particularly cerebral
- Later in life: gout, acne, kyphoscoliosis, recurrent gingivitis.

This case represents uncorrected tetralogy of Fallot. Most patients die in childhood; the rate of survival is 66% at 1 year of age, 40% at 3 years, 11% at 20 years, 6% at 30 years and 3% at 40 years.

In a (young) adult it may represent an incomplete correction. Consider the case if the patient was born outside the UK, particularly in social deprivation.

Expect symptoms of dyspnoea and a reduced exercise tolerance; they may have had cerebral abscess or stroke.

Currently complete surgical correction is attempted when patients are very young – closure of the VSD and relief of the RV outflow obstruction.

Previously, infants underwent one of three palliative procedures to increase pulmonary blood flow – all involving anastomoses of a systemic artery to a PA – thereby reducing the severity of cyanosis and improving exercise tolerance:

- Waterston anastomosis: back of ascending aorta to the right PA
- Glenn operation: SVC to right PA only
- Blalock–Taussig shunt: either subclavian artery to the respective PA.

Patients who have had a correction will have a midline thoracotomy scar, cyanosis and digital clubbing. One radial pulse will be weaker than the other; the venous pressure will be normal.

There will be a left parasternal heave, often with a displaced apex from LV volume overload (which may be diffuse because of developing failure) and a thrill with an ejection systolic murmur across the pulmonary valve; the same proviso applies as above – if the RV outflow is severely stenosed there may be no murmur.

Questions

1. What are the components of tetralogy of Fallot?

- VSD
- Overriding aorta
- Pulmonary stenosis
- RVH.

2. Children with uncorrected tetralogy of Fallot often squat when they are resting: why?

The large VSD means that ventricular pressures are equal. Right-to-left shunting of blood occurs because of the increased resistance to flow in the RVOT. As the resistance at the RV outflow is fairly fixed, changes in the systemic vascular resistance (SVR) affect the magnitude of the right-to-left shunting. Squatting increases the SVR and decreases the right-to-left shunt, improving both pulmonary blood flow and cyanosis. Furthermore the reduction in venous return, especially acidotic blood from the legs, helps mitigate infundibular spasm, which can lead to cyanotic attacks – the features of which include syncope, seizures, stroke and even death.

SCENARIO 20. COARCTATION OF THE AORTA

The patient is in SR, the rate is x (normal) and the carotid pulse prominent, but of otherwise normal character; the radial pulses are synchronous and of equal volume; the blood pressure in the arms is equal with a wide pulse pressure and hypertension (y/z mmHg).

The femoral pulses are delayed, anacrotic and weak (or even absent) compared with the radial pulses. The JVP is normal.

On palpation of the chest and precordium there are palpable collaterals over and around the scapulae and around the shoulders; the apex is minimally displaced and pressure loaded indicating LVH. A systolic thrill may be palpable in the suprasternal notch.

On auscultation there is continuous murmur heard over the thoracic spine and/or below the left clavicle. In a larger coarctation the murmur is ejection systolic. Over the collateral vessels the murmur is ejection systolic.

There may be signs of an associated bicuspid aortic valve (page 239), or more rarely a PDA or VSD. The coarctation may extend down the thoracic and into the abdominal aorta and the signs will thus be heard lower down along the spine.

If the coarctation is proximal to the left subclavian artery the patient will have differential signs in the upper limbs.

Differential diagnosis

The source of an ejection systolic murmur can cause confusion in coarctation. In contrast to aortic stenosis, the findings in coarctation are that A2 is usually loud, but not usually delayed beyond P2.

There are (broadly speaking) three types of coarctation:

1. **Infantile**: they present in the first month of life with heart failure and associated lesions.
2. **Adult** (most common): coarctation is juxtaductal or slightly postductal. Obstruction develops gradually and the patient presents in the second or third decade. Associated lesions are rare apart from bicuspid aortic valve.
3. **Pseudo-coarctation**: tortuosity of the aorta in the region of the duct with no haemodynamic significance.

Associated lesions

- Bicuspid aortic valve: about 50% and practically the most important
- PDA: the most common associated shunt:
  - postductal coarctation and PDA: usually a left-to-right shunt into the PA; if this shunt is large pulmonary hypertension can occur

  - infantile coarctation and PDA: high PVR results in a right-to-left shunt with the distal aorta, trunk and legs supplied by the RV flow through the PDA; this may result in differential cyanosis (pink fingers, blue toes) and heart failure
- VSD: in isolation or with more complex disease, eg transposition
- Mitral valve disease: stenosis or regurgitation
- Non-cardiac: berry aneurysms, renal anomalies (especially in Turner syndrome).

Clinical features

- M:F – 3.5:1
- Infantile heart failure: > 50% of preductal coarctation
- Postductal coarctation can be missed in childhood and present in adolescence or early adult life with one or more of:
  - vigorous pulsation in the neck or throat
  - hypertension, often symptomless
  - tired legs or intermittent claudication
  - subarachnoid haemorrhage from a berry aneurysm
  - infective endocarditis on the coarctation or a bicuspid aortic valve
  - LV failure
  - rupture or dissection of the proximal aorta – more common in pregnancy
  - angina, premature coronary arteriosclerosis.

Question

1. What are the broad management principles of coarctation?

Most patients die before the age of 40 years owing to complications; thus surgical correction is recommended for postductal coarctation either between 5 and 10 years or at diagnosis. If aortic stenosis coexists, the coarctation is dealt with first and the valve replaced subsequently if necessary.

Bypass surgery with a Dacron graft and balloon angioplasty has its proponents in certain settings and centres.

SCENARIO 21. PULMONARY STENOSIS

Consider the appearance of the patient:

- Rounded, plump face with isolated pulmonary valve stenosis
- Noonan syndrome – 'male Turner syndrome' (see page 273)
- William syndrome (see below).

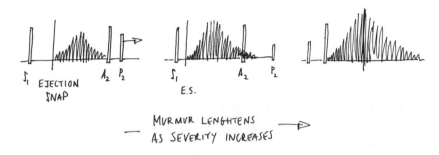

Figure 3.12   Pulmonary stenosis.

The pulse rate, rhythm and character and blood pressure are normal. The JVP is raised with large 'a' waves (see above). The apex is normal but there is a left parasternal heave – indicating RVH – and a thrill over the pulmonary outflow tract. On auscultation:

- Mild valvar stenosis: an ejection sound followed by an ejection systolic murmur. A2 and P2 are clearly heard and widely split.
- Moderate valvar stenosis: as the stenosis increases the murmur is longer and obscures A2. P2 is delayed longer and becomes softer.
- Severe valvar stenosis: with severe stenosis P2 becomes inaudible; as the valve calcifies the ejection sound disappears.

The murmur radiates towards the left shoulder and over the left lung posteriorly. In all cases, depending on the severity and how the lesion is tolerated, the following clinical features may be present:

- RVF:
  - dyspnoea and fatigue: because of low cardiac output; orthopnoea and PND do not occur
  - ascites, leg oedema and jaundice
- The competence of the tricuspid valve, presence or absence of a VSD, ASD or PDA and the maintenance of SR also affect the clinical syndrome
- Angina and effort syncope (compare aortic stenosis) as well as infective endocarditis are uncommon. The patient may notice the large 'a' wave in the neck.

As in aortic stenosis the outflow obstruction can be at several levels:

- Peripheral pulmonary artery stenosis: stenoses of the main trunk of the PA can be either localised or diffuse. Occurs as part of William syndrome or rubellar syndrome (with an associated PDA).
- Pulmonary valve stenosis (90%): 'common' isolated lesion (7% of congenital heart lesions). Also occurs in Noonan syndrome, teratology of Fallot and rubellar syndrome, and is rarely acquired, eg carcinoid syndrome.
- Infundibular and subinfundibular stenosis are rare.

The differential diagnosis is from aortic valve or subvalvar stenosis, VSD, Ebstein's anomaly, an ASD or innocent pulmonary outflow murmurs in children.

Question

1. *What are the features of William syndrome?*

Infantile hypercalcaemia, supravalvar aortic stenosis and PA stenosis with elf-like facies, intellectual impairment.

SCENARIO 22. NOONAN SYNDROME

Turner-like syndrome and should be read in concert with that condition. It can affect males as well as females.

The patient is short with characteristic facies, which have been described as elfin, or triangular, namely:

- Epicanthic folds
- Ptosis
- Hypertelorism
- Myopia
- Keratoconus
- Strabismus
- Low set and/or abnormal auricles – rotated forwards so the lobes are prominent
- Anterior dental malocclusion
- Propensity for keloid.

There is a low posterior hairline with webbing of the neck. The chest is shield like with pectus excavatum and cubitus valgus.

On examination of the cardiovascular system you may find pulmonary stenosis; septal defects occur more rarely. The cardiac lesions are more varied than in Turner syndrome and are characteristically right sided in Noonan syndrome whereas in Turner syndrome the lesions are left sided. Cryptorchidism occurs with delayed sexual maturation (as opposed to sexual infantilism in Turner syndrome). There is a degree of learning disability but it is highly variable such that Noonan syndrome is no bar to high academic achievement in any field.

Pulmonary stenosis is present in two-thirds of cases resulting from valve dysplasia.

The condition is usually diagnosed on the basis of the cardiac abnormalities so, in the absence of these, it may go undiagnosed. The karyotype is normal and the inheritance autosomal dominant, and the precise genetic abnormality has not been identified.

NEURO WORDS

ysphagia

ysartria

horea

ystonia

arapesis

ysphasia — understandin(production of
                        language

PERSONAL PRESCRIPTION PA

| ☐ TO SELF | ☐ Do | ☐ Consider | Date _____ |
| | ☐ Remember | ☐ Research | |

☐ NAG NOTE for _____ from _____

where is lesion

what is nature

| ☐ Now | ☐ This week | ☐ Next month |
| ☐ Later | ☐ This month | ☐ Someday |

BMA Library
Anytime. Anywhere.

020 7383 6625   bma-library@bma.org.uk   bma.org.uk/lib

THE NEUROLOGICAL EXAMINATION

The neurological station fills most candidates with a certain dread. Unlike the cardiology, respiratory or abdominal examination there is no standard approach to the neurological examination that will cover most cases. A full neurological examination usually takes far longer than the 7 minutes allotted in PACES; the skill is in knowing which aspects of an individual case need particular attention based on the instructions and, to an extent, the likely pathology.

You must demonstrate your ability to make a diagnosis in a limited amount of time; you are likely to be successful if you have a clear plan of action. This is easier to have beforehand than to make up on the spot. The instructions before the case have been thought out very carefully and will direct you to the most fruitful part of the examination that should enable you to answer two questions:

1. Where is the lesion?
2. What is its nature?

Finally you must screen the rest of the nervous system quickly and efficiently and keep your eyes open for systemic disease or disease in other systems.
You are likely to be asked to examine one of the following:

- Upper limbs
- Lower limbs
- Cranial nerves
- Cerebellar system
- Motor or sensory system
- Speech
- Eyes
- Gait and proceed as you wish.

You may have to pay attention to the spine and skull for injury of disease, bruits around the orbit, elsewhere on the skull or over the carotid arteries.

The case will usually have been chosen for having signs that are obvious to candidate and examiner alike. If a sign is dubious or doubtful it might be better not to mention it because it is a greater sin to mention a sign that is not there than to miss one (despite correct technique) that is.

General examination

Too often we wish to leap into the detail of the case and ignore vital clues that are present. Do not rush:

Stop → Look at the patient → And **think**

- Are the patient's dress and appearance appropriate?
- How is the handshake? Consider specifics, eg:
  - Is there myotonia?
  - Is it strong, weak, sweaty or tremulous?
  - Is there intention tremor?

As you introduce yourself there is the opportunity to ask one or two questions surreptitiously:

'Good morning I'm Dr Amarceepe; you are Mr Neuron, is that right?' or 'Can you tell me your name please?'

'Are you right or left handed?'

Try to ask this if the information is not given.

'Are you comfortable?'

Is there dysarthria or dysphasia?

Is there anything to point to a disorder of higher mental function or thought process? For example, euphoria is sometimes seen in MS (multiple sclerosis), emotional lability in pseudobulbar palsy from multilacunar states, depression or dementia.

General inspection

- Asymmetry
- Poverty of movement
- Wasting, hypertrophy, fasciculation
- The posture of the limbs, eg pyramidal posture
- Abnormal movements
- Injuries, eg fingertip burns or scars in syringomyelia; cuts, ulcers, deformed joints
- Signs of systemic disease – diabetes, acromegaly, Cushing's disease, Paget's disease.

Cranial nerves

Position the patient carefully to enable you to conduct the examination best, eg sitting over the edge of the bed.

Look very carefully for:

- Proptosis
- Ptosis
- Asymmetry
- Craniotomy scars (scalp, eyebrows)
- Neurofibromas
- Naevi: Sturge–Weber syndrome.

Olfactory (I)

You are exceedingly unlikely to be asked to examine smell, but it is prudent to enquire whether it is normal at the start of the examination. If it is mentioned then you test smell with standard bottles of smells (eg coffee), which you must smell, rather than identify as such, testing each nostril in turn.

Causes of anosmia

Bilateral	Upper respiratory tract infection
	Meningioma of olfactory groove
	Ethmoid tumours
	Basal or frontal skull fracture
	Post-pituitary surgery
	Congenital, eg Kallman syndrome
	Smoking
	Increasing age
Unilateral	Trauma
	Early olfactory groove meningioma

Ophthalmic (II)

Acuity

With the patient wearing his or her normal spectacles test each eye in turn with either a Jaeger chart (recorded right N5, left N6) or a Snellen chart at 6 m, recording the distance at which he or she stands (6/6) over the line that he or she can read (6/6). If the patient cannot read the top line (6/60) move him or her forward; if the patient cannot read at 1 m, ie 1/60, ask him or her to count fingers at 1 m – failing this, perception of movement at 30 cm and, if that fails, perception of light is assessed.

Consider the potential causes of decreased acuity.

Sites of lesions to consider when faced with decreased acuity

Cornea, eg trachoma, *Chlamydia trachomatis*
Aqueous
Lens, eg cataract
Vitreous, eg preretinal haemorrhage
Retina, eg retinitis pigmentatosa, macular degeneration
Optic nerve, eg optic neuritis
Chiasma, eg pituitary tumour
Tract ⎫
Radiation ⎬ eg stroke, tumour
Cortex ⎭

Fields

Fields are tested by confrontation, with a small red- or white-topped hat pin, brought slowly in from the periphery; using moving fingers is incredibly insensitive for abnormalities and is usually not permissible. Check each quadrant in turn, considering the patterns of abnormality; finally, map out the blind spot – it is enlarged in neuritis and papilloedema.

Test for sensory inattention in the fields.

Fundoscopy

If fundoscopy is the focus of the case, it is more usually at the eye station; however, in many cases fundoscopy can be integral to the case. Should you wait till the end of the cranial nerves to examine the fundi or do it now? Both have their merits; you do not want to have just completed the examination, 7 minutes have passed, and say 'I would like to perform fundoscopy' with no time left; thus you can find out if it is necessary by saying that you would like to look at the fundi now.

Oculomotor (III), trochlear (IV) and abducens (VI)

Appearance

In good light with the patient looking into the distance, note:

- Pupil size
- Shape
- Equality
- Regularity.

Is there ptosis (bilateral ptosis is easy to miss; see page 591)?

Is there a scar to suggest Horner syndrome?

Light reflex

The patient must look into the distance so that he or she does not accommodate; do not shine the light at the fovea because it is painful. Look for the direct and consensual reflexes on both sides; both should be equally brisk.

Relative afferent pupillary defect (Marcus–Gunn pupil)

Employ the swinging light test. Move the torch in an arc from pupil to pupil. If there is optic atrophy, neuritis or reduced acuity, the affected pupil will dilate, rather than constrict, when the torch is moved from the normal to the abnormal eye. (Shining the light in the healthy eye causes rapid constriction to both eyes. Subsequently, when the light is moved to the affected eye the impaired afferent limb results in slow transmission, allowing time for the pupils to dilate.)

Accommodation

Place your finger about 30 cm in front of the patient's eyes, just above his or her horizon, and ask him or her to look into the distance, and then to focus on to your finger. The eyes should adduct and intort, and the pupils should constrict (see page 278).

Ophthalmoplegia

There are six cardinal directions of gaze. With normal spectacles if possible, the patient should be asked if he or she sees double in a particular place (you must have established vision in both eyes). If he or she does, there are two rules:

1. If the images are side by side only the lateral or medial recti can be responsible.
2. Separation is greatest in the direction of movement of the affected muscle, or the direction in which the weak muscle has its purest action.

Move your finger like a letter H, thus allowing the action of each muscle to be assessed. If diplopia is present, at maximum separation of the object, cover the eyes in turn. When the outer image is lost this is the eye, and thus the muscle, involved. If diplopia persists with one eye covered, it may be lens dislocation, astigmatism or factitious. If the pattern of loss is complex and cannot easily be explained, always consider Graves' disease or myasthenia.

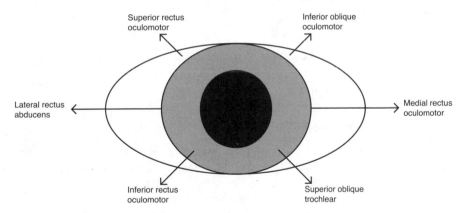

Figure 3.13

Is there internuclear ophthalmoplegia (see page 599)?

Hold lateral gaze to check for nystagmus, remembering that at extremes of gaze nystagmus (see page 606) becomes physiological and upwards for fatigability – ptosis (see page 591) may appear.

Trigeminal (V)

Inspect for wasting of temporalis and masseter. Loss of bulk is best appreciated on palpation while the patient clenches the teeth. If there is unilateral weakness on opening the jaw, it will deviate to the affected side, pushed by the intact pterygoid. The motor root runs with the mandibular division.

The jaw jerk is normally absent or just present (see Pseudobulbar palsy, page 329).

Test sensation in each division on the trigeminal nerve – ophthalmic, maxillary, mandibular (see Sturge–Weber syndrome, page 372).

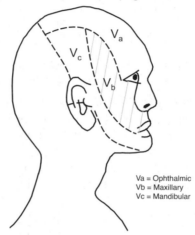

Va = Ophthalmic
Vb = Maxillary
Vc = Mandibular

Figure 3.14   Trigeminal nerve – sensory testing

Look for sensory inattention.

The mandibular division is not involved in cavernous sinus disease because it leaves the skull through the foramen ovale (see page 371).

Elicit the corneal reflex by touching, not wiping, the cornea (not the conjunctiva); the efferent limb is the facial nerve. Loss may be the first sign of pathology, eg acoustic neuroma. When zoster damages the nerve, corneal involvement is more likely if the nasociliary branch on the side of the nose is involved. Never test the central part of the cornea because, in corneal anaesthesia, to do so risks corneal ulceration and subsequent visual impairment.

Facial (VII)

See page 339.

Vestibulocochlear (VIII)

If you suspect disease inspect the external auditory meatus and drum with an otoscope.

Test gross hearing whispering: '68' or '77' (high tones) or '100' or '22' (low tones) 30 cm from the ear, at the end of expiration while moving your fingers next to the other ear.

Perform Weber's and Rinne's tests with a 256- or 512-Hz tuning fork.

If vertigo is mentioned perform Hallpike's manoeuvre

Hallpike's manoeuvre

Tell the patient what you are about to do. Ask him or her to sit up and then quickly drop back so the head is 30° below horizontal, turned 30° towards the examiner, with the eyes open looking at the ceiling. If positive, after a short pause there will be vertigo and nystagmus to the lower ear for up to a minute. It is not reproducible for 10–15 minutes and indicates benign positional vertigo. If it occurs immediately and is not fatigable, it indicates a central cause, eg brain-stem disease

---

Acoustic neurofibromas present insidiously with unilateral deafness, followed by ataxia and headache. Tinnitus is common but patients rarely complain of vertigo. The corneal reflex is lost first, and then papilloedema, nystagmus and signs of an ipsilateral cerebellar lesion occur if large. The nearby nerves VI and VII can be affected

Glossopharyngeal (IX) and vagus (X)

Inspect the palate with a torch. Is the uvula central?

Ask the patient to say 'Ah'; if there is unilateral weakness of the vagus nerve the uvula will move to the normal side.

Check the gag reflex – the sensory limb is the glossopharyngeal and the motor the vagus nerve. Thus if sensation is intact but contraction absent, this suggests a vagus lesion. The most common cause of a reduced gag is old age.

Ask the patient to speak and cough – a test of the recurrent laryngeal nerves.

The gag has little or no bearing on our ability to swallow; it gives an indication of our ability to protect the airway. Swallowing should be tested separately with a glass of water if necessary.

Taste is not routinely assessed, but you would use sugar, salt, quinine and citric acid.

Isolated glossopharyngeal lesions are very rare.

In both bulbar and pseudobulbar palsy the voice is nasal. In both, the palate fails to move when the patient says 'Ah'. However, the gag in pseudobulbar palsy is exaggerated, because it is an upper motor neuron (UMN) lesion, whereas in bulbar palsy it is absent (see Pseudobulbar palsy, page 329).

Accessory (XI)

Ask the patient to shrug the shoulders, testing the trapezius muscles, and then turn the patient's head against resistance, testing sternomastoids; feel the muscles. Damage is usually a result of inflammation or operation on the upper cervical lymph nodes.

Hypoglossal (XII)

Inspect the tongue in the mouth. The hypoglossal nerve is purely motor; in UMN lesions (eg pseudobulbar palsy) the tongue is small and immobile and, in lower motor neuron (LMN) lesions (eg bulbar palsy), it is wasted and fasciculations are seen.

On protrusion of the tongue, it will deviate to the weak side in unilateral disease.

Isolated disease is rare.

Peripheral nervous system

Observation and Inspection

When you shake hands, again specifically consider the following: myotonia, wasting of the small muscles, tremor, sweaty, firm or weak, acromegaly, fingertip marks from blood glucose monitoring.

Look around the bed: is there a wheelchair or walking sticks? Look at the shoes – callipers, built-up heels, scuffed toes?

Ensure that the patient is adequately exposed before considering the following points:

- Are the limbs the same length? In old polio there is sometimes shortening of a lower limb.
- Posture: pyramidal, with flexed upper and extended, adducted lower limbs?
- Bulk: any wasting? If so what is the pattern: distal, (eg Charcot–Marie–Tooth disease), proximal, generalised, symmetrical?
- Abnormal movements
- Fasciculation (see page 326)
- Tremor (see page 357)
- Spontaneous movements
- Skin: neurofibromas, herpes zoster, purpura, rash, lipohypertrophy.

Lower limbs

Gait (see page 359)

Ask the patient to walk in an open space such as down a corridor and do not be tempted to stick close by the side in case he or she might fall. If there is a danger of falling ask the examiner or a nurse to assist the patient; you cannot examine the gait from the patient's side. Note the stride length, arm swinging, posture, base and any involuntary movements.

Ask the patient to stand on his or her toes – a sensitive test for weakness of gastrocnemius and soleus.

Have the patient stand on his or her heels – failure to do so indicates foot drop. Is it bilateral, eg Charcot–Marie–Tooth disease (hereditary sensorimotor neuropathy or HSMN) or unilateral, as in a common peroneal nerve palsy?

Perform Romberg's test; this is truly positive only if the patient falls over when he or she closes the eyes. If you think that it might be positive, eg if the gait was steppage, ask the patient to stand with back against the wall.

A positive **Romberg's test** suggests that ataxia is sensory in nature, ie it depends on proprioception (peripheral sensory neuropathy, eg diabetes mellitus, chronic inflammatory demyelinating neuropathy; dorsal column disease, eg tabes dorsalis [neurosyphillis]). A negative Romberg's test suggests that ataxia is cerebellar in origin.

Tone

Assess the tone in the quadriceps, hamstrings and calves; much useful information can be gained by palpating the muscles alongside the more common rolling and then lifting the leg (the heel should not leave the bed). (Only by palpating the muscles of every patient whom you see can you develop this important skill. Most of us do not do it because we have not been taught how to examine the neurological system by a seasoned clinical neurologist or general physician.)

Hypertonia

Spastic or **clasp knife**: the tone is increased but is suddenly overcome, characteristic of UMN pathology
Lead pipe: there is resistance to movement right throughout the range of movement; if tremor is superimposed this is 'cogwheel' rigidity
Hypotonia: probably not a valid term because, in a fully relaxed normal person, you should be able to detect no resistance to passive movement. However, some report it as a feature of LMN or cerebellar pathology
Test for ankle and knee clonus

Power

Grade the power; it is usual to subdivide power using the MRC scale:

- 5: normal power
- 4: active movement against gravity and resistance:
  - 4+: against strong resistance

- – 4: against moderate resistance
- – 4–: against slight resistance
- 3: active movement against gravity
- 2: active movement with gravity eliminated
- 1: flicker or trace of contraction
- 0: no contraction.

The muscles to be tested are listed (the most useful*), together with their nerve and root level.

Action	Muscle	Nerve	Segmental level
Hip flexion*	Iliopsoas	Femoral	**L1, L2,** L3
Hip extension	Gluteus maximus	Inferior gluteal	**L5, S1,** S2
Hip adduction	Adductors	Obturator	**L2, L3,** L4
Knee flexion*	Hamstrings	Sciatic	L5, **S1,** S2
Knee extension*	Quadriceps	Femoral	L2, **L3, L4**
Ankle dorsiflexion*	Tibialis anterior	Deep peroneal	**L4,** L5
Ankle plantar flexion*	Gastocnemius	Tibial	S1, S2
Ankle inversion*	Tibialis posterior	Tibial	L5, S1, S2
Ankle eversion*	Peroneus longus and brevis	Superficial peroneal	L5, S1
Toe dorsiflexion	Extensor digitorum brevis	Deep peroneal	L5, S1
Cupping the sole of the foot	Small muscles of the foot	Medial and lateral plantar nerves	S1, S2

The most important roots are in bold.

As the description of *each* muscle's power can become cumbersome and confusing; you have to become adept at conveying the details of the case **quickly** and **clearly**. Thus it may be more appropriate to just say that there is a proximal myopathy, weakness in the left upper limb† in a pyramidal distribution, weakness of the small muscles of the hand or radial nerve palsy, without going into cumbersome detail about each root, nerve or muscle.

Reflexes

Strike the tendon of interest firmly and ideally once. The reflex is proportional not only to the strength of the strike but also to the stretch under which you have

---

† The arm is the portion of the upper limb from the shoulder to the elbow and the leg is the portion of the lower limb from the knee to the ankle, so it is correct to say upper and lower limbs. Some examiners prefer anatomical accuracy whereas others take exception to the needless complexity of saying 'upper limb' when 'arm' will do. There are many more instances where two people think the same thing should be said in slightly different ways; do not let it become an issue with an examiner.

the tendon. They are crucial in clinical neurology/medicine and if absent it always requires an explanation; do not accept that they are absent until Jendrassik's manoeuvre has been performed; compare the sides.

Knee jerk

L2, **L3, L4**.

Ankle jerk

S1: you must be able to demonstrate the ankle jerk confidently; it is extremely important for clinical neurology. If it is absent actively consider cauda equina pathology because it is extremely easy to miss on a 'routine' neurological examination (see page 370).

Plantar

Corticospinal tract, afferent limb is L5, S1: gently scratch a key or stick along the outer edge of the sole of the foot towards the little toe, then medially along the metatarsus. This causes contraction of the tensor fascia lata, often with contraction of the adductors and sartorius. As the stimulus increases, flexion of the toes occurs, from lateral to medial, at the metatarsus. The ankle dorsiflexes and inverts. It is never completely absent in normal individuals. Scratching medially can induce a grasp reflex, which is a different sign (see below).

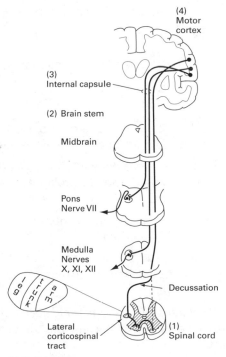

Figure 3.15   Sites of UMN lesions

An extensor response (Babinski's sign) is found only in corticospinal tract lesions and is thus pathognomic of UMN pathology. In major corticospinal lesions the area from which an extensor response can be elicited (receptive field) enlarges, such that Oppenheim's sign (pressing on the medial border of the tibia) becomes positive.

+++	pathologically brisk in UMN lesions
++	normal, particularly in young, thin or anxious people
+	normal
±	present on reinforcement; suggests LMN pathology or advanced myopathy – where the signs are usually obvious
-	absent in LMN lesions or in severe myopathy

Coordination

If the patient can walk that is the most useful test for coordination; if he or she is lying down ask the patient to run the heel up and down the other leg.

If the patient is weak it becomes more difficult – you can ask the patient to tap the foot against your palm (dysdiadochokinesia) or to make small circles at the ankle. It is very difficult to conclude anything from testing coordination when there is weakness; it often looks awful and makes you look incompetent if, for instance, you try to perform heel–toe in a patient with weakness of hip and knee flexion.

In principle it is better to ascribe incoordination, where there is muscle weakness, to that weakness unless the weakness is minimal and the incoordination gross.

Loss of proprioception can also cause incoordination (eg sensory ataxia, see page 360).

Sensation

Test the sensation in the L1, L2, L3, L4, L5 and S1 dermatomes; if there is **any** concern about the cauda test S2 – ask about perineal sensation.

Compare left and right. There is considerable overlap of dermatomes and thus an isolated root lesion, eg L5 caused by a disc prolapse at L4–5, may cause only a patch of sensory loss, in this case on the dorsum of the foot.

Test from abnormal to normal, having first demonstrated to the patient what normal feels like, usually on the anterior chest.

Note that the dorsal columns decussate in the medulla, whereas pain and temperature fibres enter the cord before crossing a few segments higher to ascend in the spinothalamic tract.

- **Light touch** (*dorsal columns and spinothalamic tracts*): dab a wisp of cotton wool. Never stroke the cotton wool because this stimulates the spinothalamic tract.

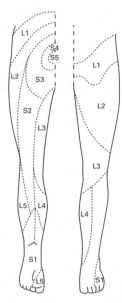

Figure 3.16   Dermatome distribution.

- **Vibration sense** (*dorsal columns*): ideally use a 128-Hz tuning fork at the great toe and, if it is normal there, it is conventional to assume that it is normal more proximally. If it is absent, move proximally to the medial malleolus, knee, iliac crest and sternum as necessary. If the patient detects the feeling of vibration ask him or her to say when it stops before deadening the fork with your fingers. Individuals can usually detect vibration for more than 10 seconds; it is useful in quantifying progressive impairment but it would depend on using the same fork each time. A bioaesthesiometer is a machine that delivers a measurable variable intensity of vibration if you need to quantify this sensation formally.
- **Proprioception** (*dorsal columns*): explain to the patient what up and down are first. Grip the toe by the sides so as not to stimulate pressure sensation. Normally a few degrees of movement is detected. Move proximally as necessary.
- **Pain** (*spinothalamic tracts*): only when you have gained the patient's confidence is it prudent to test pain; use a clean neurological pin, never a hat pin. Ask the patient to say when it feels normal or if a pin feels sharp or blunt. Is there dissociated sensory loss, eg syringomyelia?
- **Temperature** (*spinothalamic tracts*) can be tested if necessary, with test tubes of warm and cold water.
    - if a stocking sensory loss is present demonstrate that it is present right round the limb
    - if you suspect compression of the cord, demonstrate a sensory level. This is often asymmetrical.

Upper limbs

Observe outstretched hands

This can tell you so much about the nervous system analogous to examination of gait; after general examination look at the patient when the arms are outstretched *with palms up* and eyes closed. The following conditions may be suggested:

- UMN lesions: the hand on the affected side may fall while the forearm pronates; the movement starts distally and moves proximally.
- The forearm pronators are embryologically flexors, which remain stronger in pyramidal lesions.
- Cerebellar disease: the arms drift upwards and, if they are pushed down against resistance, the limbs overcorrect before finding the starting position.
- Sensory ataxia: in severe upper limb sensory ataxia (ie loss of joint position sense) the fingers display pseudoathetosis – Romberg's sign.

Tone

See Lower limbs (page 282).

In early UMN lesions you may find that the tone in the forearm pronators has a slight catch compared with the supinators – the pronator catch (compare pronator drift above).

Power

Power is graded on a scale of 1–5 as in the legs, with the same provisos.

Action	Muscle	Nerve	Segmental level
Shoulder abduction	Deltoid	Axillary	**C5,** C6
Elbow flexion (with forearm supinated)	Biceps	Musculocutaneous	C5, **C6**
Elbow flexion (with forearm midway between supination and pronation)	Brachioradialis	Radial	C5, C6
Elbow extension	Triceps	Radial	C6, **C7,** C8
Wrist extension	Extenor carpi ulnaris and radialis	Radial	C5, **C6, C7,** C8
Finger extension	Extensor digitorum	Radial	**C7,** C8
Finger flexion (index and ring)	Flexor digitorum superficialis (PIP), profundus I and II (DIP)	Median anterior Interosseous	C7, **C8,** T1 C7, **C8**
Opposition of thumb	Opponens pollicis	Median	C8, **T1**
Abduction of thumb	Abductor pollicis brevis	Median	C8, **T1**
Abduction of the little finger	Abductor digiti minimi	Ulnar	C8, **T1**
Abduction of the index finger	First dorsal interosseous	Ulnar	C8, **T1**
Adduction of the index finger	Second palmar interosseous	Ulnar	C8, T1

The most important roots are in bold.

Reflexes

Grade the reflexes, with reinforcement, as discussed above.

- **Biceps**: **C5**, C6
- **Supinator**: **C6**, C7
- **Triceps**: **C7**, C8.

The following reflexes can be elicited depending on the circumstance:

- **Abdominal reflex**: gently scratching towards the umbilicus in the four quadrants of the abdomen, around the umbilicus, causes reflex contraction of rectus abdominis in normal individuals. These reflexes are commonly lost with age, obesity or after abdominal surgery. However, it is a curious feature of UMN pathology that it can result in loss of the abdominal reflexes, so if they are unilaterally absent it can provide valuable information. The levels of the upper are T9 and T10 and lower T11 and T12.
- **Homman's sign**: in UMN lesions there is a generalised sensitivity to stretch in many of the muscles. Flicking the terminal phalanx of the index finger causes reflex flexion of the remaining digits

The **primitive reflexes** indicate frontal lobe damage:

- **Glabellar**: tap between the eyes (from behind so the patient cannot see your hand; it is positive if blinking is persistent). It is unreliable and often unpleasant for patients.
- **Snout reflex**: tapping the nose induces grimacing.
- **Sucking reflex**: stroking the lips produces pouting and sucking movements of the lips.
- **Chewing reflex**: a tongue depressor placed in the mouth produces reflex chewing.
- **Grasp reflex**: stroking the palm elicits a grasp that gets firmer as you attempt to remove your fingers.

Coordination

As above, this can be difficult to demonstrate if the patient is weak.

Dysdiadochokinesis is the failure to perform alternate movements. Thus ask the patient to tap one hand alternately with the palm then dorsum of the other hand; *listen to the rhythm*. It is natural for the non-dominant hand to be a little less coordinated.

Akinesia, seen in Parkinson's disease, is perhaps best demonstrated by asking the patient to perform piano playing movements with the outstretched fingers.

Finger-nose testing – hold the object at the extreme of the patient's reach and ask him or her to touch it and then the nose repeatedly, as accurately (not quickly) as possible. In essential tremor, the tremor on maintaining movement may persist on movement and even worsen towards an object, but only with cerebellar disease does it appear as the hand approaches the target and true past pointing occurs (see also Tremor, page 357).

Sensation

Test the sensation in the C5, C6, C7, C8 and T1 dermatomes in the upper limb (for the same modalities as in the lower limb)

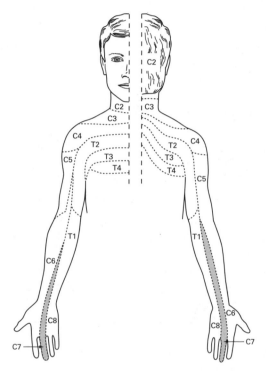

Figure 3.17   Upper limb dermatomes.

Test, as in the lower limbs, the dorsal column and spinothalamic tracts.

Consider if there is dissociated sensory loss, seen in intrinsic cord lesion (see Syringomyelia, page 345).

The common peripheral nerve lesions likely to be encountered in PACES are discussed in the peripheral neuropathy section of the neurological scenarios.

Sensory levels on the trunk are:

- nipple T5
- umbilicus T10.

Do not forget that posteriorly in the midline L1 is just below the ribcage.

Examination of speech

For those with a speech disturbance speaking is a great effort and they can become easily distressed. Sit with the patient, and make a great effort to put him or her at ease. If the patient starts to struggle, make it clear that you appreciate how difficult it is for him or her.

The patient may be reluctant to talk; engage him or her on a topic about which he or she can talk freely, eg his or her holidays or job; you want to see how the patient forms sentences so avoid asking questions that are answered 'yes' or 'no'. If the patient is still having difficulty show him or her a picture in the paper and ask for a description. You will know what it shows.

As the patient speaks pay attention to three particular aspects:

1. Are the words articulated normally?
2. Are the sentences formed normally?
3. Are the words being used correctly?

Does the patient have hemiparesis? Is there facial asymmetry? Is he or she using the right hand as much as the left? The speech centres are in the dominant hemisphere and as such dysphasia and right-sided weakness often appear together.

Look closely at the body language; patients with expressive dysphasia know that they cannot quite say what they want and find it very frustrating. They often gesture with their eyes, face and hands, or sigh, gasp and roll their eyes. By contrast a patient with dementia might be as unconcerned as he or she is uncommunicative.

There are two main patterns that you might see: dysphasia and dysarthria.

Dysphasia

See page 353. The patient has a central problem with the understanding or the production of language, spoken, written, read or even sung, and this occurs with lesions in the dominant hemisphere. The areas of concern are shown in the figure below.

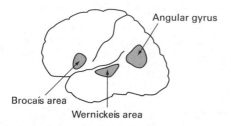

Figure 3.18   Speech areas.

Lesions in the frontal lobe, anterior to the motor cortex, cause 'motor' or 'expressive' dysphasia – the speech is non-fluent but comprehension is preserved.

Lesions in the parietal and temporal lobes cause 'sensory' or 'receptive' dysphasia – the speech is fluent but comprehension is impaired. One must note three things.

Questions

1. Is the speech fluent or not?

If non-fluent, listen to the flow of what is said: it lacks the normal melody, sentences are short and lack fillers such as 'and', 'but', 'so', 'to'; a lot of information can be given but it may sound rather abrupt – 'lots information given sounds abrupt'. The patient often appears to put a lot of effort into getting the words out.

If fluent the words flow, sentences are normal length, the melody of speech is preserved but the information content is low. What is said may sound right but the words may be wrong, ie paraphasia, of which there are three types:

1. Literal: a consonant is substituted as in 'band' instead of 'hand'.
2. Verbal: a word is changed for one with an obvious association, eg 'foot' is said instead of 'shoe'
3. Neologism: non-existent words are used such as 'narm' instead of 'house'; these usually indicate involvement of the posterior speech areas.

2. Can the patient repeat or not?

Aphasic patients often have trouble repeating phrases such as 'no ifs, and/or buts'. They may get some of it right but not the whole thing, eg 'no ifs or buts'. Words with a visual image such as 'house', 'ship', 'horse' or 'flower' may cause less trouble; they are postulated to have a wider distribution in the brain than non-picture words and hence are less susceptible to damage to the speech area.

3. Is comprehension normal?

Patients with severely impaired comprehension may give the appearance of understanding everything that is being said because they can follow non-verbal clues from those around them such that their body language can appear entirely normal, they may nod and smile during breaks in the conversation and can gesticulate so freely that their predicament may go unnoticed even by their own family. You must make allowances for the dysphasia when trying to ascertain whether the patient comprehends or not, and this can be done in one of two ways:

1. Reduce what the patient might have to say to 'yes' or 'no'. 'Do you understand what I am saying?', 'Do you know what this is?' (you hold up a watch), 'Is it a pen?', 'Is it a house?'. if the patient answers no to those questions but immediately says 'yes' when you ask 'Is it a watch?' you can

infer some comprehension, but you must be careful because there is a 50:50 chance of getting the answer right and patients also exhibit perseveration, where they repeat the same answer. Use double-barrelled questions to reveal more subtle defects of comprehension such as 'Do you put your shoes on before your socks?' or 'If the fox eats the chicken, is the chicken alive?'

2. Ask the patient to follow commands; start with one-step commands, 'Touch your knee', and gradually increase the steps to three-step commands – 'Touch your knee, then your nose then your ear' or 'Pick up the pen with your right hand then put it on the bed by your pillow'. (Beware of helping the patient, eg asking the patient to point to different things while looking quite clearly at them, or nodding the appropriate answers for the patient.) Most individuals with aphasia can follow one command but have trouble with sequences. Some patients with apraxia cannot protrude their tongue on command.

Hence when describing dysphasia do so in terms of fluency, paraphasia, repetition and comprehension, then you can use one of the common terms if you so wish – although these terms often mean different things to different people, and in the exam an awful question is 'Precisely what do you mean by …?'. (This is a recurring theme in clinical medicine and is even more troublesome with the fracturing of clinical care; as such it is something to be very much aware of in a practical assessment of clinical examination skills.)

You should ask the patient to read and write to complete the examination.

Dysarthria

Having established that the speech content and comprehension are normal assess the following:

- Repetition of words and phrases that are difficult to say:
  - artillery, British constitution, monotonous, constabulary, autobiography, according to legend, statistical analysis.
- If a simple word can be said well try to increase the complexity
  - city, citizen, citizenship
  - zip, zipper, zippering.
- Repetition of sounds testing different muscles of articulation:
  - weakness of lips – difficulty saying 'puh'
  - weakness of tongue – difficulty saying 'tuh'
  - weakness of palate – difficulty saying 'kuh'.
- Have the patient cough; a bovine cough signifies damage to the recurrent laryngeal nerve causing a vocal fold palsy.
- Examine the motor system:
  - LMN features seen in the muscles of articulation – facial weakness, wasting and fasciculation of the tongue, absent gag and palatal palsy;

these signs are consistent with bulbar palsy as part of motor neuron disease (MND)

- UMN features – brisk jaw jerk, spastic, exaggerated gag, hemiparesis, emotional lability; pseudobulbar palsy in multilacunar states or MND
- cerebellar dysfunction – nystagmus, intention tremor and gait ataxia
- extrapyramidal features – resting tremor, akinesia, rigidity, festinant gait with poor arm swinging.

Examination of the wasted hand

You may be asked to do this either in neurology as an examination of the upper limbs or in rheumatology as in, 'take a look at these hands', 'this patient has been complaining of …'.

You might be asked to comment on wasting of the hands in cases of Pancoast's tumour in a respiratory station, Horner syndrome in ophthalmology, a cutaneous vasculitis in dermatology, severe hypothyroidism or acromegaly in endocrinology, ie it is a potentially common occurrence and deserves special mention and a considered approach.

All the small muscles in the hand are supplied by the median or the ulnar nerve; their root level is T1. Thus in a root lesion all the muscles are affected and in an isolated nerve lesion there is selective wasting. Imagining that one has been asked to look at the upper limbs or the hands in front of the patient, the following is a reasonable schema.

Inspection

- **Age**: some wasting is normal as we age; it is symmetrical and mild but there is no associated arthropathy and the muscles are not weak.
- **Arthritis:** this causes wasting but little in the way of weakness. The pain from the arthritis limits movement more than there being weakness as such; there is some disuse atrophy. Subluxation of the thumb can cause thenar wasting, which can be mistaken for a median nerve lesion.
- **Clawing** of the ring and little fingers suggests an ulnar nerve lesion.
- **Scars**: over the elbow suggest ulnar nerve damage or release; at the carpal tunnel indicate decompression.
- **Size**: of the fingers, thumbs and thumb nails. Is there hemi-smallness to suggest a lesion before the completion of skeletal maturity, usually infancy, eg polio, stroke, birth trauma?
- **Pupils**: is one pupil smaller with ptosis suggesting Horner syndrome (see page 594)? On the side of the wasting this suggests a T1 root or cord lesion.
- **Fasciculations**: suggest MND.

Question

1. Which muscles are affected?

Take specific note of abductor pollicis brevis (APB), abductor digiti minimi (ADM) and the first dorsal interosseus (first DI). There are three patterns of wasting:

- Wasting confined to APB: usually a median nerve lesion, rarely a cervical rib.
- Wasting confined to ADM and first DI: ulnar nerve lesion.
- Wasting of all three: several possibilities (see Wasting of the small muscles of the hand, page 323).

Test power, etc

While you are interested in the muscles of the hand and these three muscles in particular, you must make a general assessment of overall weakness. Assess the neurology in the upper limbs (how you do this naturally depends on the station), power in deltoid, biceps, triceps, brachioradialis, wrist extension, finger extension, APB, ADM and first DI, and test reflexes, sensation and coordination. For a description of the three patterns that emerge, see page 363.

Neurological Scenarios

The number of cases that you may face, and the variety of different examination techniques that you may be required to perform, make the neurological station a peculiar challenge.

As always you must go into the station with an idea of what might come up; you must know the most common cases inside out.

1. Spastic paraparesis
2. Multiple sclerosis
3. Cervical myelopathy
4. Myotonic dystrophy
5. Peripheral neuropathy
6. Charcot–Marie–Tooth disease
7. Foot drop
8. Parkinson's disease
9. Wasting of the small muscles of the hand
10. Motor neuron disease
11A. Bulbar palsy
11B. Pseudobulbar palsy
12. Carpal tunnel syndrome
13. Ulnar nerve palsy

SCENARIO 1. SPASTIC PARAPARESIS

A good candidate

- Will look for sensory loss
- Will look for a sensory level
- Will look for cerebellar signs
- Will look for local spinal disease/tenderness.

The patient walks with a characteristic gait where both legs are held stiffly, in extension and adduction with the foot inverted and plantar flexed; the legs describe an arc as they come through – circumduction; the feet cross on each step, which is often described as scissoring. Muscle bulk is preserved, tone is increased bilaterally and prolonged clonus is present at the ankle and knee. There is a symmetrical paresis both proximally and distally, with the flexors being weaker than the extensors, ie in a pyramidal pattern. The reflexes are pathologically brisk and the plantars are extensor, ie Babinski's sign.

Questions

1. What are the causes of a spastic paraparesis?

Hypertonia, clonus and hyperreflexia tell you that the lesion lies above L1 because the pyramidal tracts end there.

- **Multiple sclerosis** is suggested by a younger patient, often a female from temperate climes with any or all of the following:
  - cerebellar signs
  - sensory loss (more commonly the dorsal columns than spinothalamic tracts)
  - brisk reflexes in the upper limbs
  - paraesthesiae on flexing the neck (Lhermitte's sign)
  - papillitis or optic atrophy
  - disinhibition
  - a history of sphincter disturbance or impotence.
- **Trauma**: a common cause and usually the history is clear on this matter, but you will look for evidence of a previous injury to the spine or deformities.
- **Cord compression**: although not the most common cause, it must always be actively considered particularly if the history suggests an acute or subacute onset with recent alteration in sphincter function; you must *always* determine if there is a sensory level.
- **MND**: a complete absence of sensory signs and a combination of UMN and LMN signs is almost diagnostic of **MND**; where those signs are in the same muscle groups at the same time it is almost pathognomonic.
- **Cerebral palsy** is suggested by intellectual impairment and behavioural problems, or a history of birth injury.

2. How would you classify cord lesions?

They are either intrinsic or extrinsic.

Extrinsic

- Lesions that are important from a therapeutic point of view are usually one of the 'three Ts':
  - tumours (primary or secondary)
  - tubercle (occasionally other infections)
  - trauma (including spondylosis).

Intrinsic

- Vitamin B$_{12}$ deficiency, being treatable, is the most important intrinsic lesion.
- Demyelination is the most common.

3. Can you relate the aetiology to the onset?

Acute or subacute

- Disc prolapse above L1–2.
- Tumours: intra- and extradural – carcinoma (lung, breast, kidney and prostate), lymphoma, myeloma or leukaemia. The most common benign lesions are thoracic meningiomas and neurofibromas.
- Cervical spondylosis.
- Infection: abscess, syphilitic myelitis, HIV infection, Pott's disease of spine.
- Rheumatoid arthritis: atlantoaxial subluxation.
- Haemorrhage: any cause of thrombocytopenia, or bleeding diathesis, arteriovenous malformation (AVM), primary intramedullary haemorrhage.
- Vascular: arterial occlusion – thrombotic, embolic, dissection, vasculitic, hypotensive.
- Inflammatory: sarcoid, SLE, MS, transverse myelitis.
- Subacute combined degeneration of the cord.

Chronic

- MS
- MND
- Syringomyelia
- Primary intramedullary and dural tumours, or indeed any cause of compression
- HTLV-1 (human T-lymphocytic virus 1): tropical spastic paraparesis
- Radiation myelopathy
- Subacute combined degeneration of the cord.

4. What are the symptoms that you would enquire about?

Weakness of the lower limbs is the most common presenting complaint.
The key questions to determine the aetiology are duration of onset, sphincter disturbance and associated features of the underlying cause.

5. What investigations would you do?

Suspicion of developing spinal cord compression is a medical emergency because, once sphincter dysfunction has been present for 24 hours, it is irreversible. Therefore the necessary investigations must be carried out as a matter of urgency – full blood count (FBC), erythrocyte sedimentation rate (ESR), chest radiograph and plain radiology of the spine can be done immediately, then ideally MRI or a CT myelogram is performed. A neurosurgeon should be contacted if there is cord compression.

What other investigations would you do in spastic paraparesis?

Considering spastic paraparesis more generally and depending on the likely differential, the following may need to be done:
- Lumbar puncture (LP): CSF for:
  - oligoclonal bands
  - culture
  - acid-fast bacilli (AFBs)
  - ACE (angiotensin-converting enzyme)
  - cytospin
- Biopsy of masses
- ESR/C-reactive protein (CRP)
- HTLV-1 serology
- HIV test
- Syphilis serology in blood and CSF (cerebrospinal fluid)
- Blood culture
- Sputum culture, early morning urine
- Vitamin B$_{12}$
- Autoantibodies
- MRI of the central nervous system (CNS)
- Electromyography
- Nerve conduction studies.

6. How would you manage cord compression?

Time is of the essence if sphincter involvement or progression is to be prevented.

Spinal cord compression with bladder or bowel involvement often requires surgical decompression. Stabilisation of the spine may be necessary. Dexamethasone and radiotherapy may suffice for malignant compression.

The main problem with benign tumours is that the paraparesis may be attributed to MS, despite the symptoms not being disseminated in time and place.

With malignancy the main danger is indecision; the condition is obviously incurable but surgical treatment at an early stage may relieve pain, minimise weakness and preserve bladder function.

Physiotherapy and occupational therapy plus specialist nursing care are likely to be necessary in any circumstance.

SCENARIO 2. MULTIPLE SCLEROSIS

An important factor for the diagnosis of MS is that there has been more than one episode affecting two or more sites (ie dissociation in time and space), so close attention to the introduction of the case is paramount.

The most common first presentation is usually monosymptomatic, eg unilateral optic neuritis, numbness or tingling in the limbs, lower limb weakness, or brainstem or cerebellar symptoms such as diplopia or ataxia.

Questions

1. What visual symptoms and signs might the patient have?

Optic neuritis

Pain on eye movement and blurred vision evolving over days, perhaps to complete blindness, or with a selective loss of colour vision, is characteristic of optic neuritis; there may be flashes of light on movement of the eye.

Hemiparetic visual loss, from lesions behind the chiasma, occurs more rarely.

The most common signs are papilloedema in optic neuritis close to the disc. Lesions further behind the eye may just show a scotoma, loss of colour vision or unilateral blindness. As damage to the optic pathway progresses optic atrophy may occur (see page 597), the first sign of which is temporal pallor.

Eye movements

Abnormalities are often found in MS, and may cause symptoms such as oscillopsia or diplopia. The most usual sign is horizontal jerk nystagmus. Weakness of the lateral rectus is more common than isolated nerve III and IV palsy. Internuclear ophthalmoplegia is often bilateral and may coexist with gaze paresis to produce the 'one-and-a-half' syndrome.

ONE-AND-A-HALF SYNDROME

This occurs with a lesion at the facial nucleus in the lower pons, where the lesion extends up to involve the ipsilateral medial longitudinal fascicle (MLF); it is extremely closely allied to internuclear ophthalmoplegia (these signs are difficult to many and no apology is made in repeating their nature).

The salient points of the normal pathway pertinent to this syndrome are:

- Attempted lateral gaze to the right is controlled by the left frontal eye field which sends axons down to the contralateral nerve VI nucleus; having decussated in the midbrain, they proceed down to the ipsilateral (right) abducens nucleus in the lower pons and into abducent motor neurons;
  - the right eye abducts normally.

- Fibres cross from the abducens nucleus (as abducent internuclear neurons) to the contralateral (left) MLF, where they ascend to synapse with the (left) oculomotor nucleus and into the oculomotor neurons;
  - the left eye adducts normally.
- The facial nucleus lies in close proximity to the abducens nucleus in the lower pons and a lesion here will cause:
  - a left facial palsy
  - a left abducens palsy.
- In 'one-and-a-half' syndrome the lesion also extends to involve the MLF and thus also causes;
  - a failure of adduction on gaze to the right, ie a right internuclear ophthalmoplegia.
- As always in an internuclear ophthalmoplegia you can demonstrate normal action of the third nerve in adduction by testing accommodation.

2. How might motor dysfunction be apparent?

Spastic paraparesis (see page 299): impaired mobility is common, usually as a result of demyelination within the spine (transverse myelitis). There is pyramidal weakness but spasticity is often more of a problem than the weakness itself.

LMN signs can occur as the dorsal motor roots leave the cord; see, in particular, Bell's palsy (page 340).

3. What symptoms and signs of cerebellar dysfunction might the patient have?

Gait disturbance, nystagmus, dysarthria and intention tremor occur (see page 357). Incoordination of individual limbs or truncal ataxia may be all that is apparent; it is usually seen in combination with pyramidal signs.

4. How might other brain-stem disease be apparent?

Facial palsy occurs (see page 339), alongside other signs such as hemifacial spasm and rippling in the muscles – myokymia. Occasionally persistent hiccup, the lateral medullary syndrome or the locked-in state can occur. Paroxysmal symptoms are brief, repetitive and persist for months before gradually remitting, eg trigeminal neuralgia with associated sensory signs and motor loss.

5. How might sensory dysfunction be apparent?

The presence of perineal numbness with disturbed sphincter function is characteristic of MS, as is Lhermitte's sign, in which disturbing pains shoot down the body, into the chest or limbs, on flexing the neck.

Unpleasant sensory symptoms often accompany damage to the posterior columns in the cervical cord, and spinothalamic damage may lead to loss of pain and temperature sensation; however, rather non-specific tingling in the limbs may be the only symptom.

On examination, signs in keeping with the above symptoms may be found; however, loss of vibration sense in the legs is occasionally seen even in the absence of symptoms.

6. Do autonomic symptoms occur in MS?

Autonomic symptoms occur in most patients with MS, bladder symptoms being the most common in women and impotence in men.

7. Describe the cognitive and affective symptoms and signs that might occur

An overall impairment of intelligence, related to the duration of disease and affecting memory rather than language, occurs. Depression is more common than expected compared with other patients with a similar level of neurological disability and, although hypomania does occur, it should not be confused with pathological laughter and crying that arise from loss of central inhibition of facial and bulbar reflexes in extensive brain-stem disease.

8. What patterns of MS are there?

- **Relapsing/remitting MS:** symptoms come and go. Periods of good health or remission are followed by sudden symptoms or relapses (80% of people at onset).
- **Secondary progressive MS:** follows on from relapsing/remitting MS. There are gradually more or worsening symptoms with fewer remissions (about 50% of those with relapsing/remitting MS develop secondary progressive MS during the first 10 years of their illness).
- **Primary progressive MS:** from the beginning, symptoms gradually develop and worsen over time (10–15% of people at onset).

9. What are the incidence and prevalence in the UK?

Between 3/100 000 and 7/100 000 of the population are diagnosed with MS each year and about 100–120/100 000 of the population have MS. From these rates it is estimated that, in England and Wales, about 1800–3400 people are newly diagnosed with MS each year and that 52 000–62 000 people have MS.

NICE (2003) guidance on making a diagnosis of MS

There is no single specific diagnostic test available, but, in practice, the diagnosis can be made clinically in most people.

- When an individual presents with a first episode of neurological symptoms or signs suggestive of demyelination (and there is no reasonable alternative diagnosis), a diagnosis of MS should be considered.

- When an individual presents with a second or subsequent set of neurological symptoms, which are potentially attributable to inflammatory or demyelinating lesions in the CNS (and, again, there is no reasonable alternative diagnosis), the individual should be referred to an appropriate expert for investigation.

A diagnosis of MS should be made clinically:

- by a doctor with specialist neurological experience
- on the basis of evidence of CNS lesions scattered in space and time
- primarily on the basis of the history and examination.

When doubt about the diagnosis remains, further investigation should:

- exclude an alternative diagnosis; or
- find evidence that supports the potential diagnosis of MS:
  - dissemination in space should usually be confirmed, if necessary, using MRI, interpreted by a neuroradiologist, using agreed criteria such as those described by McDonald et al. (2001)
  - dissemination in space may also be confirmed using evoked potential studies; visual evoked potential studies should be the first choice
  - dissemination in time should be confirmed clinically, or using the MRI criteria described by McDonald et al. (2001).

Other tests supportive of the diagnosis of MS, such as analysis of the CSF, should be used only when either the investigation is being undertaken to exclude alternative diagnosis or the situation is still clinically uncertain.

The diagnosis of MS is clinical and MRI should not be used in isolation to make the diagnosis. CT of the brain should be used only to exclude alternative diagnoses that can be diagnosed using that investigation.

Any CSF samples taken from individuals who might have MS should be tested for the presence of oligoclonal bands and should be compared with serum samples.

The evidence supporting the diagnosis and its degree of certainty should always be documented formally in the medical notes and letters discussing the diagnosis. This allows the diagnosis to be critically reviewed and reinvestigated if necessary.

Source: National Institute for Health and Clinical Excellence (2003) *CG8 Multiple Sclerosis: NICE guideline 26*. London: NICE. McDonald et al. (2001) Recommended diagnostic criteria for MS. *Ann Neurol* 50:121–7.

SCENARIO 3. CERVICAL MYELOPATHY

In the lower limbs, while the muscle bulk is preserved there is clasp knife spasticity, with clonus at the ankle (and the knee?) and weakness in a pyramidal distribution. The reflexes are pathologically brisk and Babinski's sign is present; the abdominal reflexes are absent.

The sensory symptoms may not be at all marked despite clear signs: when involved there is evidence of dorsal column loss with impairment of vibration sense and cutaneous sensation, whereas proprioception is relatively preserved; the spinothalamic tracts carrying pain and temperature are relatively spared in cervical myelopathy.

A good candidate

Will look for and, if present, note that in the upper limbs the reflexes are asymmetrical and inverted – the midcervical reflex pattern. (Inverted reflexes are the contraction of triceps when the biceps tendon is tapped and finger flexion when supinator is tapped. Biceps and supinator jerks may be absent as a result of damage at C5–6, whereas the triceps and finger jerks are brisk because their reflex arcs lie below the level of the lesion. This is the midcervical reflex pattern.) However, the signs in the upper limbs may not be marked.

Questions

1. What symptoms might the patient have complained of?

- Chronic weakness of the lower limbs, perhaps with sensory loss; the latter may continue up the trunk.
- Bladder or bowel disturbance (although not always), and men may have a loss of potency.
- The cervical spine is often painful, but not always, and there is often reduced movement.

2. What do you know about the movements of the cervical spine?

There are three movements for which the cervical spine is responsible:

1. Flexion and extension is performed at the atlanto-occipital joint
2. Lateral rotation is performed at the atlantoaxial joint
3. Lateral flexion involves the whole spine.

3. What is the likely cause?

Cervical spondylosis – a degenerative disease that is most pronounced in the midcervical region at C5–6, and the myelopathy associated with spondylosis is often maximal at this level.

4. What are the other causes of a cervical cord lesion?

The most common causes of a cervical cord lesion are cervical spondylosis and demyelination, although tumours – both intrinsic and extrinsic – and syringomyelia need consideration. The duration of onset and associated features are helpful in distinguishing them; spondylosis is a degenerative condition of the cervical spine and occurs in older patients:

- Demyelination: possibly a younger patient, look for other lesions dissociated in space. Is there anything in the history to suggest lesions dissociated in time
- Syringomyelia: dissociated sensory loss ± bulbar signs (see page 345).
- Intrinsic cord lesions: spinothalamic loss occurs earlier than dorsal column loss.

5. How will you investigate a patient with presumed cervical cord disease?

Clinical differentiation between the causes, and particularly exclusion of a tumour, are not usually possible, so the cord needs imaging. The signs in the upper limb and the sensory level help dictate where the spine is imaged. MRI is the ideal investigation or CT myelography.

Check vitamin B_{12}.

6. How will you manage cervical myelopathy?

Myelopathy at one level, if the result of a disc prolapse, or multiple levels caused by diffuse narrowing of the canal are best managed in consultation with a neurosurgeon. Manage conservatively, with a collar, only if surgery is unsuitable.

SCENARIO 4. MYOTONIC DYSTROPHY

The face is long and expressionless with bilateral ptosis, cataracts and wasting of temporalis, masseter and (invariably) sternomastoid; frontal balding is seen in men. Eye closure is weak – the sclera may remain visible in severe cases.

There is myotonia – the patient has difficulty in releasing grip, eg on handshake; you will be able to demonstrate percussion myotonia – best seen in the tongue (as teeth marks) or at the thenar eminence.

There is wasting and weakness of the peripheral muscles, initially distal – especially the forearms, sparing to a degree, at first, and the small muscles of the hands – subsequently becoming more proximal and affecting the limb girdle. Hyporeflexia and subsequent areflexia develop.

A good candidate

Will be looking for the following more unusual features:

- Myotonia disappearing as the weakness develops
- External ophthalmoplegia – rarely
- Dysphagia and dysarthria from both weakness and incoordination consequent on myotonia
- Reduced intelligence or a history of progressive dementia
- Bradycardia and cardiomegaly
- A cardiac pacemaker
- Cor pulmonale secondary to diaphragmatic weakness, with subsequent hypoxaemia or right heart failure
- Small firm testicles
- Gynaecomastia.

Questions

1. What can you tell me about the aetiology?

It is inherited as an autosomal dominant condition; the locus is at chromosome 19 q13.2–q13.3. Males are affected more commonly than females.

It exhibits anticipation whereby the features become more severe and appear earlier in subsequent generations. Presenile cataracts may have been present in prior generations before the full-blown syndrome occurred in an individual. There may have been a progressive social decline in the family in successive generations.

Diabetes mellitus occurs in 5% as a result of impaired insulin secretion.

The cardiac disorder occurs in two-thirds of cases, most often recognised on ECG rather than clinically. This is the result of disease of the conducting system rather than of the myocardium.

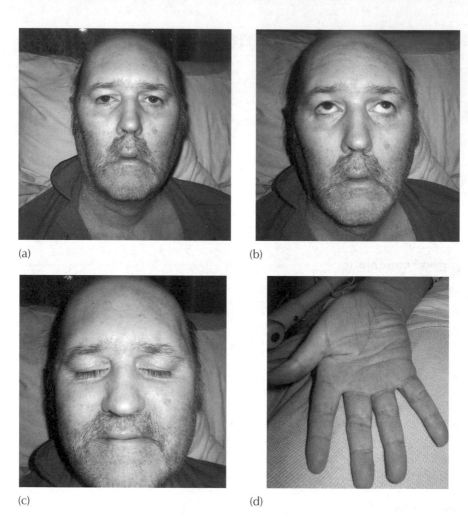

(a)

(b)

(c)

(d)

Figure 3.19   (a) Myotonic dystrophy facies (b) on upgaze (note furrowed brow); (c) weakness of eye closure; (d) wasting of abductor pollicis brevis (note flat, featureless thenar eminence)

2. *What is the differential diagnosis?*
- Fascioscapulohumeral dystrophy
- Hypothyroidism: slowness of thought and prolonged muscular contraction (see page 620).

3. *How could the patient present?*

Presentation is in the third and fourth decades, often after the gene has been passed on, before the onset of gonadal failure. Weakness of the hands and difficulty walking are the usual initial symptoms. Myotonia is rarely obtrusive initially, but the failure to release grip can become troublesome. Myotonia is often worse when cold or excited.

Poor vision, weight loss, impotence, ptosis and increased sweating are common. Later in the course of the disease, low-output heart failure consequent on bradycardia and heart block occur; hypersomnolence and drowsiness occur. Stokes–Adams attacks can occur and death usually results from cardiorespiratory failure in middle age, within 15–20 years of the onset.

4. *How will you investigate the patient?*

- Creatine kinase (CK): can be raised 2–10 times normal.
- IgG: reduced as a result of excess catabolism.
- Thyroid-stimulating hormone (TSH), thyroxine (T_4).
- FSH (follicle-stimulating hormone) raised as a result of gonadal resistance; normal testosterone.
- ECG: low-voltage p waves, bradycardia, first-degree block or more complex disorders.
- Electromyography (EMG): demonstrates myotonic discharges evoked by movement of the electrode. Myopathic potentials are recorded from weakened and wasted muscles during volitional movement. EMG will exclude McArdle's disease, in which painful and reversible contractures occur after exertion as a result of myophosphorylase deficiency, and cases of polymyositis, polyneuropathy and spinal muscular atrophy in which percussion myotonia can rarely occur.
- Muscle biopsy: frequent long chains of nuclei are seen in the middle of muscle fibres; these changes are much more marked *post mortem*.

5. *How will you manage the patient?*

- No treatment influences the progressive muscle wasting and weakness that eventually develop.
- Myotonia itself can be treated (but only if it causes functional impairment) with procainamide and/or phenytoin.
- Pacemaker for symptomatic bradycardia.

SCENARIO 5. PERIPHERAL NEUROPATHY

A good candidate

Will understand that the appearance of the feet and legs may be completely normal but look for particular signs of more severe distal neuropathy, namely:

- Deformity and collapse of the midfoot or ankle – Charcot's joint
- Healed or current pressure ulcers
- Dry, atrophic skin
- Wasting of the small muscles of the feet: evidenced by overriding toes, with evidence of increased pressure over the MTP heads and prominent extensor tendons (the flexors of the toes are in the plantar aspect of the foot and, if these are weak, the dorsiflexors, in the anterior aspect of the calf, as they are comparatively stronger, pull the toes up)
- The marked distal wasting of the muscles of the legs that is characteristic of Charcot–Marie–Tooth disease (see page 316)
- Cutaneous vasculitis (see page 520)
- Deforming arthropathy of the small joints (see page 543).

Distal bilateral sensory motor neuropathy

There is a stocking (and/or a glove) sensory neuropathy with loss of the deep tendon reflexes.

If it is severe, and depending on the aetiology, you may detect distal muscle weakness; the first muscles to be affected are often the small muscles of the feet, and is often most evident by overriding toes with prominent tendons. There is consequent pressure on the metatarsophalangeal (MTP) heads (you may see callus formation).

It occurs most commonly in the lower limbs – the nerves are longer and more susceptible to damage – than the upper limbs and, if present in the upper limbs, it is usually evident in the lower limbs.

Questions

1. What are the causes of a peripheral sensory motor neuropathy?

- Metabolic, eg diabetes mellitus, uraemia, hypothyroidism, porphyria, amyloidosis
- Malignant disease
- Collagen vascular disease:
  - SLE
  - rheumatoid arthritis (RA)
  - panarteritis nodosa (PAN)
  - scleroderma

- Deficiencies:
  - vitamin B_{12} and folate
  - thiamine (Wernicke's encephalopathy and Korsakoff's psychosis in those with alcohol problems)
  - niacin (pellagra)
- Inflammatory:
  - Guillain–Barré, syndrome
  - leprosy
  - diphtheria
- Toxic:
  - alcohol
  - drugs (isoniazid, vincristine, amiodarone, cisplatin)
  - heavy metals
- Hereditary:
  - hereditary sensorimotor neuropathy (HSMN 1) and 2, aka Charcot–Marie–Tooth disease
  - Refsum's disease
  - Freidreich's ataxia.

2. *What symptoms might the patient have?*

The following apply typically to diabetes:

- Unpleasant tingling, numbness, burning and aching in the lower legs and feet
- Mild weakness, nocturnal discomfort with a tendency to progression over many months
- Painless, punched-out, plantar foot ulcers are seen and are a major cause of morbidity.

The following are associated with diabetic neuropathy and may be sought if warranted:

- Autonomic dysfunction:
  - impotence
  - urinary retention
  - diarrhoea
  - constipation
  - postural hypotension (prudent and simple to check for)
- Amyotrophy:
  - proximal weakness
  - weight loss
  - slight sensory signs
- Femoral/sciatic neuralgia: note that, in diabetic sciatic neuropathy, straight-leg raise is normal and Lasegue's sign is absent
- Thoracic radiculopathy.

3. How would you investigate a patient with peripheral neuropathy?

Investigations are directed, by the pattern of the presentation, at the underlying cause for the precise diagnosis, but nerve conduction studies ± EMG are often helpful. Where there is a segmental demyelination, eg in diabetes, carcinoma or Guillain–Barré syndrome, abnormalities are detected with ease, but, in an axonal degeneration, eg caused by alcohol, the overall conduction velocity can remain normal despite a reduction in the number of units.

- Fasting glucose
- Serum vitamin B$_{12}$
- Protein electrophoresis
- FBC, ESR
- U&E, bone profile
- LFT and γ-glutamyltransferase (GGT)
- Chest radiograph
- Lumbar puncture (in Guillain–Barr, syndrome shows raised protein)
- Nerve biopsy: useful in a progressive neuropathy or to identify vasculitis as a cause; sensory nerves are usually biopsied.

4. How will you manage the patient?

This depends on the specific cause.

- In diabetes: rigorous control of glycaemia, often with intensive insulin regimens, can improve diabetic neuropathy, particularly if the syndrome arose acutely. Simple analgesics, tricyclic antidepressants, anticonvulsants (phenytoin and carbamazepine), oral mexiletine, intravenous lidocaine or topical capaiscin may be helpful.
- In nutritional deficiency, replace it.

Subacute combined degeneration of the cord (SCDC), if suspected, demands *emergency* treatment with intramuscular vitamin B$_{12}$

Incipient iron deficiency can be revealed with vitamin B$_{12}$ therapy

SCDC can be precipitated by giving folate for megaloblastic anaemia where vitamin B$_{12}$ deficiency is present. Thus vitamin B$_{12}$ deficiency must be excluded before giving folate.

5. How would you manage diabetic autonomic neuropathy?

Autonomic neuropathy is difficult to manage:

- Postural hypotension: helped by raising the head of the bed at night or fludrocortisone
- Vomiting: metoclopramide

- Diarrhoea: erythromycin or tetracycline is used to cure bacterial overgrowth responsible for diarrhoea
- Impotence: may require vacuum devices, intracavernosal papaverine, prostaglandin E_1 (also intraurethral) or sildenafil.

SCENARIO 6. CHARCOT–MARIE–TOOTH DISEASE

Also known as HSMN or peroneal muscular atrophy.

Type 1

This can occur in a young patient.

There is pes cavus (with or without an eqinovarus deformity) and clawing of the toes, and severe, symmetrical, distal wasting in the legs (you may see this in the upper limbs as the disease progresses) – this may spare the upper part of the lower limb (in 50% cases) causing the 'inverted champagne bottle' appearance or stork legs. Kyphoscoliosis is apparent (and in some a tremor is seen in the upper limbs)

There is weakness distally (which tends to cause bilateral foot drop) and the tendon reflexes are depressed or lost. There is a stocking sensory loss (to a variable degree) and a steppage gait.

The peripheral nerves may be thickened.

Ataxia may be present (this may be referred to as Roussy–Lévy syndrome, but it is not genetically distinct).

On examination of the gait there is foot drop and a steppage gait.

Questions

1. How do patients present?

HSMN-1 presents in the first decade with difficulty walking or with foot deformity.

HSMN-2 has a later onset, with a peak in the second decade, but many cases present in middle or even late adult life, with weakness or wasting.

It is common and affects about 1 in 2500 individuals and HSMN is the most common inherited disorder of the peripheral nervous system. It is under-diagnosed.

2. How do HSMN-1 and -2 differ?

HSMN-2 tends to be confined to the lower limbs with less severe wasting and weakness; deformity at the feet or the spine occurs much less commonly and the peripheral nerves are not palpable.

3. What do you know about the aetiology?

HSMN-1 is classified according to electrophysiology and histopathology: HMSN-1 is a demyelinating peripheral neuropathy with onion-bulb formations on histology and HSMN-2 a primary axonal neuropathy with regeneration on histology.

In most cases the inheritance is autosomal dominant but autosomal recessive and X-linked forms occur.

4. *What is the differential diagnosis?*

- **Peripheral neuropathy**: wasting is not such a feature, sensory loss is more marked and perhaps in a stocking distribution. If the neuropathy is long standing, pes cavus may occur.
- **Mononeuropathy**: may occur in the context of diabetic peripheral neuropathy or vasculitis; the common peroneal nerve may be damaged at the neck of the fibula. However, mononeuropathy is neither symmetrical nor proximal.
- **L4–5 root lesion**: may cause bilateral foot drop but inversion at the ankle is also lost and there are dermatomal sensory signs. Furthermore, adduction may be impaired and the reflexes are normal.
- **Cauda equina lesions**: must be actively considered where there are distal signs, eg an absent ankle jerk. There is saddle anaesthesia and sphincter involvement.
- **MND**: progressive muscular atrophy may cause LMN signs in the limbs but the pattern of the disease, with appearance of UMN signs, and the complete absence of sensory involvement help differentiate between the two disease processes.

5. *What management could you offer the patient?*

Orthotic appliances and sometimes surgical correction of foot deformity or tendon transfer can help affected individuals.

SCENARIO 7. FOOT DROP

Common peroneal nerve palsy

On examination of the patient's gait, there is unilateral foot drop, the foot is inverted and there is wasting of tibialis anterior; dorsiflexion of the foot is weak, as is eversion and extension of the toes. The reflexes in the lower limb are normal and there is sensory loss on the outside of the leg and across the foot, characteristic of a lesion of the common peroneal nerve.

Look for a scar or bruise at the top of the fibula.

The anatomy of the common peroneal nerve

The common peroneal nerve is a terminal branch of the sciatic nerve; it arises in the lower third of the thigh and runs downwards through the popliteal fossa, closely following the medial border of biceps. It is in a very exposed position as it leaves the popliteal fossa, crossing superficially the lateral head of gastro-cnemius, then passing behind the head of the fibula and winding laterally round the neck of the bone, it pierces peroneus longus and divides into its two terminal branches, the superficial peroneal nerve and the deep peroneal nerve.

Questions

1. What are the causes of a common peroneal lesion?

As the common peroneal nerve is vulnerable at the neck of fibula, it can be damaged with inversion injuries at the ankle, which lead to a fracture of the neck of fibula. It can also be damaged by poorly fitting cast or splints that put pressure at that site.

Deep peroneal nerve palsy (rare)

Unilateral foot drop with preserved eversion. The sensory loss is confined to a very small area on the dorsum of the foot on the lateral half of the great hallux and median half of the second toe.

The superficial peroneal nerve supplies peroneus longus and brevis, which evert the foot; in a lesion of the deep peroneal nerve these are unaffected. The lateral cutaneous nerve of the leg is also a branch of the common peroneal nerve and, as it is unaffected, the sensory loss is confined to a much smaller area.

L4, L5 root lesion

There is unilateral foot drop and, alongside weakness of dorsiflexion, there is weakness of inversion of the foot. Weakness of hip abduction may be evident. The reflexes are normal and there are sensory symptoms and signs in the L4, L5 dermatomes (see page 287).

The causes of this are lesions at the L4, L5 root of plexus such as a prolapsed intervertebral disc, a tumour in the cauda equina or obstetric injury to the lumbosacral trunk.

Foot drop, with weakness of all the muscles in the foot and preserved proximal power.

Peripheral neuropathy

Foot drop, but there may be weakness of all the muscles of the foot with normal movements at the hip and knee and a stocking sensory loss.

Sciatic nerve lesions

Foot drop, loss of the ankle jerk, extensive sensory loss and, depending on the level of the injury, weakness of hamstrings. The lesion results from pressure, trauma, vasculitis or tumour. It is rare but this author has seen it in buttock haematoma.

Root or plexus lesions

Foot drop with loss of the ankle jerk, anal reflexes, saddle anaesthesia and urinary incontinence. It can be caused by cauda equina compression from a tumour or a prolapsed disc, or plexus damage from trauma or tumour.

MND

Foot drop with wasting, fasciculation, hyperreflexia and normal sensation.

Corticospinal lesions

Paraparesis

This suggests a spinal cord lesion. Ascertain the level. Are the arms involved? Is there a sensory level?

Parasaggital lesions (eg meningioma) that damage both homunculi, leading to bilateral foot drop, are very rare.

One leg is weak.

Brown–Séquard syndrome

This is caused by lesions affecting half of the cord, eg hemisection; there is ipsilateral paralysis and loss of joint position sense below the lesion. At the level of the lesion there is ipsilateral analgesia and thermoanaesthesia but there is contralateral loss of these modalities a few segments below the lesion, ie there is dissociated sensory loss. There is hypertonia and brisk reflexes ipsilaterally. There will be sphincter disturbances. It is caused by trauma, infection, tumours, MS and degenerative diseases.

Dissociated sensory loss is a very important sign in clinical neurology.

The patient can feel the slightest touch in an affected area but is unable to distinguish one end of a pin from the other. Selective loss of pain sensation is a feature of syringomyelia, hemicord lesions (eg Brown–Séquard syndrome) and the lateral medullary syndrome.

Anterior cerebral artery occlusion

As there is frontal lobe damage, check for a grasp reflex on the ipsilateral side. The motor cortex responsible for the lower limb is supplied by the anterior cerebral artery (see below).

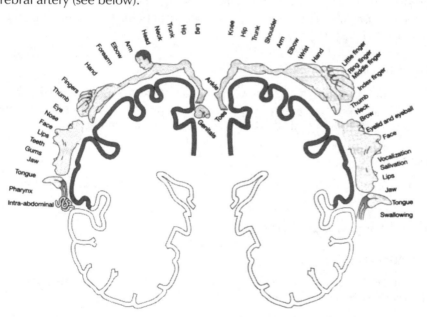

Figure 3.20   Lateral surface of the brain; arterial supply showing how the limbs are involved depending on the arterial territory.
Kind permission has been given by Continuum International Publishing Group to reproduce the diagram above taken from The Brain's Behind It by Alistair Smith, published in 2001

Cortical lesion

The arm and leg are weak on the same side – hemiparesis (see page 336). The lesion is likely to be above the cervical cord.

SCENARIO 8. PARKINSON'S DISEASE

The patient has a resting, 'pill-rolling' tremor, bradykinesia, mask-like expressionless facies with a tendency to dribble saliva. On standing the posture is stooped and there is some difficultly maintaining posture, with a tendency to fall with poor correction. On walking there is a festinant gait – shuffling, small steps on a narrow base, with little arm swinging and difficulty turning. There is dysarthria and the voice is quiet and monotonous.

In the limbs there is 'lead-pipe' rigidity, ie resistance to passive movement right throughout the range of movement; superimposed upon this is the tremor, giving the feeling of cogwheel rigidity. Ask to see the patient write.

A good candidate

Will consider the differential diagnosis and look for other neurological features of the Parkinson's disease + syndromes:

- Multisystem atrophy:
  - autonomic failure – Shy–Drager syndrome
  - ataxia – olivopontocerebellar degeneration
  - severe akinesia – striatonigral degeneration
- Progressive supranuclear palsy:
  - failure of downward gaze, pyramidal signs and dementia – Steele–Richardson–Olszewski syndrome.

Questions

1. What symptoms might the patient have?

Tremor, being very common, is to be expected; it is usually asymmetrical.

Bradykinesia is usually not noticed by the patient but commented on by relatives; it is often the most disabling feature, however. Postural abnormalities and difficulty in walking can lead to instability and falls. Constipation and depression occur.

2. What is known about the aetiology?

The aetiology is unknown, but it probably reflects a genetic susceptibility to environmental factors.

There is destruction of the dopaminergic neurons in the substantia nigra. About 85% of these neurons must be lost, with a corresponding loss of dopamine, before symptoms and signs occur. The median age of onset is 55 years.

3. What other conditions are considered when you assess the patient?

Parkinsonism is seen in the following situations:

- Pure parkinsonism
- Postencephalitic parkinsonism (encephalitis lethargica)
- Neuroleptic drugs
- MPTP (1-methyl-4-phenyl-1,2,3,6-tetrahydropyridine) toxicity
- Cerebral anoxia, caused by bilateral basal ganglia infarction.

Furthermore, parkinsonism is associated with other neurological features in:

- Wilson's disease
- Huntington's disease
- Cerebral palsy
- Progressive supranuclear palsy (Steele–Richardson–Olszewski syndrome)
- Multisystem atrophy (Shy–Drager syndrome)
- Cortical Lewy body disease.

4. How will you investigate the patient and make a diagnosis?

There is no diagnostic test, the diagnosis being clinical and needing two out of: bradykinesia, rigidity and tremor. The response to pharmacological therapy is characteristic and to all intents and purposes confirms Parkinson's disease. If there is no response to therapy consider the differential diagnoses.

5. What do you know about the management of Parkinson's disease?

Levodopa – the gold standard – may be associated with an earlier onset of motor fluctuations; thus it may be preferable to delay its use, particularly in younger patients. In older patients and in those with significant disability, it should not be delayed. It is combined with the dopa decarboxylase inhibitors benserazide and carbidopa.

- Dopamine agonist monotherapy with ropinerole may delay the onset of motor fluctuations. Other class members include the ergot derivatives, apomorphine and pramipexole.
- The role of selegiline in neuroprotection remains controversial. Entacapone and amantadine also have roles.
- Antimuscarinics reduce cholinergic activity in the brain, and are particularly useful for drug-induced or postencephalitic parkinsonism.
- Surgical therapies such as pallidotomy, bilateral subthalamic deep brain stimulation and fetal transplantation can be considered for those who fail medical therapy.

SCENARIO 9. WASTING OF THE SMALL MUSCLES OF THE HAND

Three patterns may be seen.

Weakness confined to abductor pollicis brevis

There is wasting of APB; abduction of the thumb against resistance is weak. The cause is compression of the median nerve in the carpal tunnel, ie **carpal tunnel syndrome** (see page 330).

If the lesion is at the elbow there will also be **weakness** of the following:

- **Flexor carpi radialis**: leading to weak flexion at the wrist; on attempted flexion adduction occurs caused by flexor carpi ulnaris (supplied by the ulnar nerve).
- **Flexor pollicis longus** and **flexor digitorum profundus (lateral half** – only the index finger): weak flexion at the interphalangeal joints (IPJs) of the first two fingers, while the lumbricals attempt flexion at the metacarpophalangeal (MCP) joints; on making a fist the first two fingers tend to remain straight whereas the latter two flex; the latter two are weakened, however, by the loss of **flexor digitorum superficialis**.
- **Flexor pollicis longus**: weak flexion of the terminal phalanx of the thumb.

There will be sensory loss over the lateral half of the palm, over the lateral three-and-a-half fingers and, on the dorsal surface of the hand, the tips of the lateral three-and-a-half fingers.

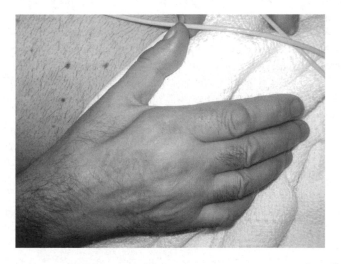

Figure 3.21   Wasting of first dorsal interosseus neuro-wasting of small muscles.

Weakness confined to abductor digiti minimi and first dorsal interosseus

There is wasting of ADM and the first dorsal interosseus (DI), and weakness of abduction of the little finger and abduction of the index finger, respectively. In both cases the muscle belly can normally be seen and felt. Look for the characteristic sensory loss. The cause is usually an ulnar nerve lesion at the elbow (see page 332).

Weakness of all three muscles

There are many causes and to get to the bottom of it may require a detailed neurological examination; check for:

- Horner syndrome
- Ptosis
- Facial weakness
- Wasting of the tongue
- Jaw jerk
- Sternomastoid wasting
- Wasting, weakness and reflex changes in all four limbs
- Sensory loss and dissociated sensory loss.

Again there are characteristic patterns:

- Unilateral wasting, weakness of finger extensors, flexors and triceps. Triceps reflex is lost. There is sensory loss on the ulnar aspect of the forearm and hand; these signs indicate problems at the C7, C8 and T1 roots or the lower part of the brachial plexus. If this is caused by a cervical rib there may be a subclavian bruit and diminished pulses in that arm; if it caused by Pancoast's tumour, Horner syndrome may be evident, with a cough, cachexia; lymphadenopathy and radiotherapy tattoos on the chest.
- Unilateral wasting of the whole upper limb with flaccid paralysis of the limb, areflexia and ipsilateral sensory loss. The usual cause is an avulsion injury to the brachial plexus, eg after a motorcycle accident. Horner syndrome may be present.
- Unilateral (or bilateral) wasting of the hand, ipsilateral areflexia and dissociated sensory loss, in a cape-like distribution on the affected side(s). Look for trophic skin on the affected side, with shiny swollen fingers and evidence of multiple small injuries or burns on the fingers. This suggests intrinsic cord pathology such as syringomyelia.
- Bilateral wasting of the hands* with spasticity in the lower limbs and a sensory level: suggests a cord lesion at C8, T1 (not cervical myelopathy[!]

---

*A common question is 'Is the weakness of the small muscles of the hand likely to be a result of cervical spondylosis?'. Obviously a trick question because T1 is not a cervical root! Furthermore, a good working rule is that wasting of the small muscles is uncommon in spondylosis and another cause should be sought.

because it is the wrong level; T1 is not a cervical root) such as trauma or a tumour.

- Bilateral generalised wasting and weakness, fasciculation, hyperreflexia and no sensory signs: suggests MND (see page 326); look at the tongue and listen to the voice.
- Distal wasting, weakness and sensory loss in all four limbs, areflexia and glove-and-stocking sensory loss – peripheral neuropathy (see page 312).
- Distal wasting and weakness in all four limbs, hyporeflexia, baldness, ptosis and cataracts: dystrophia myotonica; look for percussion myotonia.

SCENARIO 10. MOTOR NEURON DISEASE

You may see any combination of UMN and LMN symptoms and signs, and they are often initially asymmetrical. It is the coexistence of upper and lower motor signs in the same muscle groups at the same time that is pathognomonic of MND.

Three clinical patterns are initially seen, which tend to merge with time:

1. **Amyotrophic lateral sclerosis (ALS)**: there is a spastic tetraparesis (or paraparesis) (*lateral corticospinal tracts*) with added LMN signs – wasting and fasciculation (*anterior horn cells*); note that ALS often initially presents with predominant spinal UMN signs, when it is termed 'primary lateral sclerosis'.
2. **Progressive muscular atrophy**: there are predominantly LMN signs in the limbs, particularly wasting, with fasciculation and weakness in the hands and arms.
3. **Bulbar palsy**: there is LMN involvement of the lower cranial nerves shown by dysarthria with quiet, hoarse or nasal speech; there is palsy of the muscles of mastication, facial muscles, muscles of deglutition and the tongue, which is flaccid and shows fasciculation. The gag reflex is diminished or absent (in contrast to pseudobulbar palsy – a UMN lesion – where there is a small spastic tongue, exaggerated jaw jerk and gag reflex; it can coexist in MND but is less common).

Questions

1. Tell me about the aetiology of MND

There are familial and sporadic forms of ALS. In 20% of familial forms there is an identifiable mutation in the gene for copper/zinc superoxide dismutase (SOD-1) located on the long arm of chromosome 21. Genotype and phenotype correlate poorly. In most cases, however, the cause is unknown.

It is rare and tends to affect people who are middle-aged to elderly.

2. How might the patient present?

Those with bulbar palsy present with dysarthria and dysphonia, dysphagia and difficulty chewing, with nasal regurgitation of fluids, recurrent chest infections and dyspnoea; there may also be orthopnoea as a result of diaphragmatic weakness.

If MND affects the limbs it often presents with weakness of a hand or the whole upper limb, with wasting that the patient has noticed, such that the muscles may appear to have been sucked out of the hand; progressive foot drop occurs and cramps are common.

3. What other conditions must be distinguished from MND?

- **MS** and **polyneuropathies** both share features with MND but both have sensory signs, which are absent in MND.
- **Cervical myelopathy** will show UMN and LMN signs at the same time, but not in the same muscle groups and there are no cranial nerve signs.
- A pure **motor neuropathy** can be confusing because, in MND, LMN signs can dominate the presentation.
- **Cord or cauda equina compression** causes sphincter disturbance – this does not occur in MND.
- **Myasthenia gravis**: weakness of the external ocular muscles does not occur in MND.
- **Diabetic amyotrophy** is dominated by proximal lower limb weakness and wasting.
- **Cervical and lumbar stenosis**: this combination may be confusing because it can cause UMN signs in the upper limbs and LMN signs in the lower limbs.

4. How will you investigate the patient?

The diagnosis is clinical and depends on the simultaneous existence of UMN and LMN signs in the same muscle groups in the limbs and similar signs affecting the cranial nerve-innervated muscles. If there is any concern that a spinal cord lesion might be present, imaging of the spine is essential, ideally with MRI. EMG will show denervation but not its cause; surface EMG in all limbs can reveal widespread denervation before signs are evident.

5. Outline the management

The condition is progressive and the backbone of treatment is mostly supportive care, with the aim of overcoming difficulties and reducing symptoms. Speech and language therapy may help with dysarthria, dysphonia and dysphagia should they develop, and these bulbar symptoms commonly lead to malnutrition. Riluzole has been recommended by NICE for asymptomatic patients with AML; it extends the time to mechanical ventilation in this invariably fatal disease.

6. What is the prognosis?

ALS has a remorseless progression in both muscles involved and severity, with death usually occurring within 2–4 years of diagnosis, predominantly from ventilatory failure, aspiration pneumonia or choking; malnutrition also contributes. The median survival rate from onset, in those with bulbar symptoms, is 20%; only 5% survive for 5 years.

Spinal-onset disease fares better with a median survival of 29 months and 15% surviving for 5 years.

The predominantly LMN syndromes – progressive muscular atrophy (or spinal muscular atrophy) – fare better, with a more benign course than ALS.

The predominantly UMN syndromes are rarer; they start insidiously in the legs and ascend ultimately to involve the bulbar muscles. Pseudobulbar emotional lability can be distressing because cognition is normal.

SCENARIO 11A. BULBAR PALSY

There is a history of dysarthria and/or dysphagia and, as the condition progresses, there may be inhalation of foodstuffs

There is a flaccid tongue with prominent fasciculations. Palatal movement and the gag are absent.

The speech is characteristically weak.

The causes are:

- MND
- Syringobulbia
- Guillain–Barré syndrome
- Poliomyelitis
- Neurosyphilis.

SCENARIO 11B. PSEUDOBULBAR PALSY

- There is a history of dysarthria (of a more spastic type) and/or dysphagia.
- The tongue is spastic and fasciculations are absent. The gag is spastic.
- The speech is weak.

It occurs most commonly in patients with diffuse small vessel cerebrovascular disease as a sequela of hypertension. The typical presentation is difficulty in walking and progressive dementia; incontinence can occur. Examination may reveal primitive reflexes and bilateral pyramidal signs affecting the cranial nerves as well as the peripheral nervous system. The jaw jerk will be brisk and the gait may be marché petit pas (see page 360).

Other causes include MS, MND and tumours high in the brain stem.

SCENARIO 12. CARPAL TUNNEL SYNDROME

There is wasting of APB; abduction of the thumb against resistance is weak. Sensation in the distribution of the median nerve is reduced (see below); light touch and two-point discrimination are most affected, pin prick and hot/cold less affected, and proprioception is preserved. As sensation over the palm is spared, it is clear that the lesion has occurred after the deep palmar branch has left the median nerve, ie there is compression of the median nerve in the carpal tunnel, ie **carpal tunnel syndrome**.

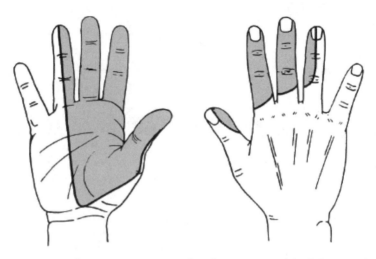

Figure 3.22   Median nerve sensory distribution. (Modified from *Aids to the Examination of the Peripheral Nervous System*).

If the compression is prolonged, weakness of APB and opponens pollicis can be demonstrated.

Tinnel's and Phalen's signs may be positive (but have little predictive value for the presence or absence of median nerve compression).

Is there a scar over the carpal tunnels?

A good candidate

Will do the following:

- Comment on the lack of involvement of the deep palmar branch of the ulnar nerve, which supplies all the other intrinsic muscles of the hand, and also comment on the features of an underlying aetiology:
  - usually idiopathic or related to repeated occupational trauma

- pregnancy
- RA
- hypothyroidism
- acromegaly
- gout
- the menopause.

Beware of a cervical radiculopathy.

Questions

1. What are the presenting symptoms?

It characteristically occurs during pregnancy and in middle-aged women, especially those who do manual work; it usually begins as pain and tingling, and eventually decreased sensation in the thumb, index and middle fingers, and radial half of the ring fingers. Symptoms may be more proximal, even up to the arm in some. It is worse at night, or first thing in the morning, and may be relieved by shaking the hand at the side.

2. What is the management?

Rest, splinting, diuretics and local hydrocortisone injection may help temporarily while an underlying cause is relieved.

Division of the flexor retinaculum will rapidly relieve symptoms; however, sensory function will return over 6–12 months and muscle power, if impaired, may return almost to normal.

3. What signs would you expect with damage to the median nerve at the elbow?

With damage to the median nerve at the elbow, the pronator muscles in the forearm and the long flexor muscles of the wrist and fingers, with the exception of flexor carpi ulnaris and the median half of flexor digitorum profundus, will be affected/paralysed. The forearm will be supine; wrist flexion is weak and accompanied by adduction. There is no flexion at the interphalangeal joint of the first two fingers on making a fist.

SCENARIO 13. ULNAR NERVE PALSY

Ulnar nerve compression at the elbow

There is wasting of flexor carpi ulnaris and the medial half of flexor digitorum profundus (the latter *may* be seen on the inner aspect of the flexor surface of the forearm); the hypothenar eminence, interossei and ulnar half of the thenar eminence are wasted. There is hyperextension of the MCP joints in the little and ring fingers with flexion of their IPJs – this is the ulnar claw hand.

Adductor pollicis is weak – ask the patient to hold a piece of paper between the thumb and a flat palm; normally on attempting to remove the paper resistance is maintained by adduction but, in an ulnar nerve palsy, with weakness of adductor pollicis, the thumb will flex under the influence of flexor pollicis longus (anterior interosseus nerve branch of median nerve in forearm); this is Froment's sign.

On attempted flexion at the wrist against resistance, the hand deviates to the radial side; you will not see the tendon of flexor carpi ulnaris as it attaches to the pisiform bone.

There will be sensory loss over the medial one-and-a-half fingers (see below). Look for evidence of surgery, osteoarthritis or a fracture at the elbow.

Points: you must examine the hand with it pressed against a flat surface because the long extensors and flexors act as abductors and adductors to some extent.

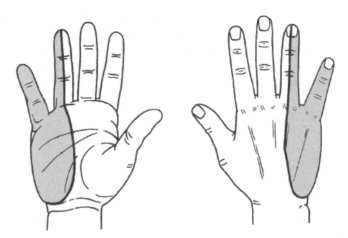

Figure 3.23   Ulnar sensory loss. (Modified from *Aids to the Examination of the Peripheral Nervous System*).

Question

1. With what might the patient present and what treatment can you offer?

There may be an antecedent history of trauma or surgery at the elbow. Sensory symptoms are not prominent but the patient may notice some numbness and tingling of the two ulnar fingers and the ulnar border of the palm. Usually attention is drawn to the palm by the muscular wasting and weakness.

If the patient's habits are responsible (eg resting the elbows on a hard surface while reading) suggest a change; in entrapment the nerve can be released from the ulnar groove and placed anteriorly.

SCENARIO 14. WRIST DROP

You are likely to be asked to examine the neurology in the upper limbs; wrist drop should be immediately obvious and it dictates what follows.

Bear in mind that wrist drop is caused by weakness of flexor carpi radialis longus (C5, C6 and the radial nerve) and flexor carpi ulnaris (C7, C8 and the posterior interosseous nerve, a branch of the radial nerve):

1. In a **radial nerve lesion** the hand will be flexed at the wrist and brachioradialis will be weak.
2. In a **posterior interosseus nerve lesion** there will be radial deviation of the hand.
3. In a **corticospinal lesion** the arm will be slow to rise and the elbow as well as the wrist may remain a little flexed.

A good candidate

Will look for the following:

- **Scars or bruises** over the spiral groove of the humerus in the posterior part of the arm
- **Facial asymmetry**
- **Muscle wasting**: particularly in the extensor component of the forearm.

Assess tone; it will be normal in peripheral nerve or root lesions and usually increased in a corticospinal lesion.

To assess abduction of the fingers in a radial nerve palsy, you must lay the hand flat on a table; it is impossible to abduct the fingers when the MCP joints are flexed.

Radial nerve palsy

1. There is weakness of extension at the wrist and of the fingers and brachioradialis. Triceps is normal, so the lesion is likely to be in the spiral groove of the humerus – this is a 'Saturday night' palsy. Look for sensory loss in the snuffbox.
2. There is weakness of extension at the wrist and fingers, and of the elbow and brachioradialis. There is sensory loss in the snuffbox, down the posterior surface of the lower part of the arm and down a narrow strip on the back of the forearm (the area is relatively small because of overlap from adjacent nerves). This is likely to result from damage to the radial nerve in the axilla, eg someone who is drunk falling asleep with the arm over a chair, or a brachial plexus lesion.

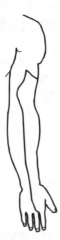

Figure 3.24   Radial nerve palsy – area of sensory loss in high radial nerve lesions.

3. If it is a root lesion affecting just C7–8, eg spondylosis or a plexus lesion, there will be radial deviation on wrist extension as flexor carpi radialis longus is not affected or brachioradialis (it must be immediately evident that the key muscle in a radial nerve palsy is brachioradialis).

Posterior interosseous nerve lesion

There is weakness of finger extension with radial deviation of the wrist on attempted extension – signifying weakness of extensor carpi ulnaris. Brachioradialis is intact. The reflexes are normal and there is no sensory loss, which results from a posterior interosseous nerve lesion; this is rare and can result from entrapment of the nerve or be part of a mononeuritis of any cause, eg diabetes mellitus.

Hemiparesis

There is generalised weakness of the muscles of the upper limb in a pyramidal distribution, ie it is most marked in deltoid, triceps, wrist extension and finger extension. This indicates a corticospinal lesion. The tone is increased and there is hyperreflexia. Look for facial and lower limb weakness.

Question

1. What will you tell the patient with wrist drop to expect and what will you do?

The prognosis is good; in compression recovery is over weeks. Even if the wrist requires splinting muscle function starts to recover 4–8 months later.

The wrist must be splinted in extension as must the MCP joints – the latter not rigidly.

SCENARIO 15. HEMIPARESIS

You will need to consider during the course of the examination whether the anatomical distribution of signs suggests a cortical lesion, a more unusual brain-stem lesion or a lesion within the cord.

While introducing yourself, consider whether the patient is dysphasic.

The patient has paucity of movement on the affected side and a pyramidal posture – that may be all that your need to say; it summarises the following two paragraphs succinctly:

- A characteristic gait if the lower limb is affected, where the leg is held in extension at the hip and knee, and adducted; it will describe an arc as it moves through and the foot may be inverted and plantar flexed such that the toes scrape the ground (look at the pattern of wear on the shoes, and, if you look at the shoes, think ahead to the possible aetiology – are there spots of precipitated glucose on the toes of a man's shoes to suggest diabetes mellitus with glycosuria?)
- The arm, if affected, may be held in flexion at the elbow and wrist, internally rotated at the shoulder and does not swing when the patient walks.

The face, if affected, shows UMN facial weakness, possibly with involvement of the palate, tongue, muscles of mastication and external ocular muscles.

The following are also present:

- Pyramidal drift
- Clasp-knife spasticity in a pyramidal distribution*
- Clonus at the ankle (and knee?)
- Weakness in a pyramidal distribution: where the flexors in the upper limb and the extensors in the lower limb are relatively stronger
- Hyperreflexia
- Upgoing plantars: Babinski's sign.

A good candidate

Will look for the following:

- Oppenheimer's sign: a firm stroke downwards on the medial side of the tibia will, in extensive pyramidal lesions, lead to an extensor plantar response.
- Hoffman's reflex: flicking or nipping the nail of the second, third or fourth finger will, if the reflex is present, cause a flexion of these fingers and maybe the thumb. Its presence indicates that tendon reflexes are hyperactive. (Occurs with any cause of hyperreflexia.)
- Homonymous quadrantanopia or hemianopia (see page 589).
- Papilloedema, which may be present if there is a space-occupying lesion.

*Clasp-knife spasticity is when there is resistance to movement up to a point and then resistance is overcome, in contrast to lead-pipe rigidity where there is resistance right throughout the movement

Check the following:

- The gag reflex on both sides of the palate
- If there is any sensory loss, eg hemianaesthesia or inattention: this would indicate involvement of the sensory cortex either in the postcentral gyrus or less commonly in the internal capsule.
- Listen to the quality of the voice and the strength of the cough and if appropriate assess the swallow.

Specifically consider the possibility of dysphasia (see page 291 and 353):

- Expressive (motor) dysphasia indicating damage to Broca's area anterior to the motor cortex: as a result of its localisation to the motor cortex, it is not unusual if the hemiparesis is caused by a cortical lesion. The speech will not be fluent but the understanding will be intact.
- Receptive (sensory) dysphasia indicating damage to Wernicke's area in posterior lesions: it is less commonly seen and implies a larger area of damage. The speech is fluent but mistakes are made with words or even syllables; when severe the speech can just be nonsense, there is little or no understanding and an erroneous diagnosis of 'confusion' can be made.

Listen to the carotid arteries for bruit – the more elderly the patient, the more you should consider the presence of atheromatous carotid artery stenosis; the younger the patient the more you should consider carotid artery dissection.

Is there a suggestion of lesions in other parts of the CNS, eg optic atrophy, cerebellar dysfunction? Is there anything in the history to suggest lesions dissociated in time? Both of these may suggest demyelination in the appropriate clinical setting.

Desirable information from the history

- What hand does the patient write with? Most right-handed people and perhaps 50% of left-handed people are left hemisphere dominant; speech is located in the dominant hemisphere and dysphasia can therefore suggest disease in the dominant lobe.
- What was the onset of the weakness? An abrupt onset of a neurological deficit with a tendency to improve, with or without preceding transient ischaemia, is almost diagnostic of stroke, particularly in the presence of cardiovascular risk factors.
- A protracted history with a slowly worsening circadian headache, drowsiness, vomiting, symptoms attributable to focal brain damage and seizures suggests a space-occupying lesion. The nature of the lesion usually dictates the speed of onset, eg meningioma or breast carcinoma metastases.

All this is designed to move towards answering the questions:

- **What is the lesion?**
- **Where is the lesion?**
- Are all the signs consistent with a unilateral hemispherical lesion?

Causes of a unilateral hemispherical lesion

- Stroke:
  - Ischaemic:
    - Thrombotic
      - Cardiovascular disease or risk factors: hypertension – particularly in lacunar infarcts
      - Prothrombotic tendencies: antiphospholipid syndrome
      - Vasculitis: internal carotid artery dissection
    - Embolic: source of emboli:
      - Cardiac:
        - Atrial fibrillation (AF)
        - Mural thrombus
        - Subacute bacterial endocarditis
      - Carotid artery:
        - Stenosis – more elderly
        - Dissection – younger and distinct clinical features (more commonly embolic phenomena rather than loss of blood flow)
        - Peripheral emboli though a persistent foramen ovale (PFO)
  - Haemorrhagic:
    - Hypertension
    - Aneurysm – subarachnoid haemorrhage
    - Arteriovenous malformation
  - Thrombocytopenia, eg severe ITP (idiopathic thrombocytopenia purpura), but rare:
    - Bleeding diathesis:
      - Anticoagulants
      - Antiplatelets
      - Thrombolysis
- Intracranial space-occupying lesion:
  - Tumour
  - Aneurysm
  - Abscess
  - Haematoma
  - Granuloma
  - Tuberculoma
  - *Toxoplasma* sp.
  - Cysts, eg cysticercosis.

If the signs are not consistent with a unilateral cranial lesion, is it a specific brain-stem syndrome (see Weber syndrome, page 372) or a more unusual spinal cord syndrome?

SCENARIO 16. FACIAL PALSY

The muscles of facial expression are supplied by the facial nerve (nerve VII). The loss of the nasolabial fold confirms a facial palsy; however, if deepened compared with the normal side it may indicate a longstanding palsy.

There are four main patterns that may be seen:

1. Unilateral weakness of all facial muscles
2. Unilateral weakness of all the facial muscles except frontalis and orbicularis oculi
3. Bilateral facial weakness
4. Weakness of one or two muscles unilaterally.

Unilateral weakness of all facial muscles

Loss of tone in the muscles leads to characteristic sagging in LMN lesions.

There is paralysis of all the muscles of facial expression on the left-hand side; the patient cannot wrinkle the forehead.

On attempting to close the eyes, you can see Bell's phenomenon (where the globe rotates up) because closure is incomplete. The nasolabial fold on the left is less distinct, the corner of the mouth is drooping slightly and the patient cannot puff out his or her cheek, whistle or evert the lip (the latter indicating weakness of platysma).

The absence of wrinkling of the forehead on the affected side indicates that this is an LMN nerve VII palsy and the most common cause is **Bell's palsy**.

A good candidate

Will look for the following:

- Loss of taste on the anterior two-thirds of the tongue: indicating that the chorda tympani is involved.
- Ipsilateral hyperacusis: indicating that the nerve to stapedius is involved.
- Evidence of corneal damage, conjunctivitis or a lateral tarsorrhaphy.
- Aberrant reinnervation, indicating a longstanding lesion: when the patient blinks does the corner of the mouth twitch? When he or she smiles does the ipsilateral eye twitch?
- Enquire about excessive lacrimation on the affected side: the punctum of the lacrimal duct is separated from the conjunctiva; the volume of tears is reduced in Bell's palsy, however, as the parasympathetic fibres in the greater superficial petrosal nerve are interrupted.

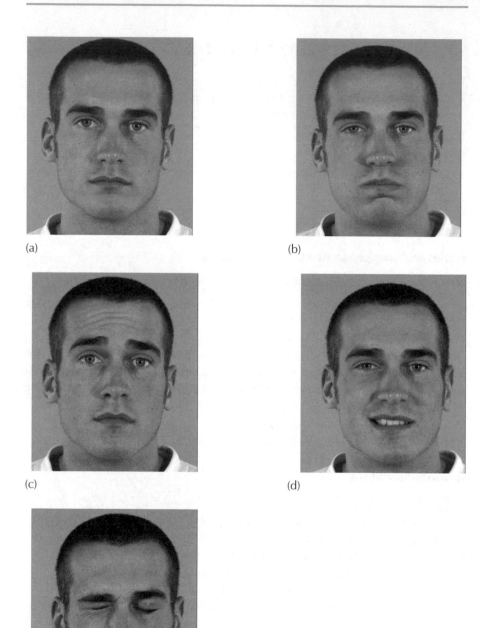

(a)

(b)

(c)

(d)

(e)

Figure 3.25   Neurology of Bell's palsy:
(a) face at rest; (b) 'Puff out your cheeks';
(c) 'raise the eyebrows' – note the symmetry
of furrows on the forehead; (d) 'Show me
your teeth'; (e) 'Close your eyes', showing
left facial weakness

Consider causes other than Bell's palsy:

- Vesicles behind the ear, within the external auditory meatus or on the palate: these indicate geniculate herpes, ie Ramsay Hunt syndrome. Vertigo, tinnitus or deafness may be found.
- Associated cranial nerve lesions:
  - compression at the cerebellopontine angle, eg acoustic neuroma or meningioma – nerves V, VI, VII, VIII
  - very rare:
    - Millard–Gubler syndrome (see page 372)
    - Foville syndrome – unilateral nerve VI or VII and failure of conjugate gaze to the affected side (cannot look at the lesion).
- Dissociated lesions in space, eg optic atrophy, relative afferent papillary defect, internuclear ophthalmoplegia or ataxia (or a history of dissociated lesions in time) – MS (the long, post-nuclear, intrapontine course of nerve VII leaves it susceptible to demyelination – see below).
- Evidence of diabetes or sarcoid (lupus pernio?): mononeuropathy.

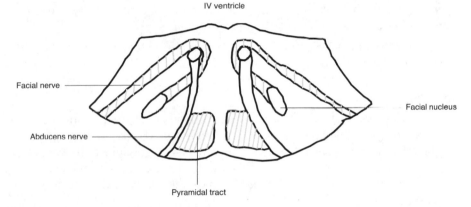

Figure 3.26   Transverse section of pons.

Unilateral weakness of all the facial muscles except frontalis and orbicularis oculi

There is no loss of tone – hence sagging is not a prominent feature. Look for ipsilateral limb weakness. Stroke or tumour is by far the most common cause.

Bilateral facial weakness

This can be very easy to miss, but look for an expressionless face. Bell's phenomenon will be seen if it is LMN, along with some sagging. The causes are the following:

- Sarcoid: parotid swelling, pyrexia and possibly rash
- Neuromuscular disease:
  - fascioscapulohumeral dystrophy
  - dystrophia myotonica (see page 309)
  - myasthenia gravis (see page 350) – ptosis and ophthalmoplegia may be present, with fatigability; the pupils are normal
- Parkinson's disease, but in truth this is more akinesia than weakness
- Multilacunar states may have bilateral UMN facial palsy along with pseudobulbar palsy (see Pseudobulbar palsy and Examination of gait), a brisk jaw jerk and exaggerated involuntary movements or expressions
- Lyme disease: erythema migrans and the appropriate geographical history
- Guillain–Barré syndrome is the usual cause if it is acute, with generalised weakness and areflexia.

Weakness of one or two muscles unilaterally

This is usually caused by aberrant reinnervation after Bell's palsy.

Rarely it may be a result of damage to the terminal branches of the nerve, eg parotid tumours, trauma, skin cancer or rarely leprosy.

Does the history mention parotid surgery or is there evidence of this or parotid enlargement on examination?

Test facial sensation

- Bell's palsy: normal. The blink reflex will be expected to be poor on the affected side in Bell's palsy but the contralateral eye blinks, indicating that the afferent limb of the reflex, ie the trigeminal nerve, is intact. (Beware of testing the corneal reflex if there is any suggestion that it may not have normal sensation because this might damage the cornea and cause an ulcer.)
- Acoustic neuroma: loss of corneal sensation, with no blinking of either eye, ie the afferent limb is affected; it might be the only sensory abnormality. The weakness can be mild and deafness is present.
- Stroke: facial hemianaesthesia
- Brain-stem lesions such as syringobulbia or glioma show dissociated sensory loss, where pain sensation is lost but light touch is preserved. This follows an 'onion-peel' pattern, quite distinct from peripheral lesions of the trigeminal nerve (see Syringomyelia page 345)
- Leprosy: anaesthesia in the cooler parts of the face, ie the nose and ears – rare.

Management of Bell's palsy

Patients commonly feel pain in or behind the ear. There can be slight alteration of sensation on the affected side of the face, which can be ignored as long as sensation is objectively intact, including the afferent limb of the corneal reflex. Loss of taste on the ipsilateral anterior two-thirds of the tongue commonly occurs and you should ask about hyperacusis and any rash that may indicate herpes zoster; ask about any recent viral infection or immunisation.

Questions

1. How would you treat Bell's palsy?

Blinking is affected and closure may be incomplete, especially at night, so consider an eye pad or taping the lid shut during sleep. The cornea can be dry so artificial tears should be prescribed. Reassurance that the patient has not had a stroke is prudent because patients are often anxious, and tell the patient that most get better and only a minority do not.

What is more contentious is the use of corticosteroids and/or aciclovir.

The most recent Cochrane Database systematic review in 2004 is quite clear in its conclusion that the available evidence from randomised controlled trials does not show a significant benefit from treating Bell's palsy with corticosteroids (Salinas et al. 2004). However, the available evidence for treating Bell's palsy with steroids (and aciclovir) is similarly well reviewed (Gilden 2004; Holland and Weiner 2004). This has again been recently tested in double blind, placebo controlled, randomised trials of patients within 72 hours of presentation with Bell's palsy who received either prednisolone (25 mg twice daily), aciclovir (400 mg five times daily), prednisolone and aciclovir or placebo for 10 days. Early treatment with prednisolone significantly improved the chances of complete recovery at 3 and 9 months; aciclovir alone or in combination offered no benefit. The gist of this is that prednisolone 1 mg/kg started as early as possible (certainly within 72 hours and definitely within a week) might shorten the course and prevent permanent facial disfigurement.

There is a close association between Bell's palsy and herpes simplex virus (HSV) infection and the limited evidence from randomised trials suggests that aciclovir (or valaciclovir) may reduce the proportion of patients with incomplete recovery 4 months after treatment (Allen and Dunn 2003).

2. What is the prognosis in a Bell's palsy?

Two-thirds of patients recover spontaneously without treatment; just over a tenth have minor sequelae. A sixth of patients are left with moderate-to-severe weakness, contracture, hemifacial spasm or synkinesis (from aberrant reinnervation).

If there is total paralysis, electrodiagnostic studies, performed 1–2 weeks after the onset, can demonstrate the 15% with axonal degeneration. This must recover by wällerian regeneration and can take many months.

If the palsy is partial, the patient is likely to fare better, with 94% making a full recovery.

In those who recover without treatment major improvement occurs within 3 weeks in 85%.

3. *What are the poor prognostic features in Bell's palsy?*

- Complete facial palsy
- No recovery by 3 weeks
- Age over 60 years
- Severe pain
- Ramsay Hunt syndrome (herpes zoster virus – HZV)
- Associated conditions: hypertension, diabetes, pregnancy
- Severe degeneration of the facial nerve shown by electrophysiological testing.

This has again been recently tested in double blind placebo controlled, randomised trials of patients within 72 hours of presentation with Bell's Palsy who received either prednisolone (25 mg twice daily), aciclovir (400 mg five times daily), prednisolone and aciclovir or placebo for 10 days. Early treatment with prednisolone significantly improved the chances of complete recovery at 3 and 9 months; aciclover alone or in combination offered no benefit.

Sullivan F.M., Swan I.R.C., Donnan P.T. et al New England Journal of Medicine 2007 Oct 18; 1598–607. PMID: 17942873

N.B. The generated correspondence is also worthy of attention.

SCENARIO 17. SYRINGOMYELIA

In the upper limbs there is wasting and weakness of the hands (APB, ADM and first DI – see page 323) and the muscles in the forearm and arm (anterior horn cells), with areflexia and dissociated sensory loss – pain and temperature sensation (spinothalamic tracts), which we conclude from the presence of multiple small injuries and scars on the fingers. The sensory loss extends onto the trunk in a cape-like distribution.

In the lower limbs there is a spastic paraparesis and Horner syndrome.

You may see scoliosis and Charcot's joints in the upper limbs.

The patient has syringomyelia, a central cord syndrome; the differential diagnosis includes intrinsic cord lesions and Tangier syndrome.

Questions

1. What signs would you expect if the syrinx extended rostrally?

Rostral extension of the syrinx into the brain stem (syringobulbia) may cause dysarthria, dysphagia, wasting of the tongue and sensory loss in the face (sparing the central areas such as the mouth and nose until last – see below).

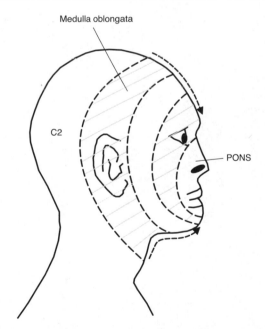

Figure 3.27   Syringomyelia.
Pattern of sensory loss seen in rostral extension syrinx into the brain stem the arrows show the progression of sensory loss.

2. What are the associations of syringomyelia and syringobulbia?

They occur commonly in association with the Arnold–Chiari malformation (cerebellar ectopia), where some of the cerebellum extends through the foramen magnum around the spinal cord. There may be associated cerebellar signs, and signs of raised intracranial pressure or cord compression.

3. Outline the management

If there is an Arnold–Chiari malformation decompression of the foramen magnum may be attempted to help the flow of CSF out of the fourth ventricle, preventing dilatation of the syrinx.

4. What are the causes of Charcot's joints?

Syringomyelia (shoulder or elbow), tabes dorsalis (knee), diabetes and leprosy.

SCENARIO 18. CEREBELLAR SYNDROME

The patient's speech is scanning, staccato (interrupted) and slurred. There is nystagmus (usually towards the side with the lesion – the direction of nystagmus is conventionally defined by the direction of the fast phase). On the side of the lesion the tone is normal and the reflexes are present (they may be + or ±). There is limb ataxia, an intention tremor, past pointing and dysdiadochokinesia. The gait is broad based and unsteady, and the patient has a tendency to fall to the affected side on walking (if this is not evident on normal walking, it can be brought out by asking the patient to walk heel to toe). Romberg's test (see page 283) is negative.

Vermal lesions may give truncal rather than limb ataxia; they can appear perfectly well until asked to stand.

A good candidate

Must be able to give a prompt considered differential diagnosis:

- A lesion in the ipsilateral cerebellar hemisphere:
  - demyelination – MS (see page 303)
  - cerebellar or brain-stem stroke – thromboembolic or haemorrhagic
  - space-occupying lesion, eg primary or secondary tumour
- Vermal or global cerebellar dysfunction:
  - chronic alcohol abuse
  - phenytoin
  - paraneoplastic
  - severe hypothyroidism
  - Friedreich's ataxia (see page 349)
  - a lesion at the cerebellopontine angle (see page 354).

The following are worthy of mention because they can present with ataxia and are treatable:

- Wilson's disease: tremor, chorea, dysarthria, mental deterioration, cirrhosis; autosomal recessive (chromosome 13) (see page 358)
- Refsum's disease: pes cavus, retinitis pigmentosa, nerve deafness, anosmia, cerebellar ataxia; autosomal recessive, as a result of abnormality in lipid metabolism – excess phytanic acid.

Questions

1. Apart from ataxia and slurred speech how could the patient present?

- Headache: many patients, even some with large tumours, present with a mild but persistent occipital headache, worse in the morning and that recurs on straining. As intracranial pressure rises the headache becomes severe and generalised with associated impairment of vision (papilloedema may occur).

- Visceral disturbances: persistent vomiting, hiccups, cardiorespiratory dysfunction and sudden death occur in this group of tumours.
- Cranial nerve dysfunction occurs from compression of the brain-stem nuclei.
- Hydrocephalus: dilatation of the lateral ventricles, especially the frontal horns, can cause intellectual and behavioural impairment.

2. *What investigations will you do?*

- MRI of the posterior fossa (or CT if unavailable); even with trivial symptoms and signs there can be a considerable mass in the posterior fossa; many are cystic and amenable to surgery
- Plasma alcohol, LFTs, GGT
- Phenytoin level
- TSH, T$_4$
- Glucose, lipids
- HIV test
- Chest radiograph: lung cancer causing paraneoplastic syndrome, or with multiple metastases
- ECG
- Maybe lumbar puncture if there is no space-occupying lesion.

SCENARIO 19. FRIEDREICH'S ATAXIA

The patient has pes cavus, kyphoscoliosis, spastic paraparesis, with extensor plantars, but areflexia as a result of an axonal neuropathy; ataxia is caused by spinocerebellar degeneration.

- Diabetes mellitus occurs in 10%
- Some have intellectual impairment
- Cardiomyopathy occurs in two-thirds.

Autosomal recessive or X linked; the onset is usually in childhood and always before age 25 years.

SCENARIO 20. ABSENT LOWER LIMB REFLEXES AND UPGOING PLANTARS

This may be the finding in a number of situations. The sensation may be normal or abnormal in the foot and lower limb depending on the cause.

The diagnoses to consider are:

- Diabetes mellitus: a peripheral neuropathy combined with a stroke; look for Charcot's joint, ulcers, hemiparesis
- Friedreich's ataxia: see above
- MND: see page 326
- Vitamin B_{12} deficiency: SCDC; a rare neurological emergency; if suspected that a patient has neurological symptoms or signs caused by vitamin B_{12} deficiency, he or she should receive parenteral replacement there and then after diagnostic bloods have been taken
- Tabes dorsalis.

SCENARIO 21. MYASTHENIA GRAVIS

There is bilateral ptosis (can be unilateral), which develops or is more evident on sustained upward gaze; the head is held back, the patient looking down the nose to counteract the ptosis; the face is expressionless and on attempted smiling you see a 'myasthenic snarl'. Muscle bulk is preserved (early in the disease).

Diplopia develops on holding the extremes of gaze; it does not correspond to an isolated nerve or muscle lesion and there is no proptosis.

On reading aloud or counting continually, the voice becomes weak and quiet. Neck weakness develops on holding the head up from the pillow and in the upper limbs proximal weakness becomes evident on repeatedly lifting a weight; shoulder weakness is greater than pelvic weakness.

Tendon reflexes and sensation are normal.

Questions

1. What do you know about the epidemiology and aetiology of myasthenia gravis?

The frequency and recognition of this rare condition are increasing; the annual incidence is between 0.25 and 2.0 per 100 000; however, there is no change in the number of patients aged under 40 who present, but there is a shift in the age-related frequency to those over 60, with a bias towards men.

The point prevalence has been estimated at between 100 and 400 per million. The prevalence of the disease is affected by the fact that 20% have spontaneous remission and 20–30% will die within 10 years of their diagnosis.

Myasthenia gravis is a heterogeneous disorder and in about 90% no cause is found, although there is likely to be a genetic susceptibility to largely unidentified environmental factors.

It is characterised by acquired weakness and the hallmark of the disease – fatigability of muscle; the heart is uninvolved. It may be localised or generalised and is caused by a defect of transmission at the neuromuscular junction.

IgG antibodies to the acetylcholine receptor are found. Immune complexes (IgG and complement) are deposited at the postsynaptic membrane, which cause interference and subsequent destruction of the acetylcholine receptor.

Thymic *hyperplasia* is present in 70% of patients aged below 40 years. These patients have an increased association with HLA-B8 and -DR3.

Thymic *tumours* occur in 10%; the incidence increases with age. These patients have antibodies to striated muscle and 30–60% of thymic tumours are associated with myasthenia gravis.

The peak incidence in men and women is in the eighth decade.

Women are affected more often than men despite the increase in male-specific incidence over the age of 60.

It may be associated with other organ- and non-organ-specific autoimmune diseases, eg thyroid dysfunction, RA, pernicious anaemia and SLE.

2. How may the patient present?

The complaint of weakness on work or the prospect of work is common, but objective weakness on exertion relieved by rest is rare. A presentation with painless, fatigable weakness is, as such, the hallmark of myasthenia gravis. However, fatigue is not always evident and can be overlooked.

The pattern of muscles involved varies between individuals but the most common initial presentation is weakness affecting the extraocular muscles, usually with ptosis (ocular myasthenia); diplopia may occur but only at the end of the day.

The proximal limb muscles, and the muscles of mastication and of speech and facial expression are commonly affected in the early stages; bulbar weakness can lead to regurgitation of fluids and importantly **respiratory weakness may occur**.

The involved groups may remain localised at the outset but become generalised with time; the condition tends to relapse and remit, and intercurrent illness, particularly infection, may provoke severe exacerbations. Pregnancy, hypokalaemia, over-treatment, change of climate, extreme emotion, exercise and certain drugs, eg penicillamine, opiates, aminoglycosides, suxamethonium and β blockers, can also provoke deterioration

3. How would you investigate the patient?

The diagnosis can be made clinically in many cases.

The most useful diagnostic test is acetylcholine receptor antibodies with 90% sensitivity and 100% specificity,* such that you usually do not have to resort to a Tensilon test.

On EMG there is a characteristic decrement in the evoked muscle action potential after stimulation of the motor nerve.

The chest radiograph may show a mediastinal mass but CT is necessary to look for a thymic mass.

---

*Two syringes are prepared, one with 10 ml 0.9% saline, the other with 10 mg edrophonium to a volume of 10 ml. A blinded observer must comment on the effect of a test dose of 2 ml of each intravenously (reactions can occur so resuscitation facilities, with atropine, must be present). After 30 s give the remainder of both syringes. The observer comments on the effect of both. It is positive only if edrophonium improves muscle power. It is often not dramatic; eye movements may in particular be difficult.

4. What do you know about the management?

Pyridostigmine, an anticholinesterase, is the drug of choice because of its sustained duration of action at a dose of 60 mg 3–16 times/day; atropine can be given for muscarinic side effects.

Overdose of pyridostigmine can cause a cholinergic crisis; although the weakness can be indistinguishable from myasthenia gravis, the cholinergic symptoms of hypersalivation, lacrimation, sweating, vomiting and miosis are characteristic. If there is this uncertainty about whether a patient's weakness is caused by cholinergics or myasthenia gravis a test dose of Tensilon can be given, with an anaesthetist and resuscitation equipment standing by.

Pyridostigmine does not alter the natural history of the disease.

Thymectomy is likely to benefit all patients, especially those under 40 years and those who have had the disease for < 10 years. After thymectomy 60% of non-thymoma cases improve. Thymomas require surgical excision because they may be malignant; however, the myasthenia gravis tends not to improve.

Immunosuppression with corticosteroids or azathioprine may offer an improvement for 70% of patients who have incomplete response to anti-cholinesterase.

Finally plasmapheresis – by removing the circulating antibody – can be tried in emergencies.

Myasthenic crises are life-threatening episodes of respiratory or bulbar paralysis. The onset of respiratory difficulty can rapidly become an emergency, and the facility to intubate and ventilate should be available. Respiratory muscle weakness is best measured by forced vital capacity (FVC) rather than peak flow.

SCENARIO 22. SPEECH DISTURBANCE

Expressive dysphasia

The patient with this has a paucity of movement on the right side in the upper limb and there is an UMN nerve VII palsy. The speech is not fluent with little melody, the patient appears to be putting great effort into his speech and the information content is high although there are sparse filler words and no paraphasias; the patient can repeat normally (the more global the defect the more likely this is to be impaired) and his or her comprehension is normal. This is a motor or expressive aphasia indicating damage to Broca's area in the frontal lobe, which is completely in keeping with the evident right hemiparesis; as Broca's area lies in front of the motor cortex of the left hemisphere, a stroke or a tumour is likely to be responsible.

Receptive dysphasia

The patient with this has fluent melodious speech; however, the information content is low and there are literal and verbal paraphasias and neologisms. The patient cannot repeat and has impaired comprehension. On further examination, I find that the patient has a homonymous hemianopia affecting the vision to the right. These signs are all in keeping with damage to Wernicke's speech area in the parietal lobe or the left cerebral hemisphere; a stroke or a tumour is the likely cause.

A good candidate

In either case, a good candidate must be able to give reasonable anatomical localisation for the lesion as well as the cause, ie where is the lesion? And what is the lesion?

Dysarthria

The patient with this has slurred speech but the actual content is normal, indicating a problem with articulation.

The causes of this depend on the associated features:

- LMN features seen in the muscles of articulation: facial weakness, wasting and fasciculation of the tongue, absent gag and palatal palsy; these signs are consistent with bulbar palsy as part of MND.
- UMN features: brisk jaw jerk; spastic, exaggerated gag; hemiparesis; emotional lability; pseudobulbar palsy in multilacunar states or MND.
- Cerebellar dysfunction: nystagmus, intention tremor and gait ataxia.
- Extrapyramidal features: resting tremor, akinesia, rigidity, festinant gait with poor arm swinging.

Is it just dysarthria? Beware a patient with a right hemiparesis who might have non-fluent dysphasia.

SCENARIO 23. CEREBELLOPONTINE ANGLE LESION

This causes the following ipsilateral signs – deafness and a facial palsy. The patient may complain of a sense of imbalance.

Later on, there is ipsilateral loss of the corneal reflex and then of sensation on the face and some weakness of the muscles of mastication occurs. Nerves IX, X, XI and XII may be affected with a decreased afferent and efferent limb of the gag and a hoarse voice, weak sternomastoid and trapezius, and weakness of the tongue such that it protrudes to the side of the lesion. Eventually long tract and cerebellar signs can occur from compression of the brain stem and cerebellum, respectively, with subsequent hydrocephalus.

The likely cause is an acoustic neuroma.

Unilateral deafness and tinnitus should always alert the clinician to the possibility of an acoustic neuroma; old age, noise injury or ototoxic drugs usually affect both ears.

The imbalance is often mild because the damage to the vestibular division of nerve VIII is slow and the other labyrinth has time to compensate. Contrast this with the crippling vertigo, nystagmus, nausea and vomiting that occur in vestibular neuronitis.

SCENARIO 24. FASCIOSCAPULOHUMERAL DYSTROPHY

There is facial, neck and limb girdle wasting and winging of the scapulae. The deltoids may be spared but the wasting of pectoralis is prominent. The upper limb reflexes are absent (see page 289).

Pelvic weakness occurs in only half of patients but the lower limbs are not severely affected – though foot drop might be seen. Lordosis with a protruding abdomen occurs.

It is an autosomal dominant condition in 75–90% of patients and sporadic in the rest.

It does not shorten life.

A good candidate

Will know the discriminant signs against a diagnosis of myotonic dystrophy, namely:

- There is no myotonia, balding or gonadal failure.
- The age of onset is younger, between the first and third decades; 95% show some signs by 20 years of age.
- Intelligence is normal.

Question

1. How does the patient present?

Initially weakness occurs in orbicularis oris and oculi and zygomaticus; the patient may have difficulty whistling or drinking through a straw. The extraocular muscles and the pharynx are spared. The weakness progresses downwards such that shoulder weakness is a presenting finding in over three-quarters.

CK is not significantly elevated.

SCENARIO 25. LIMB GIRDLE DYSTROPHY

There is shoulder and pelvic weakness with winging of the scapulae; atrophy is prominent. The hip girdle weakness is marked in gluteus maximus and the adductors and in the abdominal muscles; consequently the gait is wide based and the patient very lordotic. The tendon reflexes, apart from the ankle jerk, are absent.

It is inherited as an autosomal recessive condition, so it appears in both sexes. Patients present in their late teens and early 20s and although progressing slowly they have a reduced life expectancy.

CK is normal or only just modestly elevated. Facial weakness and wasting do not occur.

SCENARIO 26. TREMOR

Look at the patient as a whole and consider: is it a resting, postural or intention tremor?

What parts of the body are involved?

Specifically, are there any signs of Parkinson's disease?

When is the tremor maximal and is it coarse or fine?

Resting

There is a coarse, resting tremor of the hands. This is characteristic of Parkinson's disease (see page 321), where it is often unilateral at first and remains asymmetrical. It disappears on movement. The writing is small and cramped – micrographia.

Proceed to look for Parkinson's disease:

- Tone: cogwheeling rigidity throughout the range of movement.
- Bradykinesia: difficulty starting and stopping motor 'programmes'. Ask the patient to pretend to play a piano with the fingers; if the patient finds it difficult check the power. This will be normal in Parkinson's disease.
- Gait (see page 359): this is perhaps the most useful test. Look at the arms – do they swing? If the tremor persists during walking it is very suggestive of Parkinson's disease.
- Speech: quiet and the words tend to run into each other.

Postural

This type of tremor is more marked with the hands stretched out in front of the body.

- Essential tremor: coarse, more marked in one hand than the other; often confused with Parkinson's disease. The patient may spill the tea and writing may be illegible; however, unlike Parkinson's disease, it does not diminish in size. It is often improved by alcohol, (to which they can become addicted) or β blockers.

Proceed to try to exclude Parkinson's disease – an essential tremor can be resting and many patients with Parkinson's disease have a postural tremor!

- Look at the patient walk; the gait should be normal in essential tremor.
- The face is expressive and the patient's gestures are normal. The voice may be tremulous but of good volume. There may be tremor in the lips, tongue or chin.
- Physiological tremor: fine tremor, symmetrical; enhanced by anxiety, β_2 agonists and thyrotoxicosis.

Proceed to look for thyrotoxicosis and ask about drugs.

Intention

There is an intention tremor affecting the right hand; this indicates a lesion involving the right cerebellar hemisphere.

An intention tremor appears only as the hand approaches its target, unlike in essential tremor where the tremor can be present throughout all phases of movement and indeed worsen as the hand approaches the target.

Look for confirmatory signs of cerebellar disease (see page 347).

Coarse bat-wing tremor

This is seen in Wilson's disease. It is worth inspecting the cornea, illuminated from the side, or viewed from the side with an ophthalmoscope, for Kayser–Fleischer rings.

SCENARIO 27. ABNORMAL GAIT

Hemiparetic

One leg is held stiffly and describes an arc round the other leg as it is brought through with each stride – circumduction. The foot is inverted and the lateral aspect/toes scrape the ground. The ipsilateral arm does not swing and is flexed at the elbow. This is a hemiparetic gait. The most likely aetiology is a lesion in the contralateral hemisphere such as a stroke or a tumour.

A good candidate

Will want to demonstrate what other areas of the CNS have been affected. Where in the CNS is the lesion – the motor cortex, lacunae, brain stem or spinal cord?

Are there contralateral cranial nerve signs to suggest a brain-stem syndrome (see page 372)?

Spastic paraplegic

Both legs are held stiffly and circumduct; the feet are inverted and may cross – described as scissoring (see page 299).

Always consider if the presentation is in keeping with spinal cord compression.

Cerebellar

The base is broad, the pattern of walking is irregular, the patient has a tendency to veer to one side or the other (or both) and stagger on turning (compare page 347).

To see if the patient consistently veers to one side (suggesting an ipsilateral cerebellar hemisphere lesion) have him or her march on the spot with the eyes open and closed, walking heel to toe or round a chair.

In vermal lesions the patient may stagger in any direction and may wobble if he or she sits – truncal ataxia

Bilateral foot drop

Both feet are lifted high off the ground when walking and produce a slapping sound as they hit the ground. This high stepping gait is most commonly caused by bilateral foot drop seen in, for example, hereditary sensory motor neuropathy (Charcot–Marie–Tooth disease – see page 316) (such a patient would have difficulty walking on toes or heels).

Sensory ataxia

Both feet are lifted high off the ground when walking; the base is broad and the patient watches the feet and the ground intently while walking. Explain that you would not test Romberg's sign because you may expect the patient to fall without making any attempt to correct him- or herself. Joint position sense is absent in the feet ± knees.

The history may suggest that the patient has trouble walking in the dark. Causes of sensory ataxia include:

- Sensory neuropathy
- Tabes dorsalis
- Spinocerebellar degeneration
- Subacute combined degeneration of the cord
- MS.

Unilateral foot drop

One leg is lifted higher than the other during each stride. The affected foot hangs down while it is elevated. The patient can walk on the toes but not on the heel on the affected side. The patient cannot dorsiflex the foot against resistance; this is a result of unilateral foot drop and is usually caused by a unilateral common peroneal nerve lesion (see page 318).

Parkinsonian

The patient is stooped, the steps are small and festinant on a narrow base (compare marche petit pas), there is little arm swinging, turning is laborious and freezing may occur. In early disease the only feature may be one arm that does not swing.

Marche petit pas

Literally – walk with a small step.

The gait is very similar to a parkinsonian gait but, although the steps are small, the base is broad, the posture is normal, ie upright, and there is normal arm swinging. This gait is seen in normal pressure hydrocephalus (dementia, gait dyspraxia and incontinence very early in the course of the dementia) and multi-lacunar infarcts (dementia with bulbar palsy and emotional lability).

Waddling

The shoulders swing from side to side in an exaggerated manner. The patient lifts the feet off the ground not only by flexing the knee and hip but by tilting the trunk; this is a waddling gait. Go on to perform Trendelenburg's test.

Causes: any cause of a proximal myopathy. In an adult it is likely to be caused by a myopathy (see page 366) or osteoarthritis of the hips. In a child consider muscular dystrophy or congenital dislocation of the hips.

Antalgic

The good limb rushes through so as to decrease the time that the antalgic limb bears the weight; the antalgic limb strikes the ground softly and may buckle slightly to reduce the pressure put through it. It is usually associated with arthritis of the hip, knee, ankle or foot.

SCENARIO 28. PROXIMAL WEAKNESS OF THE UPPER LIMB

The main proximal muscles that are tested and are of interest to you are the following (main roots are in bold where appropriate).

Muscle	Movement	Nerve	Root
Deltoid	Shoulder abduction	Axillary	**C5**, C6
Biceps	Elbow flexion, forearm in supination	Musculocutaneous	C5, C6
Triceps	Elbow extension	Radial	C6, **C7**, C8
Brachioradialis	Elbow flexion, forearm midway between supination and pronation (with the thumb pointing at the shoulder)	Radial	C5, **C6**

Pectoralis major, shoulder adduction, being supplied by many roots is not a very useful localiser. As becomes clear below, you may want, in certain circumstances, to test the following.

Muscle	Movement	Nerve	Root
Supraspinatus	First 20° of shoulder abduction	Suprascapular	**C5**, C6
Intraspinatus	External rotation of shoulder	Suprascapular	**C5**, C6
Trapezius	Shoulder elevation	Spinal accessory	C3, C4
Serratus anterior	Scapular fixation and rotation	Long thoracic	C5, C6, C7

Deltoid can work only if the scapula is anchored by trapezius and serratus anterior.

The range of movement of the shoulder is increased by rotation of the scapula.

Unilateral weakness confined to the proximal upper limb is usually caused by a lesion of the cervical roots, brachial plexus or peripheral nerves.

In corticospinal lesions all the upper limb extensors, proximal *and* distal, are weak. Bilateral proximal weakness of the upper limbs is probably a result of a myopathy.

Have the patient remove all clothes on his or her trunk and upper limbs and consider the following:

- Skin: heliotrope rash around the eyes, or scaly erythema below the fingernails and on the elbows and knees, suggesting dermatomyositis
- Joints: subluxation of the humerus – damage to axillary nerve

- Wasting: particularly obvious at the deltoid where the shoulder will appear squared off; look at the patient from behind for winging of the scapula – paralysis of serratus anterior
- Face:
  - unilateral ptosis – Horner syndrome suggesting an avulsion injury of the cervical roots and T1
  - bilateral ptosis – mytonic dystrophy (see page 309), myasthenia gravis (see page 350) or myopathy
  - facial droop – with hemiparesis.

Tone will be normal (or decreased) in peripheral disorders of nerves or muscles and may be increased in corticospinal lesions.

Test power, coordination and reflexes looking for the following patterns:

1. Deltoid weakness alone: as biceps and brachioradialis are spared this cannot be a C5, C6 root lesion. If the scapula does not move on abduction (ie trapezius and serratus anterior are working) this is an axillary nerve lesion. The reflexes are normal; you might find a patch of sensory loss below the shoulder on the lateral aspect of the upper arm (where a scout/soldier's patch might be).
2. Deltoid, biceps and brachioradialis weakness: this suggests a C5, C6 or plexus lesion; consider the following to take the case further:
   - C5, C6 cord lesion – biceps and brachioradialis reflexes will be absent but triceps and the lower limbs (being below C5, C6) will be brisk. Is there an inverted supinator reflex? The vibration caused by tapping for the brachioradialis reflex excites finger flexion (the muscles for finger flexion arise below the lesion at C7, C8 and can be easily excited). Some flexion is normal but if it occurs on tapping the supinator, and brachioradialis is absent, this is the 'inverted supinator reflex' and is a strong suggestion of a C5, C6 cord lesion. Test tone and power in the lower limbs and look for a sensory level (see Cervical myelopathy, page 307).
   - C5, C6 root or plexus lesion – biceps and brachioradialis reflexes will be absent but the triceps and lower limb reflexes will be normal. The precise level of involvement can be defined by which muscles are involved along the C5, C6 root. Proximal lesions will cause weakness of all the muscles; more distally the long thoracic nerve and serratus anterior will be spared, and a little further still within the brachial plexus the suprascapular nerve to supraspinatus and infraspinatus will be spared; more distally are the axillary nerve to deltoid, musculocutaneous nerve to biceps and radial nerve to brachioradialis.
3. Weakness of all the muscles in one upper limb with:
   - absence of the reflexes in the limb: if the rest of the examination is fine then this is likely to be a brachial plexus lesion. Check for Horner

syndrome and the sensation in C5–T1. Is there dissociated sensory loss? If so consider an intrinsic cord lesion, eg syringomyelia (see page 345).
- hyperreflexia: look at the face and the lower limb to ascertain if this is a hemiparesis and what the extent of that hemiparesis is.
4. Proximal weakness in both upper limbs: this is likely to be a myopathy or a disorder at the neuromuscular junction. Power and reflexes in the lower limbs will be crucial. The following are characteristic patterns:
   - Weakness of all the proximal muscles in both the upper and lower limbs. Reflexes are normal or reduced. Sensation is preserved. This suggests a myopathy; consider polymyositis, especially in an elderly patient, if the muscles are tender or if there is a rash suggesting dermatomyositis. Myasthenia is also possible so check for fatigability. Check for weakness of neck flexion – it is characteristic of myopathies such as polymyositis.
   - Selective weakness and wasting of proximal muscles of the upper and lower limbs. In this situation certain muscles are wasted and weak whereas an anatomical neighbour – supplied by the same root – is normal, eg brachioradialis (C5, C6) is wasted whereas deltoid (C5, C6) is intact. Look for winging of the scapula; these findings suggest muscular dystrophy. Test the facial and eye movements. The patient will tend to be young. If there is areflexia consider spinal muscular atrophy (see page 326).
5. Weakness of serratus anterior and/or trapezius: this occurs when it seems that deltoid is weak, although deltoid is intact but you are instead causing the scapula to rotate. Check:
   - Are the shoulders symmetrical? One may be lower in unilateral weakness of trapezius.
   - Compare the bulk of trapezius; it is easy to see wasting and feel it in the muscle bulk.
   - Look at the sternomastoids: the spinal accessory (nerve XI) supplies both sternomastoids and trapezius.
   - Have the patient push extended arms against a wall to look for winging of the scapulae – where the vertical border of the scapula lifts away from the thorax ('wings') if there is weakness of serratus anterior. Isolated damage to the serratus anterior can occur after damage to the long thoracic nerve, eg cervical gland biopsy.

Shoulder abduction can be weak as a result of impairment of the action of deltoid or because serratus anterior or trapezius does not fix the scapula. Hence, when testing shoulder abduction with one hand feel the tip of the scapula with the other – if it moves then there is, at least in part, a problem with trapezius or serratus anterior. To test deltoid in isolation, hold the scapula as the patient abducts.

Brachioradialis is again shown to be important (see Radial nerve palsy, page 334). It helps diagnose C5, C6 root lesions and define the extent of radial nerve damage, and can be selectively weak in muscular dystrophy. When testing elbow flexion, with the forearm between supination and pronation, be aware that biceps alone is up to the task, but one can feel brachioradialis during flexion – if it is weak it will remain soft or fail to contract at all.

SCENARIO 29. PROXIMAL WEAKNESS IN THE LOWER LIMB

'This patient has some difficulty walking', 'Examine the lower limbs/ legs' or 'Weakness of the legs'.

The main proximal muscles that are tested and are of interest are (main roots are in bold where appropriate):

Muscle	Movement	Nerve	Root
Iliopsoas	Hip flexion	Femoral	**L1**, **L2**, L3
Quadriceps	Knee extension	Femoral	L2, **L3**, **L4**
Guteus maximus	Hip extension	Inferior gluteal	**L5**, **S1**, S2
Hamstrings	Knee flexion	Sciatic	L5, **S1**, S2
Hip adductors	Hip adduction	Obturator	**L2**, **L3**, L4

Weakness confined to the proximal muscles of the lower limbs is usually caused by a myopathy or a problem at the neuromuscular junction, eg myasthenia gravis. Weakness of both the proximal and distal muscles is seen in MND. Unilateral proximal weakness is often the result of a femoral nerve lesion.

Inspect the patient for the following before checking the tone:

- Gait:
  - waddling with exaggerated shoulder sway in any cause of proximal weakness or in hip joint problems (see page 360)
  - antalgic (see page 361)
  - hemiparetic (see page 359).
- Weakness: have the patient rise from a crouch; those with proximal weakness cannot do this; a child with muscular dystrophy may use the arms to 'climb up' him- or herself (Gower's sign).
- Wasting in quadriceps: easiest to see when the patient is standing. You may want to compare the circumference of the thighs at a defined distance above the knee, but practically it is difficult; often, a more enlightening sign is seeing whether one trouser leg slides up further than the other, suggesting wasting on that side.
- Fasciculation.
- Look at the back: scars in the lower spine or buttock wasting.

Power, coordination and reflexes will reveal one of the following patterns:

- Weakness of iliopsoas and weakness and wasting of quadriceps: knee jerk reduced or absent; the adductors are normal* – the patient has a femoral

---

*Both quadriceps and adductors are supplied by L2, L3, L4 – but quadriceps is the femoral nerve and the adductors are the obturator nerve

nerve lesion. Is there sensory loss over the thigh and medial aspect of the shin? The nerve can be damaged by an abscess as it winds round the lateral border of psoas, by haemorrhage into psoas from anticoagulants, by a hernia as it passes into the thigh, by traction during hip surgery or by catheterisation of the femoral artery. However, the most common causes are diabetes mellitus where it can be painful in diabetic amyotrophy, zoster or vasculitis.

- Weakness of iliopsoas, quadriceps and the hip adductors: the knee jerk is reduced or absent – this indicates involvement of the L2, L3, L4 roots or a femoral/ lumbar plexus lesion. Dermatomal sensory loss is to be expected:
  - If the cauda equina is damaged the signs are likely to be bilateral. The most likely causes are:
    - a tumour, either primary or secondary – prolapsed discs are unusual at this level
    - pelvic malignancy ·
    - obstetric injury
    - neuralgic amyotrophy.
- Weakness of one leg in a pyramidal distribution, ie most marked in hip flexion, knee flexion, ankle dorsiflexion and eversion, hypertonia and hyperreflexia. This is a corticospinal lesion causing a hemiparesis. Look for other evidence of a hemiparesis: is there dysphasia (see page 291 and 353)?
- Weakness of both lower limbs in a pyramidal distribution: this is a corticospinal lesion but it is a paraparesis and the lesion is likely to be in the spinal cord. Look for a sensory level and consider whether the history suggests spinal cord compression.
- Diffuse weakness of the lower limbs proximally. Check the upper limb power and reflexes, if there are also signs in the upper limbs then the reflexes become the decisive factor:
  - reflexes preserved or reduced: consider myopathy, eg muscular dystrophy or polymyositis, or myasthenia gravis – fatigability
  - reflexes are lost: consider spinal muscular atrophy or myasthenic syndrome (Lambert–Eaton myasthenic syndrome). The reflexes are lost in Guillain–Barré syndrome but the weakness is distal as well as proximal
  - hyperreflexia: consider MND. Are there fasciculations, wasting and fasciculation of the tongue all with normal sensation? Are there other causes of a quadriparesis such as a multilacunar state. Look for the characteristic gait, jaw jerk, bulbar speech, spastic gag and emotional state. Finally, consider cervical myelopathy where the cranial nerves will be normal with reflex loss in the upper limbs.
- Other rarer patterns: isolated adductor weakness suggests an obturator nerve lesion, usually caused by obstetric injury. Sciatic nerve lesions cause distal weakness of the leg with or without hamstring weakness.

SCENARIO 30. ABNORMAL MOVEMENTS

An important practical differentiation between tremor and the abnormal movements is that the former is rhythmical and regular in its timing, the latter not so.

Tardive dyskinesia

The usual manifestation of tardive dyskinesia is **orofacial dyskinesia** where you see a variety of chewing, pouting and lip-smacking movements, **combined** with a discrete dystonia, or choreiform movements and, sometimes, rocking trunk movements.

Tardive dyskinesia is the most distressing side effect of neuroleptic treatment; it occurs only after 6 months of continuous administration. Withdrawal of the drug leads to a gradual improvement in about half of cases, with resolution taking up to 3 years. In some, however, there is no improvement and in a small minority there will be a relentless progression, resistant to all treatment, despite stopping the offending drug.

Be aware that drugs with neuroleptic properties, eg metoclopramide and prochlorperazine, are commonly prescribed, so a detailed drug history is essential in all patients with extrapyramidal disease.

Tics

There are rapid, repetitive, sometimes semi-purposeful movements. The patient may be able to suppress the movement partially but this leads to increasing anxiety and eventually a resumption of the movement.

Chorea

There are irregular jerky movements, of varying amplitude (usually), involving all the limbs, the trunk and sometimes the facial muscles, although not all together. Causes of chorea:

- Sydenham's chorea
- Chorea gravidarum
- Chorea with the oral contraceptive pill
- Huntington's disease
- Drug induced:
  - neuroleptic drugs
  - phenytoin
  - alcohol
  - levodopa
- With systemic disease:
  - thyrotoxicosis
  - polycythaemia rubra vera
  - encephalitis lethargica
  - SLE
  - hypocalcaemia
  - hypernatraemia
- Hemiballismus or hemichorea:
  - infarction
  - tumour.

Myoclonus

There is rapid, irregular jerking movement of the body (or part of the body).
A sudden bodily jerk when falling asleep, or when surprised, is the most common form of myoclonus occurring in normal people. In an exaggerated and generalised form – flexion myoclonus – it can be a manifestation of cerebellar degeneration.

Dystonia

This refers to the situation where a part of the body adopts an abnormal posture for a variable duration. It is often not static but associated with slow writhing movements of the affected part – athetosis.

Causes of dystonia:

- Focal dystonia:
  - writer's cramp
  - spasmodic torticollis
  - cranial dystonia
  - hemiplegic dystonia caused by:
    - strokes
    - tumours
    - encephalitis
    - trauma

- Generalised dystonia:
  - drug-induced acute and tardive dystonias:
    - antiemetics – prochlorperazine, metoclopramide
    - neuroleptics
    - levodopa and dopamine agonists
  - torsion dystonia
  - dystonia with other cerebral diseases:
    - hereditary:
      - gangliosidoses
      - metachromatic leukodystrophy
      - Wilson's disease
      - Huntington's disease
      - homocystinuria
    - acquired:
      - cerebral palsy
      - encephalitis lethargica
      - mitochondrial cytopathy.

SCENARIO 31. CAUDA EQUINA COMPRESSION

The following may be in the history: weakness of the legs, difficulty walking, incontinence of urine and/or faeces, back pain, buttock pain or pain radiating down the lower limbs.

The clinical signs will be LMN weakness in the lower limbs dependent on the roots that are involved, but if only the lower regions of the cauda are compressed you may just have incontinence of urine and/or faeces.

The signs can be extremely easy to miss on a 'routine' neurological examination that stops at the ankle jerks and does not involve the testing of sensation on the back of the leg (S2) or the buttocks and perineum. In the examination it is unlikely to be appropriate to examine the perineum in every single case, but where there is any suggestion of cauda equina compression a per rectum examination is obligatory and, in a 'routine' neurological examination, it is prudent to examine sensation on the back of the leg and enquire specifically about perineal sensation.

Any candidate, when faced with this situation, will be expected to understand that time is critical when cauda expression is developing (and of course the examiners can present the case any way that they see fit); once bladder or bowel dysfunction has been present for 24 hours it is usually permanent. If the diagnosis is not considered/recognised, investigated and treated within that time we may condemn the patient to incontinence for the rest of his or her life; as there is a consequent risk of renal damage this can prove fatal. As such imaging of the cauda needs to be performed, the best test being MRI. CT may provide some useful information if MRI is unavailable and CT myelography is a more favourable alternative to MRI than plain CT.

A good candidate

Will understand the problem arising from this and be able to discuss it. You can 'suspect' cauda equina compression on every working day and in some senses the suspicion demands imaging. However, if every suspicion were to be imaged there would be no space in diagnostic imaging to investigate those who really did need it. Thus we must be always suspicious but tie this in with good clinical skills and judgement (see introduction page viii). Get your senior to re-examine the case, discuss with diagnostic imaging, and gather any other information that may strengthen or weaken the case for the imaging being necessary (see Spinal cord compression, page 299).

SCENARIO 32. CAVERNOUS SINUS SYNDROME

The patient has ptosis and a complete ophthalmoplegia with numbness over the face in the territory supplied by the ophthalmic and maxillary divisions of the trigeminal nerve; the corneal reflex is absent on the affected side.

The ophthalmoplegia does not have to be complete. It may be bilateral.

A good candidate

Will do the following:

* Examine the acuity and fields: the cavernous sinus can be invaded by a pituitary tumour which may also compress the optic chiasma or optic nerve, or a metastasis (for example) in the cavernous sinus may extend anteriorly towards the superior orbital fissure and involve the optic nerve.

The most common cause of a cavernous sinus syndrome is an intracavernous aneurysm of the internal carotid artery; the third nerve is affected more often than the fourth or sixth and it is often accompanied by pain, paraesthesia and/or numbness in the distribution of the ophthalmic and occasionally the maxillary division of the trigeminal nerve.

Superior orbital fissure syndrome

A tumour involving the superior orbital fissure may cause a complete ophthalmoplegia with pain and/or numbness in the distribution of the ophthalmic division of the trigeminal nerve, but with proptosis because of obstruction of the ophthalmic vein.

SCENARIO 33. JUGULAR FORAMEN SYNDROME

There is a unilateral LMN paralysis of muscles supplied by the vagus and accessory nerves. There is involvement of the glossopharyngeal nerve ipsilaterally, because on testing the gag there is no direct or consensual reflex.

In the jugular foramen syndrome, because nerves IX, X and XI all leave the skull together, damage affects them all (nerve XII exits very close by in the hypoglossal foramen). The syndrome is more common than isolated lesions of the individual nerves. It can occur in nasopharyngeal carcinoma, trauma, Paget's disease, meningitis, basilar aneurysms and the rare glomus jugulare tumour.

SCENARIO 34. BRAIN-STEM SYNDROMES

Lateral medullary syndrome – Wallenberg syndrome

History of acute vertigo and nausea or oscillopsia and nausea.

It occurs most commonly with dissection or occlusion of the vertebral artery with consequent ischaemia of the posterior inferior cerebellar artery. In dissection there may be pain in the neck or occipital headache, or rarely the hemicranium or whole head.

The following are seen:

- Ipsilateral:
  - limb ataxia – cerebellar involvement
  - Horner syndrome – descending sympathetic tract
  - dysphagia and paralysis of the ipsilateral vocal fold and diminished gag reflex – nerves IX and X
  - numbness and impaired sensation in half of the face – involvement of the nucleus and descending tract of nerve V.
- Contralateral: impaired pain and temperature sensation over half the body and possibly the face.

Weber syndrome

Ipsilateral nerve III palsy with contralateral hemiparesis.

This occurs with a lesion as nerve III leaves the brain stem at the base of the midbrain (see figure below).

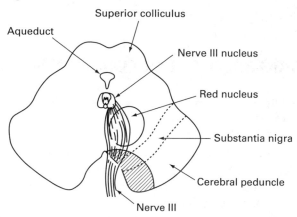

Figure 3.28   Weber syndrome

Millard–Gubler syndrome

Ipsilateral nerve VI and VII palsies with a contralateral hemiplegia.

STATION 4

The Communication Skills and Ethics Examination

COMMUNICATION SKILLS STATION

The ability to communicate effectively with a colleague, patient or relative is a fundamental part of practising medicine and the communication skills stations test your ability to do this. As with history taking, many candidates feel that they are already skilled in this aspect and do not prepare adequately for this station. The aims of the station are to explore the candidate's ability to engage in a two-way form of communication, to listen and respond to patients' concerns, and to impart information in a clear manner and upsetting news in a sensitive and empathic manner. The exam scenarios often require the candidate to have some knowledge of both medical ethics and medicolegal issues pertaining to everyday clinical practice. In addition, candidates are asked to explain procedures and obtain consent for specific situations. The following section discusses these issues and offers some guidelines as to how to break bad news and to communicate sensitive matters, before discussing 20 scenarios, which cover the vast majority of clinical situations that a candidate may be expected to deal with.

Scenarios that you are likely to encounter in the exam

Breaking bad news

This scenario is the classic communication skills station. It requires practice, but the eight-stage approach described later works for most scenarios. The cases vary from telling a family member that a relative has died suddenly, to giving patient results of a genetic test. Breaking bad news scenarios accounts for only 34% of all cases and just under half of these involve a discussion with a relative rather than the patient.

Explaining a procedure and obtaining consent

These cases occur less frequently than the other two scenarios (23%). The most common scenarios are explaining cardiac and gastrointestinal (GI) procedures to patients. Candidates should be aware of both how these are performed and the side effects associated with them. These cases often have an ethical dilemma or difficult situation associated with them.

Dealing with a difficult situation and/or ethical dilemma

These cases account for the remainder of the scenarios encountered (46%). Over half the cases involve talking to a relative rather than the patient. The relatives are usually unhappy, often about the care of their family member. It is usually a misunderstanding that is resolvable. Cases that are commonly encountered include:

- Dealing with a disgruntled relative
- Discussing a mistake made by the medical team with the patient or relative
- Confidentiality issues
- Resuscitation and organ transplantation issues
- Allocation of resources.

Here is a spectrum of examples of difficult situations that commonly occur in exams and will be covered in the text later in this chapter:

You are seeing a man in clinic after a recent admission to hospital. He has discovered that he had microcytic anaemia from a discharge summary, which was not investigated on the recent hospital admission. He is unhappy and wants to complain. He has also read on the internet that haematuria can give anaemia and is keen to discuss this.

You have been asked to have a discussion with the daughter of an elderly woman with dementia (mental test score or MTS 0/10) who is not eating or able to care for herself. You have been told by the nursing staff that the family wanted PEG (percutaneous endoscopic gastrostomy). Please discuss the situation with the family.

The son of an elderly patient has asked to discuss the health care of his father. The patient has renal failure, confusion and bladder cancer. He wants to discuss future treatment and resuscitation specifically.

Mr Jones has been exposed to asbestos in the past and has a mass on the chest radiograph, but does not want to have any further investigations. Please discuss his further management.

You are due to see Mr Smith in the clinic. He has been investigated for a mass on a radiograph and probable liver metastases on ultrasonography. Unfortunately the biopsy sample has been lost and there is no result. Please discuss with the patient whether or not further biopsy is required and whether it would alter treatment.

Background

The communication skills and ethics station in PACES is about imparting information on a subject in a clear and coherent manner. It aims to assess the candidate's ability to guide and organise the interview with the patient, with whom interaction is essential. It is not a test of medical knowledge. It is more important to put the patient at ease, establish a good rapport and understand the anxieties and needs, rather than devising a brilliant management plan.

In this part of the exam it is much more important for candidates to understand the needs of a patient, and to build a good rapport with him or her, than knowing the thirteenth cause of diabetes insipidus. Coming across as sensible and level-headed is more important than knowing all the answers to the questions. This section is designed to weed out candidates who, despite being extremely bright, are poor at discussing sensitive issues at the appropriate level.

By the time that candidates arrive at this stage of the exam they have already proved sufficient knowledge of the subject matter in the written part. The importance of the oral part of the exam is to demonstrate competence in translating this knowledge to the clinical setting and applying common sense to an individual situation. It is exactly this that makes the communication skills station such a valid and discriminatory part of PACES.

The paternalistic approach to consultation is out of step with society currently and does not fit well with clinical governance. Establishing a relationship of trust and mutual respect with the patient is of utmost importance. It should be remembered that, ultimately, the patient is in a position to make discussions about his heath care. However, you cannot forget that at times succinct advice and information must be given, perhaps not even in a sympathetic manner. The goal of the truly complete doctor is to be all things to all people, and is clearly unattainable.

Format of the station for PACES

The communication skills station of the exam is split into three parts in this exam.

Part 1

You will have 5 minutes outside the room to read the provided instructions. Read them very carefully.

Establish the key issues, which must be conveyed, and the take-home messages from the consultation, which the patient must have understood. Patients rarely remember more than two or three pieces of information from a consultation.

Only after the consultation has started, and the expectations and knowledge of the patient have been established, can the candidate work out the most appropriate way of conveying these messages.

The written scenario will contain the information about the problems surrounding the case. Further history-taking questions should be unnecessary – the information given should be taken as complete.

Consider the medical, legal and ethical issues around the patient. These are areas of specific concern to the examiners and marking is geared towards your ability to discuss them.

Consider the important issues of the consultation but do not set the direction in stone – the direction depends entirely on the interactions of the patient and doctor. It is important to remain flexible.

However, your approach should follow the 'pyramid' structure so it is wise at this stage to establish the foundation of your approach (usually establishing the patient/relatives' expectations and knowledge) and consider how you will build on this.

Part 2: The interview

You will have 15 minutes (including 1 minute to gather your thoughts at the end).

Introduction

- Introduce yourself and explain your role
- Ensure that the positioning of the furniture is correct
- Try to put the patient at ease.

The discussion

- Candidates should try to strike a balance between appearing knowledgeable and confident and appearing considerate and approachable.
- The consultation should be pitched at the correct level for the patient.
- Allow the patient to speak openly and freely but be prepared to direct the consultation.
- Establish the expectations and knowledge of the patient with open questions, eg 'We have not met before. You have come today to talk about your kidney problems. What do you understand about what is going on?'
- Why has this particular patient presented to you at this time?
- Explain to the patient the options from here, and the implication of these options.
- Try to give the patient choices rather than instructions.
- Allow pauses for patients to digest information.
- If a part of the consultation has gone badly, it is reasonable to go over that specific part again. Under these circumstances stop and ask: 'I have said quite a lot. Do you want me to go over some of it again before we move on?' There is little point in moving from one area to another, covering all of the information required, if the patient is taking none of it in.
- It is far better for the patient to have secured one or two key facts rather than a huge jumbled blur of information.
- Although you are following instructions and working to an agenda, to fail to do anything well in the hope of covering everything (albeit poorly) will result in failure.
- Under certain circumstances it is reasonable not to cover all the possible information from the instructions, eg there may be a lack of time (rushing through lists of information is not good communication), or the patient may have heard enough, eg 'I would rather come back with my family before we discuss this more'.
- It may not be appropriate to cover all the information once the patient's expectations have been assessed, eg discussing resuscitation in a patient who is clearly in shock after breaking bad news.
- If all the information has not been covered, do not panic; tell the examiners why this has happened during your discussion with them. If you can defend your conduct in a professional manner success is likely.

Before the finish
- Summarise the consultation
- Have a management plan for the future
- Ask if the patient wants anything repeated of if he or she has any questions
- Ask if there are any important issues that have not been covered
- Arrange another appointment if necessary.

Gathering thoughts (1 minute)
- Order the information in your mind
- Anticipate the likely discussion points with the examiners.

Part 3: The discussion with examiners (5 minutes)

The following issues are likely to be discussed:

- How you think it went: good areas and bad areas
- Things that could be done differently
- What you think the patient has understood
- How you would approach follow-up consultations
- The areas that were not covered
- Have the needs of the patient been met?
- Legal and ethical issues surrounding the case
- Further management and follow-up arrangements.

During this period with the examiners the candidate should remain flexible. No consultation is the same and sometimes one approach works better than another. It is reasonable to say that with hindsight you would have done things differently, and in follow-up consultations would readdress areas that were covered badly or not at all.

Once again detailed medical information is not required; the examiners are much more interested in the following:
- Was the patient put at ease?
- Were the questions open and at the right level?
- Did the candidate strike a balance of appearing confident, knowledgeable and approachable?
- Were the key issues discussed openly?
- How did the candidate handle sensitive issues?
- Were the key messages conveyed well?

Breaking bad news

Individuals are influenced by social, cultural and religious beliefs, so there is no one approach to breaking bad news that will satisfy all patients. However, a uniform, well-practised method with flexibility, dependent on the situation, can calm these choppy waters.

In reality doctors will often have known the patient for some time, making the consultation easier. For PACES this is not practical.

Classic Worst-case Scenario

> Doctor: 'So how long have you been on this treatment for your prostate cancer?'
> Patient: 'No one's told me I've got cancer.'

Never assume anything.

The eight steps to breaking bad news

1. The right information
2. The right place
3. The right people – ask the patient if there is anyone he or she would like present
4. Introduction
5. Establish what the patient knows
6. Informing the patient
7. Questions
8. Finishing.

The key to breaking bad news is in the preparation.

The right information

- Check all the information yourself, eg the histology/CT scans – do not rely on hearsay.
- Ensure that all the information needed is present before starting.
- Speak to the nursing staff looking after the patient to ascertain what the patient knows and expects.
- After breaking bad news, the patient is likely to ask about management plans for the future. Doctors should have management options for the patient before starting

The right place

- Chose a quiet location where a conversation cannot be overheard. Turn off the bleep, pager or mobile phone.
- Do not conduct the consultation across a desk, or an intervening barrier.
- Do not appear rushed; conduct the consultation in a calm, reassuring, sympathetic manner.

The right people

- Ask the nursing staff involved with the care of the patient if they would like to be present. They may have had time to form a useful relationship with the patient.
- If the patient has visitors it is often best to come back later.

- Before starting, ask the patient if he or she would like anyone present, eg friend or family. It is often helpful to have a close friend or relative present to offer emotional support. Under stressful situations the patient often retains very little of the information given.

Introduction
- Introduce yourself to the patient
- Explain your role in the medical team
- Maintain good eye contact.

Establish what the patient knows
- 'What have the other doctors told you about what is going on?'
- 'Do you understand why we have been doing these tests or suspect what might be wrong?'

Patients tend to fall in to two main groups: those who have a pretty good idea of what is going on and those who do not.

Informing the patient

PATIENTS WITH INSIGHT

- These patients will usually say something like: 'Yes, we were looking for multiple sclerosis, what do the tests show?' This is the easy group.
- Tell the patient in broad terms – details are often forgotten in this stressful situation
- Avoid medical jargon
- Talk slowly and clearly
- Use pauses to allow the patient to react
- Never lie or guess
- Ask if there is anything that the patient did not understand or wants repeated
- Keep the tone sympathetic but positive
- Summarise what has been said.

PATIENTS WITHOUT INSIGHT

- This is a more difficult consultation and is the scenario where most of the problems arise.
- The key is to give warning shots, eg 'Your condition appears to be quite serious' or 'Some of the test results are not good' – with small nuggets of information, allowing sufficient pauses for the patient to comprehend and respond. Then ask if he or she wants more information.
- If so, continue with another small amount of information and ask if the patient wants to know more.
- If not, explain that you will come back later, and if the patient thinks of any questions to ask them then.

- Suggest that it might be helpful to have members of the family present for support.
- Often the patient is just not fully prepared in him- or herself at that point and the consultation is often easier on the second occasion.
- The second consultation should start where the previous conversation left off, recapping on ground already covered.

It must be stressed that this is by no means the only way to break bad news. Any well-rehearsed and successful method is clearly acceptable.

Questions

Before leaving ask the patient if there is anything that he or she would like to ask. The most common question is 'How long have I got?'.

PROGNOSIS

It is impossible to convey all the information in one sitting, and discussing prognosis is usually best left for follow-up consultations. Prognosis varies enormously from one individual to another and depends on the response to treatment. However, it is perhaps prudent to avoid prognostication at all costs because it is so fraught with uncertainty.

If asked a question directly and you do not know the answer, never lie or guess. Explain that you will attempt to find the correct answer for the next consultation or later that day, as appropriate.

- If the doctor knows the prognosis, response to treatment and outcomes of the disease: 'No one knows what will happen in the future, and so I do not like to give exact figures. Everybody is different and some people do much better than others. However, we should probably think in terms of months rather than years, but once again no one really knows.' (If the prognosis is months.)

The next question often relates to cure: 'But there is a chance I will get better isn't there doctor?' The patient is now looking for hope, and it is important not to quash this completely. However, it is essential to prepare the patient for the inevitable in a delicate manner.

- A useful phrase to introduce the concept of a terminal illness is 'I do not think this disease will ever go away completely. Do you understand what I am saying?' Allowing time for patient reaction is important.

Do not necessarily tell palliative patients to give up smoking or drinking. The horse has already bolted.

Finishing

- Summarise what has been said.
- Ask if the patient has understood everything
- Ask if the patient wants anything repeated
- Ask if the patient has any further questions
- Give a contact number
- Make a follow-up appointment.

STATION 4

Communication Skills Scenarios

1. Breaking bad news: organ donation
2. Breaking bad news/ethical dilemma
3. Breaking bad news: multiple sclerosis
4. Explanation of results
5. Breaking bad news to a relative
6. Difficult situation: addressing patient's concerns – 1
7. Difficult situation: addressing patient's concerns – 2
8. Consent for a GI procedure – 1
9. Consent for a GI procedure – 2

SCENARIO 1. BREAKING BAD NEWS: ORGAN DONATION

As a medical registrar, you have been looking after an 18-year-old boy on ICU since he was knocked off his bicycle a week ago. He has been on a life support machine since admission. You have agreed with the father (the sole carer) the need to do brain-stem tests and he has made an appointment with you to discuss the results. The tests have confirmed that his son is brain-stem dead.

Please inform the father of the results and discuss organ donation with him. The son did carry a donor card (which is over 10 years old), but had no advanced directive.

Preliminary thoughts

This case covers important issues about how to define death and the process of organ donation. The case has appeared on a number of occasions in examinations. It can be very difficult, in that the father's reaction is unpredictable. If the father is struggling with what he is being told, progressing to a discussion about organ donation would be inappropriate, despite the text above.

- What brain-stem tests are (see page 418)
- Legalities of declaring someone dead
- What organ donation entails and the need for consent from the next of kin/relative (see page 420)
- Which organs? – speed, need, number of patients who will benefit
- Rules surrounding donor cards/advanced directives
- Will the father need other family members present to help make a decision? In an exam it is very unlikely that the father will say, 'Yes I would like my sister to be here', because the exam will come to a standstill. However, the question is worth asking in an exam, because it is what good doctors would do and candidates will be rewarded for it in the exam.

A good candidate

- Will approach the situation very carefully establishing the father's knowledge of the situation
- Will ask if other family members should be present for the discussion
- Will discuss organ donation on this occasion only if it appears appropriate.

If organ donation is not discussed, a good candidate will explain to the father that he would like to have a further discussion in the next hour.

Goals for consultation

- The father understands that his son is dead
- An informed decision to be made relatively soon about organ donation.

Key points in the consultation

- Introduce yourself and establish a good rapport
- Ask if he would like anyone else there for the discussion
- Explore and confirm the father's understanding of his son's condition
- Confirm his acceptance of the son's dependency on life support machines and why the tests were done.

The subsequent direction of the consultation depends on the father's acceptance of the previous point.

Directions of the consultation

Scenario A

> The father is unaware or does not accept that his son might be dead.

This is a difficult situation; the doctor should go through the information piece by piece, starting at the beginning when he arrived in the intensive care unit (ICU). The doctor should pause frequently to allow the father time to think and ask any questions. Ultimately it is essential that the father know that his son is dead. He may need more time to take this in and it may be inappropriate to discuss organ donation at this stage (see page 420).

The father should therefore be given some time to discuss the situation with family and friends, and a subsequent discussion about organ transplantation would then be appropriate.

Scenario B

> The father is aware of the reasons why the tests are being performed and their significance.

- Inform him of the test results, ie brain-stem death. Confirm that there is no hope of recovery; the son is being kept in his current state by the ventilator.
- Explore the father's knowledge of organ donation.
- Did the son ever discuss his feelings about organ donation? Did he know that he carried an organ donation card?
- Offer details about organ donation and the benefits to a number of other individuals. The shortage of hearts, lungs, kidneys, for example, which may enable other people to live who would otherwise die.
- Remember that this is not an all-or-nothing situation – relatives, who are legal guardians of the body, may specify which organs are acceptable or unacceptable.
- Offer him the opportunity to have a further discussion with other members of the family; arrange to meet again in the next few hours.

Finishing

- Ask the father if there is anyone else he would like to inform
- Ask if he has any questions
- Ensure that all staff involved in the case are aware of the father's decision.

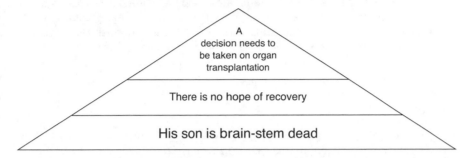

Discussion

- The examiners may discuss the difference between brain-stem death and persistent vegetative state (see page 418).
- Discussions with relatives are often best done in a group to ensure that consensus is reached. Focusing on one relative may lead to jealousy and resentment. However, if it becomes apparent that different views are held by different members, you may need to deal with a 'spokesperson' who will act for all family members.
- Advanced directives are legally binging. An organ donor card gives an indication only of what an individual felt on a specific day in the past and is not legally binding.
- This case raises the issue about whether all the information given in the text should be discussed in the exam. Clearly, in this case, if the father is inconsolable, it may not be possible to discuss this within the time limit of the exam. Under these circumstances candidates should say to the father that they would give him some time to gather his thoughts and come back in a few minutes. He may even want to wait for more of his family to arrive.

SCENARIO 2. BREAKING BAD NEWS/ ETHICAL DILEMMA

An 80-year old man, previously alert and independent, has been brought in with a massive haemoptysis. He has been resuscitated and bronchoscopy has revealed a probable bronchial carcinoma, but histology is awaited. Ultrasonography shows multiple liver metastases but an enhanced CT head scan is normal. He remains acutely confused but his wife is understandably anxious and wishes to know what is going on. She has as yet been given very little information.

Please discuss her husband's condition with her.

Preliminary thoughts

- Legal versus pragmatic issues with regard to the patient's confidentiality and when it can be broken. In this case you can act in the best interest of the patient, which will involve telling the wife (see page 415).
- Prognosis:
  - short-term prognosis – moderate (he will probably recover from the bleed)
  - medium-term prognosis – very poor if he does indeed have lung cancer.
- A need to reassure the wife about her husband's care.
- Prepare her for bad news, remembering that there is uncertainty about the diagnosis. Therefore telling the wife that he has lung cancer is potentially untrue.
- Does he have an advanced directive?

A good candidate

- Will give some assurance that there is some short-term reversibility in the condition
- Will not 'jump in' with a cancer diagnosis but explain that further investigation is required
- Will explain the confidentiality issues and the fact that her husband is not aware because of his confusion.

Goals for consultation

- The wife must be made aware that he is very unwell, although exact details of his condition may not be necessary.
- To ensure that the wife has faith in the medical care her husband is receiving.

Key points in the consultation

- Introduce yourself and establish a rapport.
- 'Ideally, we would have this discussion with your husband too, but it is not possible. You must be very anxious.'

- What has she been told already?
- Establish the wife's knowledge of her husband's condition and why she thinks he is in hospital. Often patients pick information up from the nursing staff, etc. I am aware of a patient, who spoke no English, who discovered her diagnosis of bladder cancer from a cleaner who also spoke Spanish!
- Inform her that he has had a large haemoptysis, but that this has been treated and he should recover from his confusion.

The subsequent direction of the consultation depends on the understanding and expectations of the wife. The doctor should now pause to let the wife ask questions.

Direction of the consultation

Scenario A

The wife has no comprehension of how serious the condition may be.

- Under these circumstances the wife should be informed that her husband is unwell. It should be impressed on her that the situation is serious and that further discussion with her and ideally her husband will be required in the near future.
- Allow her to ask any questions. Answer these as honestly as possible. It should be remembered that the histology is still awaited and a diagnosis of cancer, although likely, has not been confirmed.
- Discussing the diagnosis of cancer without histology is hazardous and best avoided.
- It is never appropriate to force information on patients or relatives.
- Although discussing her husband's details is technically breaking patient confidentiality, most clinicians would agree that discussing with the wife is the correct ethical thing to do. The amount of detail will of course depend on her questions and reaction to the answers:
  - legally, this is permissible as the clinician is acting in the best interests of the patient because she may be aware of his wishes in situations such as this
  - it would also be generally accepted that it is humane to let his partner know of his condition.

Scenario B

It is clear from talking to the wife that she is aware that something is seriously amiss; the thought of cancer may have crossed her mind.

- Remember that the diagnosis has not been confirmed and that the patient's confusion is likely to improve. Predicting the future is difficult and best avoided.

- Doctors should attempt to maintain a degree of confidentiality in telling the wife what she wants to know (eg 'One of the tests show there is something suspicious in his lungs; it may be a serious problem, although we are not absolutely sure of that yet').
- In view of the lack of definite histology, the authors feel that discussing resuscitation with the wife at this stage is inappropriate and the patient should remain for resuscitation. However, if the wife volunteers that her husband would not like further intervention if something went suddenly wrong, this should be considered, together with the subsequent results of the histology.

Finishing

- Summarise the consultation
- Ask if she has any questions
- Arrange a further meeting
- Inform the nursing staff of the conversation – they should ideally have been present.

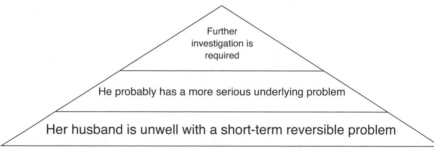

Further investigation is required

He probably has a more serious underlying problem

Her husband is unwell with a short-term reversible problem

Discussion

As with many communication skills scenarios, particularly those relating to imparting bad news, the wife dictates the direction, pace and flow of the consultation.

SCENARIO 3. BREAKING BAD NEWS: MULTIPLE SCLEROSIS

A 33-year old woman has a consultation with you to discuss the results of her recent MRI, which you had organised at her previous neurology appointment. She has a 3-year-old daughter but is actively trying for a second child. For the last 3 months she has noticed several episodes of visual disturbance and intermittent weakness of her legs. Her MRI is consistent with the diagnosis of multiple sclerosis.

Please discuss this result with her.

Preliminary thoughts

- The course of multiple sclerosis (MS) and its variable nature
- Morbidity and mortality of MS
- Implications with regard to pregnancy
- Treatment options including interferon-β and the NICE guidelines
- Inheritance of MS.

A good candidate

- Will explore the patient's knowledge of why she had the tests and MS
- Will not take all hope away and will explain the variable nature of MS.

Goals for consultation

For her to understand:

- The diagnosis and its implications
- The need for a multidisciplinary approach
- The variable nature of progression of the disease; few patients progress rapidly
- Treatment options.

Key points in the consultation

- Introduction and establish a good rapport
- Ask if she wishes for anyone else to be present.
- Explore the patient's understanding of her condition and expectations/suspicions of what may be wrong: 'Did the previous doctors tell you why they were doing the MRI or what they thought was causing the weakness?'

Directions of the consultation

Scenario A

The patient has never heard of MS and has no idea of its implications.

- The patient should be given small pieces of information in a logical manner; pauses are essential and give the opportunity for questions.
- Patients can be given too much information in one consultation after receiving bad news. It is preferable to establish one or two key points.
- Further consultations can address more detailed information. They may choose to bring a friend or relative.

Scenario B

The patient is suspicious that MS is the cause and knows a great deal about it.

- A discussion about exactly what she understands and expects is important. The press tend to report the more disabling end of the disease spectrum, heightening patient anxiety.
- Emphasise the variable progression of the disease. Often remitting/relapsing. There can be long periods with few symptoms. Few patients progress rapidly.
- Discuss available treatment options such as steroids and interferon-β (in outline only) – see page 168.
- Discuss the implications for pregnancy and whether this should be pursued – MS has no effect on fertility and does not affect pregnancy outcome.
- Reassure her that it is not hereditary.

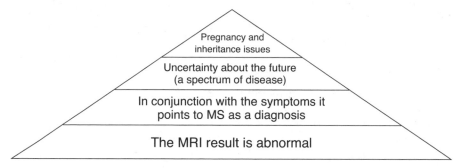

What does he understand might be wrong?

Finishing

- Summarise what has been discussed
- Ask if there is anything that she would like repeated or if she has any questions
- Arrange follow-up and put her in touch with relevant support groups.

Discussion

- Patients do not absorb masses of information from consultations. This is worse in stressful, anxious situations. For this reason it is preferable to give and repeat a little information well, to write it down if possible and to arrange to discuss issues further at the next appointment. Having a relative or friend present is reassuring and helps in the amount of information recalled.

- It is best to give a little information well rather than a lot badly.
- It is not necessary to discuss all of the details of MS in the first consultation.

SCENARIO 4. EXPLANATION OF RESULTS

You are the SHO in the endocrine clinic and the biochemical results on the next patient, a 32-year-old woman, confirm the clinical suspicion that she has Graves' disease, with a grossly elevated free thyroxine (T_4) and suppressed thyroid-stimulating hormone (TSH) with strongly positive anti-thyroid antibodies. She has moderate exophthalmos and is a smoker.

Please discuss with her the subsequent management of her condition.

Preliminary thoughts

Explanation of test results occurs frequently in communication skills scenarios (about 25%). They require a certain amount of medical knowledge. However, it has been argued that these cases do not test communication skills well, but focus more on medical knowledge. This is not the case. Remember that most of the marks in these stations are obtained for demonstration of good communication skills, allowing the patient to talk and addressing the questions. There are not that many marks for knowing the detailed side effects of the drug, for example. We suggest that candidates should approach this in the same way as a breaking bad news scenario, ie explore what the patient thinks might be wrong and what he or she has been told about the reason for the test.

It is possible that being over-burdened with detailed knowledge about specific diseases may actually impede the ability of a candidate to do well in a communication skills station, in that the candidate tends to impart enormous amounts of information without allowing the patient to take part in the consultation.

In addition, you should remember that patients may be very worried about the tests that they are having and the possibility of the results, so these cases should be handled sensitively. I have spoken to candidates who have been confronted by this type of case and have said how surprised they were about how upset the patient became. It is possible that this is because, when you think of breaking bad news in communication skills, you think of cancer, genetic disease and neurological disease, so other less major issues, such as Graves' disease, does not really count and should be a 'piece of cake'. This is a bit like pitching up to the Neu camp, to play Barcelona at football with a reserve team, after a big night out on the town – especially when you remember that actors are involved in the examinations.

- Treatment options of thyrotoxicosis and the pros and cons of each:
  - medical – carbimazole, propylthiouracil
  - radioiodine
  - surgical
- Involve her in discussion
- Fertility issues.

A good candidate

- Will explore her knowledge of why she has had the tests performed and what she knows about the management of Graves' disease
- Will allow the patient to take part in the consultation and give time to ask questions.
- Will allow the patient to make an informed decision about treatment options.

Goals for consultation

- Explore her knowledge of why she has had the tests done and what she expects
- Inform her about her disease and discuss the management options
- To agree appropriate treatment strategy
- For her to understand the seriousness of her condition and need for regular monitoring.

Key points

- Introduction and establish a rapport
- Explore her knowledge of thyrotoxicosis
- Explain the results of the blood test: the nature of an overactive thyroid and the pathological consequences of untreated disease
- Discuss the treatment options: her symptoms will improve with treatment, but may take months to resolve completely
- If medical therapy, warn of the potential side effects, especially agranulocytosis; this must be both verbal and in writing
- Establish her LMP (last menstrual period), wishes for pregnancy, and any current children
- Emphasise need for regular review.

Finishing

- Summarise what has been said
- Provide written information
- Ask if she has any questions
- Arrange follow-up with blood tests.

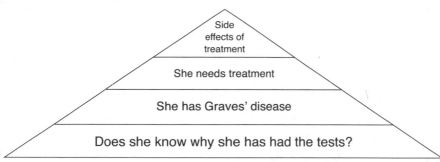

Discussion

- There are three potential treatment possibilities for thyrotoxicosis of varying appropriateness.
- The pros and cons of each modality should be discussed.
- However, initial discussions will be influenced by her thyrotoxic anxiety; informed consent is often difficult in a thyrotoxic patient (see page 617).
- For an initial presentation of Graves' disease, most endocrinologists would recommend a course of medical therapy, eg carbimazole 40 mg once daily (initially) with additional β blockade to cover/mask the sympathetic activity. Eighteen months of therapy may lead to remission in 50% of patients. The dose of carbimazole should be titrated according to thyroid function tests. An alternative regimen is to 'block and replace'. If recurrence occurs definitive treatment may be necessary.
- It is medicolegally essential to record that patients started on either carbimazole or propylthiouracil have been warned of the side effects such as rash (1 in 200) and agranulocytosis (1 in 2000), and to attend for a blood count if they experience a sore throat within the first 3 months on medication.
- Early radioiodine (^{131}I) is an alternative after the patient is rendered euthyroid. Radioiodine is obviously contraindicated in pregnancy and conception should not occur within 6 months. Close contact with small children is forbidden for a several days after ingestion.
- Surgery offers a definitive cure, but leaves a scar and the possibility of recurrent laryngeal nerve damage, as well as hypoparathyroidism (more common with total thyroidectomy).
- The last two treatments may render the patient hypothyroid requiring hormone replacement for life.
- Thyroid disease in pregnancy is the realm of specialists. Thyrotoxicosis decreases the chance of conceiving and increases the risk of spontaneous miscarriage. In Graves' disease, the stimulating antibodies can cross the placenta causing fetal thyrotoxicosis or, alternatively, both carbimazole and propylthiouracil can cross causing fetal hypothyroidism and goitre formation.

SCENARIO 5. BREAKING BAD NEWS TO A RELATIVE

As a medical SHO, the on-call team informs you that a 73-year-old man under your care died during the night. He was admitted 48 hours earlier with pneumonia and appeared to be stable. Unfortunately he deteriorated suddenly overnight and had an asystolic arrest. Attempted resuscitation was unsuccessful. The cause of death remains uncertain, although progressive pneumonia or pulmonary embolus is suspected. The daughter has been in close contact with her father during his admission, but was non-contactable last night. She has arrived on the ward and has been given a cup of tea in a private relatives room; she is unaware that her father has died.

Please explain to her what has happened and enquire about the possibility of a postmortem examination.

Preliminary thoughts

This is a case that appears difficult and candidates fear. However, if you learn and follow the accepted way of approaching this (see Breaking Bad News, page 379), it is actually straightforward. Deviating from this path, eg 'Hello Mrs Jones, when did you last see your father alive', is usually risky.

- Was she aware that her father might die in hospital?
- Active management was attempted but unsuccessful.
- The cause of death is uncertain, so a postmortem examination is desirable.
- If you are unsure of the cause of death, a coroner's opinion should be sought. He or she may be happy to have a death certificate completed without a postmortem examination.
- If a death certificate can be completed she can refuse a postmortem examination.
- Need to discuss with the nursing staff about the daughter's relationship with her father and her expectations. Also enquire about other relatives and family dynamics.
- Ask the nursing staff to attend a consultation.

A good candidate

- Will find out if she knew how ill her father was before telling her what happened
- Will make sure that she has someone with her or somewhere to go after the consultation.

Goals for consultation

For the daughter to understand the following:

- Her father has died despite the best efforts of the medical and nursing staff.
- The cause of death probably relates to a respiratory disease.
- The exact cause remains uncertain, making a postmortem examination potentially desirable.

Key points in the consultation

- Ensure that you will not be disturbed; give your pager to a colleague
- Introduction and establish rapport
- Discover and remember the surname
- Ask her if she would like anyone else present at this point
- You must break the news about her father's death early on, and provide necessary background for this grave news, so:
  - explain the seriousness of pneumonia
  - explore the daughter's knowledge and expectation of her father's illness, eg 'How was he when you last saw him?' is a good starting point.

Directions of the consultation

Scenario A

She is under the impression that all is well and he is likely to make a full and complete recovery.

- It is important to stress that her father's condition, although stable, was serious and deteriorated suddenly over night. Attempts were made to contact her. It is now worth waiting once again for her reaction.
- She should be informed of the events that took place. The word death should be used.
- She should be informed that full and active treatment was attempted, but was ultimately unsuccessful.
- During the consultation talk slowly, with empathy and appropriate pauses.
- Ask her if she would like some time alone or to contact friends/relatives.

Scenario B

She is aware that her father's condition is serious and was worried that he may deteriorate.

- Under these circumstances she should be informed that attempts were made to contact her last night.
- He deteriorated suddenly, resuscitation was attempted; however, they were unsuccessful and he died last night.

- If his death was swift and painless convey this to the relatives. Knowing that the father did not suffer may be some comfort.
- It may or may not be appropriate at this point to discuss the postmortem examination depending on her state of shock.

If she would like to go on and discuss the postmortem examination further:

- Explain that the doctors looking after her father would like to know exactly what caused the sudden deterioration. Performing a postmortem examination can do this.
- The relatives need a general understanding of the procedure. Specific details are neither helpful nor necessary.

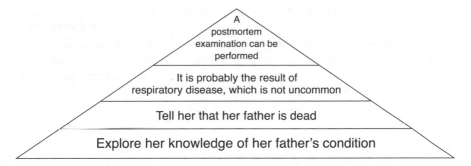

A postmortem examination can be performed

It is probably the result of respiratory disease, which is not uncommon

Tell her that her father is dead

Explore her knowledge of her father's condition

Finishing

- Give her your condolences
- Ask if she has any questions
- Ask if she would like to contact someone
- Make follow-up arrangements to speak to her or other members of the family again, if necessary.

SCENARIO 6. DIFFICULT SITUATION: ADDRESSING PATIENT'S CONCERNS – 1

You are the respiratory SHO. The next patient is a 39-year-old woman with poorly controlled asthma who has been placed on long-term oral steroids by your consultant. The patient is very worried about the steroids because she has read that they will make her put on weight and they do 'terrible things to your body'. The patient also has type 1 diabetes.

Please explain steroid therapy to the patient.

Preliminary thoughts

It is not clear where her information has come from. Data from previous candidates who have taken communication exams suggest that the patients/actors usually get information from a non-medical source such as the press, a friend or the internet. A sympathetic approach appears to be successful in most cases. Clarification of the issue is usually all that is required. The patient/actor is not looking for a confrontation but reassurance:

- Benefits vs side effects of steroids (short and long term)
- Implications with regard to diabetes
- Need for clear information
- Possible alternatives to steroids
- Legal and ethical issues: patient has the right to refuse treatment.

A good candidate

- Will attempt to discover where the information came from.
- Will know the side effects of treatment and the severity of them
- Will explain in a clear and sympathetic manner
- Will respect the patient's opinion.

Goals for consultation

- She should understand the overwhelming benefit of steroids.
- She should accept the medical advice with a minimum of compromise, because this may lead to serious adverse consequences.

Key points in the consultation

- Polite introduction and establish a rapport.
- Establish this patient's understanding of her disease and the need for steroids.
- Determine specifically why she does not want to take them and her anxieties about future use.
- Emphasise the need for steroids to prevent attacks and the consequences of poorly controlled asthma.

- Explain the possible long-term side effects of steroids:
  - weight gain
  - thin skin
  - bruising
  - possible hypertension
  - acne
  - osteoporosis

  but that these will be minimised by ensuring that her dose is tailored to her condition. Osteoporosis can be minimised by concomitant bisphosphonate therapy.
- Explain the following about the steroid therapy:
  - it will result in adrenal suppression and the absence of endogenous cortisol production
  - she should never stop the tablets suddenly
  - she must never miss a dose
  - the need for a steroid card, MedicAlert bracelet and emergency hydrocortisone pack (for parenteral self-administration if unable to take oral medication).
- Explain the effects on her diabetes and possible worsening of glycaemic control. She will probably need to increase her insulin dose, in liaison with her diabetologist/diabetic specialist nurse.

Finishing

- Ensure that the patient understands what has been said and ask if she has any questions.
- Summarise what has been discussed.
- Arrange follow-up.

Discussion

The key to this is compliance with medication. A one-sided teacher/student discussion is unlikely to result in good compliance. The doctor and patient should work together as a team. Ultimately a discussion about reducing the dose to ensure compliance may be appropriate.

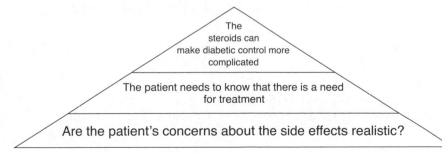

The steroids can make diabetic control more complicated

The patient needs to know that there is a need for treatment

Are the patient's concerns about the side effects realistic?

SCENARIO 7. DIFFICULT SITUATION: ADDRESSING PATIENT'S CONCERNS – 2

A 45-year-old woman with metastatic renal cancer has come to the clinic. A new drug has become available over the last few years that delays progression of disease and has a 2-month survival benefit. The drug has a licence and is used widely throughout Europe and in the private sector. It has been turned down by NICE both initially and on appeal because it was felt that it was not viable in terms of cost (£30 000/annum) vs quality of life (no benefit) and increased life expectancy (2 months). Consequently, the drug is not available at your hospital. She is currently not receiving any treatment for her cancer because she has progressed on all previous treatments. She wants to know why she was not told about this drug earlier and if it is available on the NHS

Preliminary thoughts

In broad terms this seems like a very difficult case. However, this is not necessarily true. Candidates need to peruse the principles of clinical governance – honesty, accountability and transparency – together with the reality of limited resources in the NHS:

- The drug is not available.
- The issue has been reviewed at the highest level (NICE).
- The candidate is not informed why the patient was not previously told about the drug: all you can do here is apologise and say that you will air her concerns with the consultant. There is of course an issue about whether telling a patient 'A new drug seems to work, but you can't have it' is of benefit. However, this is rather a paternalistic view and should be discouraged, especially in an exam setting, because it does not comply with clinical governance. In addition, the patients may want to write to her MP or try to fund the drug independently. Patients should not be denied this opportunity.
- Are there alternative funding possibilities? Currently, doctors can write to primary care trusts (PCTs) on an individual basis for funding under exceptional circumstances.
- Are there any ongoing clinical studies in which this patient will receive a developing treatment?

A good candidate

- Will not antagonise the patient
- Will follow the guidelines of clinical governance
- Will not attempt to make excuses about why she was not told earlier
- Will explore other options for the patient.

Goals for consultation

- She needs to be aware that the issue has been addressed at a higher level and rejected.
- She needs to leave the consultation with some trust in the medical team; it did not directly decide against funding this drug.
- The most complicated issue may turn out to be why she was not told about this drug earlier. Candidates are advised to be honest and say that they will discuss the case with the consultant in charge.

Key points in the consultation

- Polite introduction.
- The patient must be given a chance to speak without interruption.
- Defending the decision not to give the drug on an individual basis is a very hazardous route to take. Phrases such as 'the results are not that good' are counterproductive. It may be better to take the discussion to a more utilitarian level.
- Under no circumstances question the results of the clinical study.
- Explaining that these rules apply for the whole of the UK will be helpful.
- It is important not to take on individual blame for decisions made by others (NICE).
- The patient must be made aware of the possibility of the complaints procedure.
- Candidates should not try to cover up for previous colleagues when considering why she was not told earlier. This issue should be discussed with the consultant.
- The candidate should say that he or she will discuss the case with the consultant, to see if there are any other ways of getting the drug.
- The possibility of a drug study can be approached: this may require a future appointment at a cancer centre.

Finishing

- You should try to show some sympathy with the patient.
- Explain that you will discuss the case with your consultant.
- Make it clear that there are complaints procedures that can be followed.
- Ask if she has any further questions.
- Arrange follow-up.

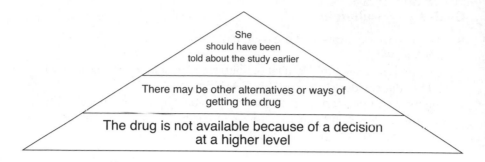

Clinical studies

Candidates are not asked directly to recruit patients into clinical studies for obvious reasons. Only a limited knowledge of clinical studies is required. They follow a principle of good clinical practice, which has been harmonised throughout Europe. It requires a number of checks at all stages of the studies from conception to statistical analysis. They exist to protect the patient, ensure that a relevant question is being asked and make sure that the study is being conducted safely and honestly. Many of these principles go back to the principles set out at the Declaration of Helsinki. Clinical studies have a sponsor, such as a university, drug company or NHS trust. If things go wrong the sponsor is ultimately responsible and individuals will have an opportunity to claim compensation.

SCENARIO 8. CONSENT FOR A GI PROCEDURE – 1

A 55 year-old man has returned to the gastroenterology outpatient clinic for a review of his ulcerative colitis. He has had this for more than 10 years, during which time he has had numerous courses of oral steroids for exacerbations and is on long-term azathioprine. Over the last 6 months he has had worsening diarrhoea and currently opens his bowels about 10 times a day. A recent colonoscopy has revealed active pancolitis. He is increasingly fed up with his condition. The multidisciplinary team has decided that a colectomy is in his best interest.

Please discuss his management with a view to recommending total colectomy.

Preliminary thoughts

- Long-term symptoms and complications of ulcerative colitis (UC) and prognosis:
  - carcinoma/bowel obstruction
  - toxic megacolon.
- Risks of surgery: although this is a surgical rather than a medical procedure candidates should know in broad terms the risks, ie anaesthetic risks, surgical risks and the presence of a stoma after surgery. However, candidates will not lose marks for explaining that the patient will have the opportunity to speak to the surgical team before surgery. Do not attempt to guess the details of a colectomy, even if it seems rather straightforward.
- Practicalities of a stoma: discuss with stoma nurse. A stoma may or may not be necessary
- Legal and ethical issues: competent individuals have the right of self-determination and this must be respected (Mental Health Capacity Act – see page 414).

A good candidate

- Will not assume that the patient has any knowledge of colectomy as a treatment option
- Will not spend excessive time discussing previous medical treatment – candidates must assume from the text that all medical options have been explored
- Will admit that they do not know all the details about colectomy (if they do not), and that the patient will need to speak to the surgical team.

Goals for the consultation

- The patient should understand why colectomy is the most viable option.
- He should be aware of the benefits and risks of surgery.
- He should gain sufficient knowledge to make an informed decision, although not necessarily immediately.

Key points in the consultation

- Introduction and establish rapport.
- Establish patient's understanding and knowledge of his condition, its severity and long-term complications. He is unlikely to be aware of the multidisciplinary team (MDT) decision.
- Establish patient's expectations (cure/incurable).
- Explain the severity of his condition and its increasing unresponsiveness to medical therapy (compare Breaking Bad News, page 379).
- Explain the risk of colonic carcinoma and toxic 'megacolon' in long-term active pancolitis.
- Introduce the idea of a total colectomy: discuss:
  - benefits of symptom relief and a more normal lifestyle
  - drawbacks of permanent stoma and bag, but potential for an ileoanal pouch anastomosis.
- Discuss patient's fears:
  - surgery
  - permanent colostomy
  - psychological implications.
- Discuss the help available, eg stoma nurse, self-help groups.

Direction of consultation

Scenario A

He accepts what has been said.

- He should be allowed time to make a decision after consultation with other members of his family, if requested.
- Arrange a follow-up appointment or telephone discussion over the next day or so.

Scenario B

He is unwilling to have the procedure

- Ultimately it is the patient's decision and under these circumstances he will continue to receive the best medical management without a colostomy.
- Ask him if he would like to talk to someone else about the decision.
- Perhaps reach some form of compromise: 'We will give steroids one more go, and then reconsider matters.'
- Ensure that he understands the implications of his decision and that colostomy is still an option for the future.
- Offer him time to discuss the issue further with family and friends. Candidates should not force a decision.

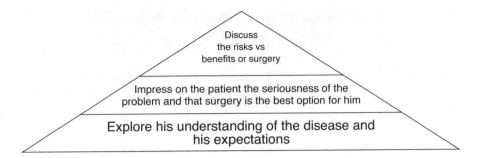

Finishing

- Ask if he has understood everything that has been said and if he has any questions.
- Contact the MDT for his next appointment.
- Make an appointment with the stoma nurse and/or other patients who have had a colectomy.

SCENARIO 9. CONSENT FOR A GI PROCEDURE – 2

Ms Jones is a 55-year-old woman who was admitted with obstructive jaundice; ultrasonography and MRCP suggest that gallstones are the cause. She has been booked for an ERCP on tomorrow's list. She will have a cholecystectomy in the future. There are no contraindications. Please discuss the ERCP procedure with her.

Points to consider

- She has gallstones and is fit for the procedure; it is a given fact that there is no point in discussing her symptoms in an investigational manner, eg is the pain worse after meals?
- It is not clear if she knows her diagnosis – assume that she does not.
- This appears straightforward, provided that candidates know what is involved.
- Candidates who have taken the exam previously, and passed, have said that they have finished this sort of case well within the time.
- The temptation is to take a history to look for a 'trick' or contraindication. This is not the aim of the section.
- Once the jaundice has settled she will have a cholecystectomy; the candidate has not been asked to discuss this with her specifically. However, the future plan (surgery) should be discussed as a long-term solution to the problem. If the candidate does not know the details about cholecystectomy he or she will not be penalised, unless he or she gives incorrect information.

A good candidate

- Will not assume that the patient knows the results of the previous investigations
- Will not dwell on the history of the gallstones: 'Is the pain worse with food?'
- Will know how an ERCP is performed
- Will explain the side effects – especially the serious ones – without causing unjustified anxiety.

Approach to the patient

- Introduce yourself.
- Ask her if she wants anyone else present.
- Tell her to interrupt and ask questions at any point.
- Ask her how she is, using phrases such as 'I have read that you have been unwell'.
- Ask her if she has been told what is wrong.
- Explain that you are here to discuss her results with her and her future management.

- Explain that she will need an ERCP to treat the gallstones in the short term, but will need an operation in the long term.
- Tell her that you have come to discuss the first part of this procedure, which is due tomorrow. Tell her that a tube will be passed through her mouth, then through the stomach to the bile duct. The procedure will unblock the duct, wash out the system and remove the stones. In addition, a stent may be inserted and the orifice between the bowel and the bile duct enlarged (sphincterotomy). A small amount of sedation will make the procedure less traumatic. The patient will make a quick recovery once the sedation has worn off and she will need to be nil by mouth before the procedure.

Complications of ERCP

- Death: diagnostic 0.21%, therapeutic 0.49%
- Haemorrhage 1.13%
- Perforation 0.57%
- Pancreatitis 1.8–7.2%
- Cholangitis 0.57%
- Desaturation > 50% (in the presence of airway disease in patients > 70 years).

Explain that the gall bladder will be surgically removed once it has settled down. There is an ongoing debate about side effects that patients need to know. The disadvantage of telling all the details of risk is that it can frighten the patient. An unwritten rule is that patients need to know serious risks such as death even if they are rare (< 1%) and common side effects even if they appear trivial.

An approach to discussing death in this situation would be 'Many thousands of these procedures have been done safely throughout the world. Very occasionally serious complications occur; these can usually be treated. However, once in about every 200 procedures patients do not recover from these complications. There is no reason to think that this will occur with you, and overall we feel that the benefits of this outweigh these very small risks'.

Below are a number of other diagnostic procedures that candidates have been asked to discuss with patients.

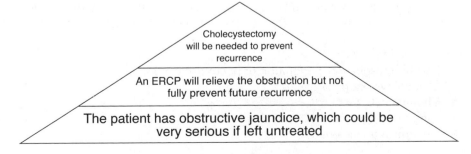

Cholecystectomy will be needed to prevent recurrence

An ERCP will relieve the obstruction but not fully prevent future recurrence

The patient has obstructive jaundice, which could be very serious if left untreated

Diagnostic OGD

Patients need to know that they may have some mild sedation (such as mid-azolam), which will make the procedure less traumatic but is associated with oxygen desaturation. However, many patients require no sedation and lido-caine throat spray is adequate. They need to be nil by mouth before the procedure. A tube will be passed down into the mouth, which may be uncomfortable. It will take less than 15 min.

COMPLICATIONS

- Death 0.001%
- Perforation 0.03%
- Mallory–Weiss tear 0.1%
- Oxygen desaturation < 90%: 45%.

Therapeutic OGD: oesophageal dilatation

This procedure is very similar to a diagnostic ODG although the risk of per-foration is increased. There is also a potential discussion about upper GI malig-nancy. Candidates are advised to avoid a detailed discussion about this issue without histology. There is no evidence that the use of dilating balloons is asso-ciated with a lower rate of complications compared with wire-guided, push-type dilators.

PERFORATION

- Benign strictures 0.4%
- Malignant strictures 10%
- Caustic strictures 14%
- Achalasia 1.6%
- Gastric outlet strictures 4–6%
- Haematemesis 0.8%.
- (Otherwise as diagnostic OGD.)

Therapeutic OGD: oesophageal stent insertion for malignant obstruction

Plastic stents have now been superseded by expanding metal stents, which are safer.

Data suggest highly variable rates of complications. Even under these circum-stances you should not assume that the patient knows the diagnosis.

COMPLICATIONS

- Death (by aspiration, perforation or haemorrhage) 3%
- Maldeployment/blockage 20%
- Chest pain 40%
- Tumour overgrowth 15%
- Stent migration about 5%.

Therapeutic OGD: variceal banding, adrenaline injection, electrocoagulation and heater probe

Variceal band ligation is used for variceal bleeding. Ulceration to the banding site is a common side effect. These other procedures are designed to stop bleeding.

There is an increased risk of perforation (up to 5% with a heater probe).

Once again, having a protracted discussion during a bleeding peptic ulcer is unlikely to occur in the setting of a communications exam.

Therapeutic OGD: PEG insertion

This case has occurred on a number of occasions in the communication skills exams, and has tended to occur in stroke, dementia and terminal cancer patients. The examination has tended to focus on ethical issues surrounding quality-of-life issues and the management of dying patients. Cases have often focused on a split or angry family. It is important to focus on the wishes of the patient or the presence of a living will. Details of what actually takes place during the procedure are usually a secondary issue. Data suggest that PEG benefits stroke patients with good rehabilitation potential. However, PEG for the hypophagia of dementia does not improve longevity or quality of life. Prophylactic antibiotics significantly reduce infection rates. Long-term patency depends on catheter size. Buried bumper syndrome is a rare complication of PEG. The condition results from excessive tension between the external and internal bumpers, resulting in migration of the internal bumper through the abdominal wall.

During the procedure an endoscope visualises the catheter being pushed into the stomach. The endoscope is used to pull a wire fed through this catheter out of the mouth, where the PEG tube is attached. It is then pulled back down into the stomach – a flange at one end stops it from being pulled out of the abdominal wall entirely, and secures it to the muscle of the stomach wall.

COMPLICATIONS

- Death 1%
- Pneumoperitoneum 38% – usually benign
- Peristomal pain 11%
- Haemorrhage 3% -
- Failure to place 5%.

Diagnostic colonoscopy/flexible sigmoidoscopy

Colonoscopy is usually well tolerated and is mostly performed with sedation. Patients require bowel preparation, which takes place the night before. There are data to suggest that screening for colorectal cancer with colonoscopy is of benefit to patients. Flexible sigmoidoscopy requires no sedation and the bowel is prepared with a phosphate enema before the procedure.

COMPLICATIONS

- Death 0–0.019%
- Perforation 0.02%
- Cardiopulmonary 0.1%.

Transhepatic portosystemic shunt (TIPSS)

This procedure is performed for patients with diuretic-resistant ascites and/or variceal bleeding. It is used when banding has been unsuccessful and it is performed in order to prevent further bleeding. It is often used as a stopgap to prevent bleeding before transplant surgery. However, it is associated with a high rate of encephalopathy.

COMPLICATIONS

- Death: procedure related 1.2%
- Failure to deploy 4.6%
- Blockage at 1 year 54.6%
- Blockage at 2 years 74%
- Hepatic encephalopathy (HE) 29.9%
- New encephalopathy 11.5%
- Death at 3 years: all cause 60.4%.

During the procedure a line is passed through the internal jugular vein to the hepatic vein. From this a stent is then passed from through the liver to the portal vein.

ETHICAL AND LEGAL ISSUES IN MEDICINE

Although communication skills are of paramount importance in a patient consultation, it is also essential that doctors are aware of the legal and ethical issues surrounding a few difficult issues. It is impossible for a candidate to discuss these issues if he or she is unaware of these rules that govern them. It should be remembered that, in real life, making difficult legal or ethical decisions alone is usually a mistake; involving other professionals makes the process easier and gives a more balanced opinion. Medical defence organisations offer legal and ethical advice 24 hours a day to members.

Although your cultural background and personal beliefs influence your approach to a patient when discussing ethical issues, it is vitally important to be able to put these to one side and to respect an individual's legal rights. These rights have changed over the years, but in the UK are currently defined by the Human Rights Act 1998. There are numerous articles within this convention, including the right to liberty and the right to respect a private life. It is also clearly stated that it is unlawful for a public authority, such as the NHS, to contravene this convention.

Consent

The philosophy that 'doctor knows best' is a thoroughly outdated way to practise medicine; patients have the right to self-determination and, after an informed two-way discussion, can refuse any suggested treatment except where covered by the Mental Health Act.

In order to obtain consent, an individual must be deemed competent to understand and retain the information, using it to reach a reasonable decision. This decision requires a patient to be accurately informed as to the nature and risks of the planned procedure. Legally, any non-consensual contact is the tort of battery.

How much does the patient need to know?

In the UK, patients do not necessarily have to be informed of every side effect or risk from a specific treatment. Patients should understand 'in broad terms' the nature of the events; doctors can withhold information from a patient on the grounds of 'therapeutic privilege' (*Chatterton v Gerson* 1981). It is not always deemed to be in the best interest of the patient to discuss extremely unlikely side effects, because it may lead to undue anxiety and poor decision-making.
In general terms patients should be told of all common side effects, even if not serious, and all serious side effects, even if rare.

Situations where consent is not possible

Unconscious patients are unable to give the necessary consent required for treatment. Under these circumstances doctors can give emergency treatment if it is in the best interests of the patient – the 'doctrine of necessity'. There has been recent upheaval in the law about this issue. It is called the 2005 Mental Health Capacity Act. The following is a summary of this act:

- It makes advanced directives legally enforceable. However, patients can direct only future treatment opinions and cannot stipulate specific wants, eg 'I want to be treated at the Hammersmith' is not enforceable, whereas 'I don't want to be treated at Bart's' is.
- It makes it a criminal offence to take advantage of someone with impaired capacity.
- There is a new process for allocating management of financial affairs.
- There is a new code of practice that applies to all health professionals who will need to know how to assess capacity (no longer the remit of psychiatrists) and who must document how it has been assessed, if the patient is deemed to have impaired capacity.

The Department of Health have separated it into five sections (www.dh.gov.uk):

1. Adults have the right to make their own decisions and must be assumed to have capacity to do so unless it is proved otherwise.
2. Individuals must be supported to make their own decisions – people must be given all appropriate help before anyone concludes that they cannot make their own decisions.
3. Individuals must retain the right to make what might be seen as eccentric or unwise decisions.
4. Anything done for or on behalf of people without capacity must be in their best interests.
5. Anything done for or on behalf of people without capacity should be the least restrictive of their basic rights and freedoms.

Advanced directives are made prospectively in order to convey our wishes on specific matters in case we are unable to give subsequent consent as a result of incompetence for whatever reason. They are recognised in law and must be respected as long as completed by a competent, witnessed adult. Patients should seek the help of a medical practitioner when completing an advanced directive. Review of advanced directives is recommended periodically.

If mental impairment is confirmed – defined as any disability or disorder of the mind or brain, whether permanent or temporary, which results in impairment or disturbance of mental function – the patient is unable to give consent. Doctors should still act in the best interests of the patient if there is no clear direction from the Mental Health Capacity Act (ie no living will). These decisions should be consistent with a reasonable body of medical opinion – this is known as the Bolam test (*Bolam v Friern Hospital Management Committee* 1957).

Detainment of patients against their will under the 1983 Mental Health Act is aimed at controlling patients who are a danger either to themselves or to others as a result of temporary or permanent mental illness. They can be detained/restrained for varying periods, depending on the clause of the Act, and can be given treatment, but only for their mental illness, that is deemed in their best interest or the best interests of the public.

Relatives have a legal influence with regard to giving consent in only two situations: in minors who are not 'Gillick competent' and after death.

The Family Law Reform Act of 1969 defines a minor as below 18 years of age. However, for the purposes of medical treatment a patient achieves adult status at 16. A competent young person aged between 16 and 18 years can therefore give valid consent to any surgical, medical or dental treatment, regardless of parental opinion. Where the age of 16 and 17 is important is in cases of mental incompetence, in which situation a parent can act for them until they come of age.

Children under the age of 16 can give consent for medical intervention, or refuse it, if they are deemed to be of sufficient maturity and intelligence to understand the implications of the treatment. This is referred to as 'Gillick competence' (*Gillick v West Norfolk and Wisbech AHA* 1985), eg prescribing the oral contraceptive pill to a 14-year-old girl without the consent of the parents is allowed only if the child has sufficient maturity to understand the implications of the treatment.

Parents must act in the best interests of their child in order to give valid consent. If it is deemed by the medical staff that this is not the case, the child can be made a ward of court and treated without the parents' consent. However, this should be the last course of action. Acting against the parents' wishes will usually result in a breakdown in the doctor–patient/parent relationship, and may ultimately compromise the health care of the individual. Often, taking time to explain the situation, and building a trusting relationship with the people involved, is an easier way to proceed.

Confidentiality

In order to maintain a good patient relationship, consultations should be carried out in confidence. We must, by law, breach confidence in certain circumstances and at other times we may breach confidence if deemed in the best interest of the patient. The latter situations are more common and potentially more difficult from an ethical perspective.

Contrary to a widespread belief by both medical practitioners and the public, relatives, other than parents of a child, are not privy to any medical details of an individual in any circumstance. However, in order to act in the best interests of a patient, confidence must occasionally be broken. For example, if a patient is unconscious it may be in his or her best interest to break confidence not only to obtain more information, but also to relieve the anxiety of the relatives. It may become impossible to manage a patient effectively without allowing the relatives on board. Striking a balance of keeping relatives happy and obtaining as much information as possible while respecting the rights of an individual is difficult.

Confidentially is often breached in hospital for the purposes of cross-specialty care; patients may rarely need to be made aware of this. It is accepted by patients that health-care professionals will have access to medical notes, but confidentiality must at all times be maintained.

Situations where confidentiality must be broken

- Notifiable diseases (eg TB, plague and food poisoning)
- Under Section 18 of the Prevention of Terrorism Act 1989
- If a warrant from a circuit judge has been obtained
- Individuals who have been involved in a road traffic accident (RTA): a doctor who suspects that a patient has been involved in an RTA is under a duty to give information to the police, but only in order to identify the driver (*Hunter v Mann* 1974).

Situations where confidentiality can be broken

- Where someone is acting in the best interests of the patient (only if unconscious, or confused).
- Acting in the best interests of society:
  - eg AIDS is not a notifiable disease and individuals have the right to confidentiality. Although the patient should be strongly encouraged to inform others at risk, he or she does not have to do so. However, in exceptional circumstances, where it is considered to be of benefit to society, disclosing information can be done without the express consent of the patient. You are acting to prevent potential harm to other individuals.
  - while the courts in England are reluctant to make A liable for the crimes of B, the extent of a doctor's duty to a third party in England would appear to be this. A doctor must not ignore the risk to others created by a patient, but weigh up duty to society against duty to an individual.

Situations where confidentiality should not be broken

In cases of sexually transmitted infection and abortions confidentiality must be maintained.

This respect of confidentiality also applies after a patient has died.

> I will respect the secrets which are confided in me even after the patient has died – Declaration of Geneva (as amended by Sydney 1968).

Negligence

Three separate issues are involved in demonstrating negligence in the UK:

1. A duty of care between the doctor and patient must be established, eg a doctor is not obliged to help someone in distress on the street because no duty of care has been established.
2. A breach of this duty of care must be demonstrated. The patient must show that the treatment was not in accordance with a reasonable body of medical opinion (see Bolam test above). This is an area of controversy and allows doctors to self-regulate. In light of recent events in the UK and subsequent press interest, self-regulation may become a thing of the past. The future points towards an independent body, with members of the public involved in the regulation of the medical profession.
3. This breech of duty of care caused harm. The claim should be bought within 3 years of the action occurring, unless under exceptional circumstances.

In the UK financial reward for a successful claim is aimed at compensating the individual or family rather than punishing the guilty parties. The Woolf reforms (2000) made the process of a claim quicker and easier. Most cases should be settled out of court and a claim should be acknowledged within 21 days.

Complaints

From 1 September 2006, changes to the NHS complaints regulation came into force. The changes are designed to make the complaints procedure clearer and easier to access for those who need it.

Three bodies can be approached for help:

1. The Independent Complaints Advocacy Service
2. The Patients' Advice Liaison Service (PALS)
3. NHS Direct.

An individual can complain if he or she feels that the NHS directly adversely affected his or her life or care. Someone can complain on another person's behalf with his or her consent. This should take place within 6 months of the event and the first stage is to complain locally. These complaints can usually be dealt with quickly. It should be done by writing to the complaints manager of the specific institution. Patients will receive a response within 25 working days. If patients are unhappy with the result of this, they can ask for an independent review from the Heathcare Commission.

Hospital notes

Patients have the right to see their medical notes and computer records, which are subject to the Data Protection Act 1998. If a patient asks to review his or her notes it should be done with a member of the medical team, to explain medical terms.

Individuals not directly involved in the health of the patient must obtain consent to see the medical records.

Life and death

From a legal point of view, life ends when brain-stem death occurs. There is a series of tests that must be carried out to confirm this. It is possible for respiration to be supported artificially, even once brain-stem death has occurred (ie ventilation). Withdrawing artificial support once a diagnosis of brain-stem death has been made requires a series of steps, detailed below. These patients are often candidates for organ donation.

Diagnosing brain-stem death

- Deep coma with absent respiration
- Absence of hypoxia, hypothermia, hypoglycaemia, acidosis, abnormal biochemistry and sedative drugs.

Tests include:

- Fixed dilated pupils, absent corneal response and vestibulo-ocular reflex
- No gag reflex or motor response in the cranial nerves
- No respiratory effort on stopping the ventilator and allowing the $Paco_2$ to rise to 6.7 kPa.

The tests should be performed by a consultant or his deputy in the presence of another doctor. They should be repeated after at least a 24-hour interval.

In the USA an EEG is required to confirm brain death.

Persistent vegetative state

Patients whose brain-stem function persists despite loss of cortical function are described as having a persistent vegetative state (PVS). Their quality of life is at best uncertain, and their life depends on artificial feeding. However, it is possible to withdraw this feeding only via a court order. The test case for this was that of Tony Bland, who was diagnosed with PVS after the Hillsborough disaster. The test case was heard by the House of Lords – the doctors and relatives involved felt that feeding should be stopped, their Lordships agreed and feeding was subsequently withdrawn.

Euthanasia

Competent patients have the right to refuse any active treatment that may prolong their life. However, euthanasia – the process of accelerating death by active artificial intervention – is viewed in a different way. Currently active euthanasia is illegal in the UK. Test cases have been unsuccessful in altering this premise (*R v Cox* 1992). The only country to allow active euthanasia is the Netherlands, but it is subject to strict guidelines. The USA remains against active euthanasia.

Under present legislation in the UK, doctors performing an intervention to terminate life are guilty of manslaughter, despite the wishes of the patient.

Whether accelerating the death of a terminally ill individual is in best interests is open to debate. The termination of life contradicts many firmly held religious beliefs across a wide spectrum of faiths, resulting in heated debate. These decisions on euthanasia should be made by society as a whole and reflected in legislation. Doctors must act within the law and may need to compromise their own personal beliefs.

Doctors can administer symptomatic treatment that has known adverse side effects. This is the 'principle of double effect'. A classic example is increasing doses of opiates to control pain of terminally ill patients but that may also hasten the process of death. From a medical point of view it would be generally accepted that the paramount objective is to alleviate suffering by relieving the pain, and administration of large doses of opiates is acting in the best interests of the patient. Do not take decisions of this magnitude alone; discuss with colleagues, nurses, patient and family as appropriate, and carefully document all decisions and discussions in the medical notes.

Once a duty of care is established doctors must act in the best interests of the patient. Omitting treatment that may prolong suffering does not necessarily break that duty of care, eg not prescribing antibiotics for infections. This omission of treatment is called passive euthanasia. Any ongoing treatment that is futile should be stopped in terminally ill patients. Administering an ineffective treatment with symptomatic side effects is not in the best interests of the patient because the side effects outweigh the benefits.

Resuscitation

Discussing resuscitation status with the patient is strongly encouraged and this should be done wherever possible or reasonable, a view supported by the General Medical Council (GMC). However, common sense governs the timing of such a discussion, eg it is probably inappropriate with relatively fit young patients where it would lead to unnecessary anxiety. Patients remain for resuscitation until a decision has been made. Resuscitation should be attempted if there is any uncertainty about the decision of the patient or the nature of the disease. If a competent patient does not wish to be resuscitated this should be respected.

Resuscitation should not be performed if it is deemed futile, or not in the best interests of the patient. Resuscitation can be an inhumane act under certain circumstances. If a decision not to resuscitate has been made, it should be clearly documented in the medical notes.

If the patient is unconscious, discussion with the relatives may give an impression of what the patient might have wanted. We do not consult relatives for their opinion on the right course of action, although this should be respected. The opinion or wishes of relatives about resuscitation has no legal standing. Living wills/advanced directives must be respected.

Gynaecological issues

Infertility treatment and abortion are areas of intense legal and ethical debate. For the purposes of PACES we do not dwell on them, because they are unlikely to be featured in the exam. However, having some general knowledge is reasonable. The 1967 Abortion Act states that a pregnancy can be terminated if the pregnancy has not exceeded 24 weeks, provided that continuing the pregnancy does not pose a risk to the mental or physical health of the mother, or existing children.

Alternatively termination may be carried out if deemed necessary to prevent grave permanent injury (mental or physical) to the mother. It can be carried out up to term if the baby is physically or mentally handicapped. Termination of pregnancy remains illegal in Ireland and the sanctity of life is one of the corner-stones of the Catholic Church.

Ownership of body parts

The Nuffield Report 1995 states that any consent to medical intervention implies that tissue removed is regarded as abandoned. Any tissue donated is regarded as a gift.

Organ donation

If the patient expressed a wish to donate organs after death this should be respected. Relatives must give consent for donation and must be consulted; they can refuse donation even if the deceased's wishes were well known. After death the next of kin have lawful possession of the body. If you die and there are no next of kin the hospital has possession. Once transplantation has taken place the organs are the possession of the recipient.

Although advanced directives are legal documents, organ donor cards are not, and give only an impression of what the deceased wished at the time of completion.

Organ donation from a live donor must not be detrimental to the health of that individual. The donor need not be an adult, eg matched, related, bone marrow donation.

Once donated, the organ is the possession of the recipient.

Organs cannot be legally bought or sold in the UK. If a donation is to take place between two unrelated individuals it must be referred to the Unrelated Live Transplantation Authority.

Research

A research project should start only after the approval of a research and ethics committee has been given. It is unlawful to carry out research on patients who are unable to give consent. Samples taken cannot be used for research retrospectively if consent was not given specifically when the samples were taken, although these samples are not deemed the property of the patient.

Allocation of resources

Individuals would like to have the health care that is most appropriate to them at the most optimal time. However, limited resources inevitably result in rationing and society decides what it can and cannot afford. Care is often delivered from a waiting list, with emergency intervention taking priority.

In the UK, the National Institute for Health and Clinical Excellence (NICE) assesses treatments for their clinical and financial effectiveness. This method of allocation is known as a utilitarian approach, which roughly translates as providing the greatest utility for the greatest number of people.

Deontological theory views ethical issues from a different angle, and is based on the optimal treatment for the individual regardless of resources. These two theories often contradict each other. For example, an expensive drug may not be approved by NICE despite showing a benefit to certain patient groups. Under these circumstances NICE would argue that the cost outweighs the benefit to society as a whole, and the resources may be better placed elsewhere.

Table of cases

Bolam v Friern Hospital Management Committee [1957] 1 WLR 582.

Gillick v West Norfolk and Wisbech AHA [1985] 3 All ER 402.

Hunter v Mann [1974] 2 All ER 414.

R v Cox [1992] 12 BMLR 38.

Ethical and Legal Issue Scenarios

A number of cases, which appear in communication skills exams, require the application of the legal and ethical issues described above to negotiate a difficult situation. Although a sympathetic attitude, a smile and positive attitude are helpful, it is not enough in many of these communication skills cases, especially in those cases involving legal issues. An ability to communicate within the framework of medical law is required. Therefore a familiarity with the previous pages, before launching into the following cases, is required.

1. Ethical dilemma: difficult situations
2. Ethical issues: driving regulations
3. Ethical dilemma: difficult situation – DNAR Orders
4. Ethical dilemma: clinical governance
5. Ethical dilemma: advanced directives
6. Ethical dilemma: consent to HIV testing
7. Ethical dilemma: difficult situation
8. Legal issues with regard to driving after a first fit

SCENARIO 1. ETHICAL DILEMMA: DIFFICULT SITUATIONS

The daughter knows that her mother has cancer but does not want you to tell her.

Legal and ethical issues

- The duty of care is to the mother.
- The daughter should not have found out – although there is nothing that you can do about that now.
- The daughter knows the patient much better than you and might be right.
- Ultimately both the patient and health-care team may rely on the daughter to support the patient; breakdown in the relationship with her would therefore be a disaster.

A good candidate

- Will acknowledge the daughter's fears and concerns
- Will explain their duty of care to the mother non-confrontationally.

Approach to the daughter

- As above, check the information; speak to the other carers looking after the patient.
- Take the daughter to a quiet room.
- Ask how she knows the diagnosis.
- Ask how she knows that her mother does not know.
- Ask why she does not want her mother to know.
- Explain that you appreciate that she knows her mother much better than the doctors. However, having seen this situation many times before, telling the mother the truth is usually what she wants and is best in the long term.

  'Deep down most people know when there is something seriously wrong, and finding out can be a relief.'

- Explain to the daughter that you need to be sure that her mother does not want to know her diagnosis.
- Explain that you will talk to the mother and give her a small amount of information, and will answer questions truthfully leading from that.

  'If she does not want to know I will not tell her.'

Follow the breaking bad news approach for patients with no insight, giving only small amounts of information at a time (see earlier).

Patients who have been previously misinformed before your consultation.

Common examples

- Patients who have been told that curative treatment is available, when it is not.
- Patients told that surgery will be next week, when the waiting list is much longer.
- Patients given the wrong diagnosis/prognosis/treatment.
- Patients informed that results will be available, when they are not.

A good candidate

- Will attempt to shift the focus of discussion from past errors to current and future choices
- Will remain calm.

What to say

- Check that the information that you have is correct.
- Explain that the previous information is not correct.
- Explain that whatever has happened in the past is out of your control now.
- Explain that the key now is to look to the best treatment for the future.
- Make an attempt to find out why things went wrong in the past.
- Offer the patient a second opinion if he or she wants one.
- The chances are that the patient will be angry with the medical profession as a whole, and you are the person available to vent anger on.
- Even though you are not responsible an apology may well be appropriate.
- An over-defensive, or aggressive, approach from you will be counterproductive.
- The best approach is to weather the storm and remain calm. Once the patient has expressed his or her opinion, suggest that you will find out what went wrong in the past to stop it happening again, but now you must try to focus on the future and the current medical problems.

Admitting your own mistakes to patients and other doctors.

It is very easy to make a mistake in medicine; admitting to it is slightly more difficult.

The key is honesty with patients and colleagues at an early stage. Any attempt to lie or cover up may backfire in a most dramatic fashion.

A good candidate

- Will apologise
- Will explain how the error will be prevented in the future.

Approach to the patient

- Most patients understand that nobody is perfect and that applies to doctors too
- Be honest and apologetic
- Tell the patient at the first available opportunity
- Explain what the plan was and what went wrong
- Explain what the options are in the future (including seeking a second opinion)
- Explain how you will try to prevent the same mistake happening again
- Listen carefully to what the patient has to say.

Surprisingly most patients will take the issue no further, proving that they feel that the explanation is satisfactory, and individuals are truly apologetic.

Most formal complaints or litigation issues are the result of a breakdown in the doctor–patient relationship and poor communication skills, rather than the mistake itself.

SCENARIO 2. ETHICAL ISSUES: DRIVING REGULATIONS

A 48-year-old taxi driver who has type 2 diabetes is attending your diabetic clinic. He has had multiple laser photocoagulations for pre-proliferative retinopathy and now has a fixed field defect that does not fulfil DVLA requirements for driving. He says that he cannot afford to give up driving because he is the only income earner in the family and has three small children.

Please discuss this with him.

Preparatory thoughts

This is one of the most common cases to appear in communication skills exams, a bit like valvular heart disease in the examination section. It is a good test because it investigates candidate's knowledge and communications skills, making it discriminatory. Therefore it is very important to know the rules about driving.

- His legal obligation to inform the DVLA
- The ethical reasons why he should stop driving – danger to others
- Your ethical and legal obligations as a doctor
- Social implications – alternative careers
- His right to ask for a second opinion.

A good candidate

- Will be very clear about the legal issues surrounding driving
- Will explain the ethical issues as well as the legal issues surrounding the case
- Will maintain the patient's trust and discuss the potential alternatives.

Goals for consultation

- Impress upon him the need to stop driving (legal and ethical issues)
- Maintain the doctor–patient relationship, so that he will return to the clinic
- He informs the DVLA.

Key points in the consultation

- Introduction and establish a rapport
- Establish the patient's expectations and understanding of diabetes and driving
- Explain the results of his visual field tests and their implications
- Approach the consultation in a manner of the doctor and patient working together as a team
- Establish why the patient 'cannot afford' to stop driving

- Look for a possible compromise, eg enlist Social Services support for alternative careers and financial support
- Impress on him the danger to himself and others if he continues to drive
- If necessary, raise issues of family and social obligation
- Inform patient of his legal obligation to inform the DVLA; if he will not, you will have to.

Finishing

- Write careful records of all the discussions in the notes
- Summarise the consultation
- Ensure that he understands what has been said
- Ask if he has any questions
- Arrange a follow-up appointment.

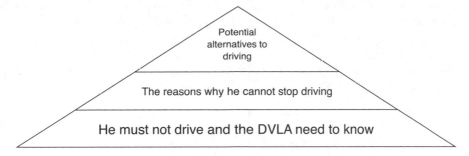

Discussion

In this scenario, the worse case is if the patient leaves the consultation and continues to drive illegally and does not return. You need to strike a balance between firmness and empathy. This scenario again emphasises the need for candidates in PACES to be familiar with the law about driving and the common medical conditions that legally prevent driving (www.dvla.gov.uk – see page 173). The same DVLA rules apply to taxi drivers as to other motor vehicle users, although they are additionally subject to restrictions from the Public Carriage Office/local authority.

SCENARIO 3. ETHICAL DILEMMA: DIFFICULT SITUATION – DNAR ORDERS

You have admitted a 74-year-old man to a general medical ward with a chest infection; he is not recovering as quickly as expected. He has known pre-existing ischaemic heart failure (New York Heart Association or NYHA class 3), for which he is receiving optimum medical therapy. The staff nurse has bleeped you to clarify his resuscitation status, because there is no written record.

Please discuss this issue with your patient.

Preliminary thoughts

These cases are disproportionately common, and should be practised with colleagues before the exam. It is relatively easy as an examiner to see which candidates have good experience of this scenario, making it a discriminatory case. The approach should be relatively slow, exploring the patient's understanding of his or her health. This should give the candidate some expectation of what the patient wants. The consultation should be directed appropriately. It is possible that a discussion about resuscitation within the time frame is totally inappropriate, although this is unlikely in an exam setting.

- Resuscitation (see page 419):
  - risk vs benefit
  - his irreversible medical condition with limited life expectancy
  - low likelihood of success
- Legal and ethical issues: the best practice is that a patient's resuscitation status should be discussed with him or her whenever possible (a view endorsed by the GMC); a possible exception to this is when resuscitation is deemed futile
- Does the patient have a living will?
- Discussion should take place in the presence of a nurse and careful documentation should be performed.

A good candidate

- Will approach the discussion asking question and in a discrete manner
- Will allow the patient to talk about his expectations for the future; clearly if he thinks that he is going to be alive and well in 5 years, there is not much point in discussing do not resuscitate (DNAR) orders – a realistic discussion about heart disease may be more appropriate
- Will be able to judge where the patient lies on the issue and guide the consultation appropriately.

Goals for consultation

- The patient makes an informed decision
- Other members of the medical and nursing team are informed of this decision.

Key points in the consultation

- Introduction and establish rapport
- Ensure that you are in a correct setting – patient on his own, with staff nurse present
- Establish patient's understanding of his underlying condition and reason for admission
- Emphasise that he is on maximum medical therapy, which will continue
- He should be aware that there will be a relentless decline in his cardiac function, which ultimately will be serious
- Explain that you want to talk about what might happen in the future
- What does he think will happen in the future?
- Ask him if he wants to talk about what might happen in the future if things were to go suddenly wrong while in hospital and he was not able to make decisions for himself.

At this point pause and allow the patient to reflect on the discussion. Before progressing the patient should be asked if he wants a family member present, knowing that the discussion is going to be a serious one.

Directions of consultation

Scenario A

The patient is unaware of the seriousness of his underlying condition and still hopes for an improvement.

- Although this may be unrealistic, the patient's views should be respected.
- Gently ensure that he is told of the seriousness of his condition.
- If he feels strongly that he would like every medical attempt made to prolong his life, that should also be respected.
- The issue of resuscitation should be addressed directly, once the patient understands his serious and progressive condition. 'We should address what you would like us to do if your health was to take a sudden turn for the worse and you were unable to make decisions fro yourself.'
- Hopefully by this stage the doctor and patient will have established a rapport, not making the question seem out of place.
- It may be that he continues to want to remain for resuscitation. If that is the case it should be carefully documented. It is difficult to argue that resuscitation in this case is futile.

Scenario B

The patient understands the seriousness of condition, but is unsure whether resuscitation would be appropriate.

- Often the patient will ask: 'What do you think doctor?'
- The patient should be informed of the relatively poor outcome of resuscitation and the often undignified manner of death (risks vs benefits).

Scenario C

The patient has thought about his condition and does not want resuscitation.

- His view should be respected and documented in his notes.
- The patient should be asked if he has discussed it with his next of kin, although this is not legally necessary.

Scenario D

The patient may leave the decision in the hands of the doctor.

- If this is the case the medical and nursing team should make a decision together.
- The patient should be asked if he or she wants relatives involved or even told.

Finishing

- Summarise the consultation
- Ask the patient if he has understood the discussion and if he has any questions
- Ask the patient if he wants the medical staff to tell family members of his decision
- Inform the nursing staff
- Document the decision carefully in the notes.

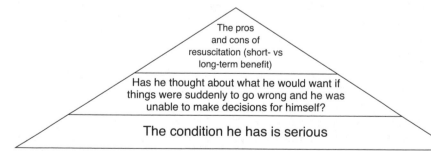

Discussion

Decisions about cardiopulmonary resuscitation (CPR) status of patients should be made whenever possible in full consultation with them.

It should be borne in mind that for every patient there comes a time when death is inevitable and failure of cardiac or respiratory function will occur. It is essential therefore to determine for each patient whether CPR is appropriate.

Detailed up-to-date guidelines are provided by the Resuscitation Council of the UK (www.resus.org.uk/pages/dnar). The principles are that effective, sensitive communication with patients should be undertaken in advance, keeping in mind that the circumstance of every patient is unique. Information about CPR and the chances of successful outcome should be realistic. A DNAR order should be given only after full consultation with the patient and the medical team. Situations in which it is not necessary to discuss with patients include those where attempting CPR will not be successful, or where there would be no benefit, eg coexistent severe morbidity.

SCENARIO 4. ETHICAL DILEMMA: CLINICAL GOVERNANCE

As a general medical SHO, you discover that one of your patients with pyelonephritis was given too much gentamicin for the pyelonephritis, over the weekend, by the on-call team, despite documented levels being toxic. She has since developed ototoxicity and deteriorating renal function, but is unlikely to need dialysis.

Please discuss the situation with the patient.

Preliminary thoughts

In this case is it would be easy to explain to the patient that the documented side effects of the drug include renal impairment and hearing loss, and it appears that they have occurred in this case. It is very likely that the patient will accept this and no more will be heard of the issue. However, this approach would be a mistake. It is very important to explain to the patient that she may have been given too much of the drug which could have made some of the side effects of the drug worse. The consultation is relatively easy from here. Mistakes get made and they need to be investigated. Tell the patient that she will be kept in the information loop and give her the opportunity to ask questions. These may include complaints (see page 417).

- Above all do not lie
- Most patients understand human fallibility and that mistakes occur
- Potentially, expect a stormy consultation; it is important to keep calm and not rise to the challenge
- This is not about apportioning blame or pointing the finger but more to do with risk management (why did the error occur and how can it be prevented?).

An incident form needs to be completed and the consultant needs to be informed.

A good candidate

- Will know about clinical governance and risk management
- Will come across as honest and transparent
- Will not be evasive.

Goals for consultation

- To have a frank and truthful discussion
- For the patient to feel:
    - that the matter is being dealt with appropriately and adequately
    - that plans are being made to prevent it happening again.

Key points

- Introduction and establish a rapport (including the patient's name)
- Tell the patient that there has been a problem with one of the drugs that she was given
- Explain the known side effects of the drug
- Explain the concept of a therapeutic range for gentamicin and the need to monitor levels
- Explain what happened
- Apologise for the error
- Emphasise openness and truthfulness
- Natural history: renal function will probably recover, but the ototoxicity may not
- Explain the steps that you have taken to determine the cause and to prevent it happening again (incidence form and risk management)
- Inform her that you will arrange for an ENT and renal opinion
- Need for continuing medical care for the pyelonephritis
- Possibility of further action for her to take in the future, eg formal complaint and PALS.

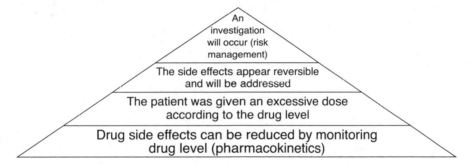

An investigation will occur (risk management)

The side effects appear reversible and will be addressed

The patient was given an excessive dose according to the drug level

Drug side effects can be reduced by monitoring drug level (pharmacokinetics)

Discussion

In circumstances of medical malpractice there are several key issues. The most important, above all, is to be apologetic and truthful. Do not:

- lie
- cover up
- be evasive
- alter notes
- point the finger

but give the impression of a failure of a number of safety steps, which need further investigation.

Although it may be tempting to try to tell half-truths or cover up mistakes in a patient's management, the truth should be told. Two erroneous ways in which to lead this scenario are either to try to pretend that an error was not made – 'We have got the levels of the gentamicin back now. They were a little bit high and that might have caused some of the problems' – or to point the finger at someone else: 'Someone has made the most terrible mistake and there is going to be a huge investigation.'

Clinical governance

This is a framework through which NHS organisations are accountable for continuous improvement of the quality of service. It must be seen as a systematic approach to quality assurance and must work at a local level.

Clinical governance will be upheld by a statutory duty on primary care trusts to monitor the quality of the heath care that they provide.

In order for it to be successful it is felt that the following must be upheld:

- Open culture: not a blame culture
- Education and sharing of good clinical practice
- Multidisciplinary approach to medicine
- Regular discussion of quality issue
- Breaking down the barriers between professional groups.

The pillars of clinical governance include:

- Clinical audit
- Clinical leadership
- Complaints
- Clinical risk management
- Application of information technology
- Continuing education.

SCENARIO 5. ETHICAL DILEMMA: ADVANCED DIRECTIVES

As a medical SHO, you are looking after a 74-year-old man who was admitted with a gastrointestinal bleed. Subsequent endoscopy has shown that this was the result of an underlying gastric carcinoma and a CT scan has demonstrated widespread metastatic disease. He is a widower who has repeatedly stated that he does not want any intervention. The psychiatrist has reviewed him and has stated that he is not depressed and is able to make informed decisions. He has now had a further GI bleed and is alert but clinically shocked. He is still refusing further intervention.

Please discuss this further with him.

Preliminary thoughts

- Does the patient understand the gravity of the situation?
- Does he have a living will/advanced directive (see Mental Heath Act 2005, page 414)
- Legal position of patient: informed consent and the right to refuse treatment, eg blood transfusion
- Legal position of doctor: treating a patient against his or her will is battery
- Treatment options available: palliative (no treatment should be given to accelerate death; however, treatment for symptoms, with side effects, can be given, eg morphine)
- Is there anyone else he would like contacted?

A good candidate

- Will ensure that the patient is making an informed decision
- Will understand and respect the patient's decision
- Will discuss the plan to tell family and sort out personal issues.

Goals for consultation

- Patient understands the seriousness of the condition.
- Patient makes a truly informed decision.
- Ensure that other members of the medical and nursing team are aware of his decision.

Key points in the consultation

- Introduction and establish a good rapport
- Explore the patient's feelings as to why he refuses treatment
- Explore patient's understanding of his underlying diagnosis and prognosis

- Explore patient's understanding of what refusal will entail, ie probable death within hours
- Explain the possible treatment options:
  - immediate for the bleeding – transfusion, sclerotherapy or laser photocoagulation; surgery is not a viable option
  - pain control, anxiolytics
- Inform the patient that you will comply with his wishes, even if he becomes unconscious
- Complete a DNAR with the patient
- Ask the patient if he has told other members of the family, or if he would like them to know of his decision; this is actually very important, as there is a good chance that he has not told his first-degree relatives
- Ask if he has sorted out his affairs at home because things may get suddenly worse
- Ask if there is anyone he would like to be informed or contacted
- Inform your registrar/consultant, nursing and on-call teams.

Finishing

- Document carefully the discussion in the notes (including a DNAR form)
- Summarise what has been discussed
- Ask if he has any questions
- Ensure that all has been done to improve his symptoms.

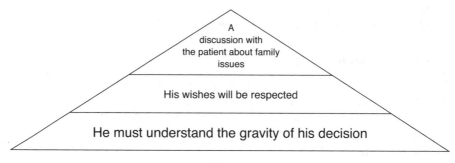

A discussion with the patient about family issues

His wishes will be respected

He must understand the gravity of his decision

Discussion

This scenario tests your understanding of informed consent, and you need to consider how an advanced directive would affect the situation (see page 414). You are not being tested on the emergency treatment of a shocked patient.

SCENARIO 6. ETHICAL DILEMMA: CONSENT TO HIV TESTING

As the SHO in infectious disease you are asked to see a 27-year-old female prostitute who had unprotected sex with her boyfriend a few nights ago. She has subsequently discovered that he is HIV positive and has now attended the walk-in genitourinary medicine (GUM) clinic for an HIV test and advice.

Please discuss these issues with her.

Preliminary thoughts

Candidates either do or do not know the process of HIV consent and testing. Clearly, having no idea about the interval between exposure and testing positive will make this consultation difficult. However, even under these circumstances the case can be salvaged. A discussion about previous potential exposure to HIV, hepatitis B and C and other sexually transmitted infections (STIs), prostitution with an unknown HIV status and financial/drug issues also need to be addressed. These are likely to take much more than 15 minutes.

- Has she had an HIV test before?
- How does she know this other person has HIV?
- It takes 2 months to test HIV positive after exposure. A p24 antigen test or PCR test may give a result sooner.
- Hepatitis B and C should also be considered (as well as other STIs).
- She should have an accelerated course for hepatitis B immunisation if she has not already received it.
- Has she put herself at risk of HIV before – unprotected sex with clients or intravenous drugs?
- She should be tested for HIV and hepatitis B today and again in 2 months. Rapid antibody testing (if available) can give a result within 30 min, but does not exclude infection in the past 3 months if negative.
- She may benefit from receiving 2 months of prophylactic highly active antiretroviral therapy (HAART) – this depends on whether or not she knows that her partner is HIV positive; as antiretroviral medication carries an appreciable morbidity and mortality this should be discussed with an HIV physician.
- Hepatitis C should be tested for now and in 10 days – interferon-α will help clear viral antigen in acute infection.
- Is she pregnant?
- What would she like to happen if she is unable to pick up her test result (next-of-kin issues)?

A good candidate

- Will know details of HIV testing
- Will not be judgemental about her lifestyle
- Will discuss other STIs and drug issues
- Will impress on her the ethical issues of potentially being HIV positive in her line of work. She needs to refrain or practise safe sex at least.

Goals for the consultation

- The patient should be aware that there is an interim period of 2 months between exposure and testing positive. She should not put others at risk in this period.
- To discuss other viruses – hepatitis B and C.
- She should be aware of safe sex.
- For her to understand that she will require prophylaxis against HIV.

Key points in the consultation

- Introduce yourself and try to establish a good rapport.
- The patient must be aware that confidentiality will be respected. However, confidentiality can be broken if she is knowingly putting others at risk.
- Discover the patient's knowledge about HIV, how it is transmitted and its prognosis.
- Depending on your rapport, try to ascertain why she is a prostitute – this may be important in terms of her future, eg intravenous drugs and coercion.
- Determine her use of intravenous drugs.
- How does she know her boyfriend is HIV positive – is there confirmatory evidence?
- Avoid being judgemental.

Directions of the consultation

Scenario A

She is not prepared to discuss her private life – she just wants the test.

- Do not attempt to force information from her.
- She should be aware of the risk factors for becoming infected with HIV, and attempt to modify her lifestyle accordingly.
- Transmission rates for heterosexual sex are thought to be low in the UK and she should be relatively reassured.
- She should be counselled about the implications of testing positive:
    - lifelong infection
    - without treatment, relatively short life expectancy as a result of immune suppression, and increased risk of a variety of infections and cancers

- – new drugs have revolutionised the treatment with a marked improvement in life expectancy
- – however, there is no cure
- – explanation that she will also be tested for other viruses that she might be at risk of – hepatitis B and C
- – that having an HIV test may have implications for future life assurance, employment, etc, but it will be up to her to disclose this
- – emphasis on her medical records being strictly confidential
- – that, if the test is positive, she will have to declare this on any future application if asked, or it will be invalid.
- She should understand the rationale behind 2 months of prophylactic HAART and its side effects (common – rash, diarrhoea, allergy; uncommon – lactic acidosis, hepatitis, pancreatitis).
- She should be aware that she may be putting others at risk of HIV if she continues to have sex with others until the result of the test is known. This may be difficult because it is her source of income.
- In any event, she should be told always to practise safe sex.

Scenario B

She is happy to discuss her life.

- Discuss her understanding of HIV infection and its risk factors.
- The relatively small chance of picking up HIV infection through this episode may be a low priority compared with other issues (intravenous drugs, accommodation, violence or sexual abuse). If appropriate offer involvement of the Social Services and a multidisciplinary approach.
- Consent for an HIV test (see above).

Finishing

- Summarise what has been said
- Ask if she has any questions
- Make follow-up arrangements
- Contact Social Services if required.

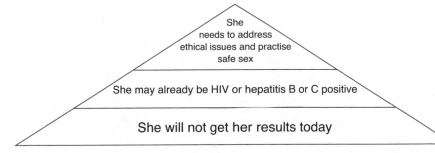

Discussion

Remember that this is a test of communication skills. It is more important to appear sympathetic and non-judgemental than to know great details about the best combination of antiretroviral therapy.

Some patients develop constitutional symptoms during seroconversion that may be worth discussing.

SCENARIO 7. ETHICAL DILEMMA: DIFFICULT SITUATION

An 84-year-old man had been admitted having been found collapsed and confused at home. He lives alone in a warden-controlled flat. On admission 2 weeks ago he had an MTS of 1/10, but after treatment of his urinary tract infection he now has an MTS of 8/10. The medical and nursing staff think that he is safe to go home and he has been assessed by the occupational therapist and physiother-apist with a successful home visit. The patient wishes to return home, but his daughter is extremely concerned about him and 'refuses' to let him home. The daughter has made an appointment to see you to discuss her father.

Please discuss the situation with her.

Preliminary thoughts

The 'unhappy relative' is disproportionably common in exams. This is probably because actors find it much easier to be relatives than patients, because they do not need to know symptoms and signs. Remember that, unless the patient has filled out an advanced directive/living will, candidates should get permission to talk to relatives from the patient. This information should be given in the text. It is not unreasonable to confirm with the examiners that this consent has been given before the interview begins. This case is straightforward and no real medical training as such is required. Start by listening to her concerns. Explain where the medical opinion lies. Attempt to find some common ground. If necessary, arrange a follow-up appointment. Previous candidates who have done well with this sort of case have remained calm and usually the actor has had a specific problem that was easily soluble. Those who have done less well attempted a more aggressive and arrogant approach: 'It's not up to you, he is going home.'

- Avoid antagonising the daughter (a foolproof way of failing the exam).
- Keep calm in a non-confrontational manner and act in the best interest of the patient.
- What are her concerns/worries?
- Flexibility and compromise will ultimately lead to common ground.
- Legal and ethical issues: the daughter has no legal rights over the care of her father (without an advanced directive), although she may be heavily involved at home. It is important to respect her opinion but, ultimately, the decision must be made in the best interests of the patient, not the daughter.

A good candidate

- Will build up a good rapport with the relative, to aid further discussion
- Will listen to the relative's concerns and try to resolve them
- Will discuss confidentiality issues with the examiners.

Goals for consultation

- To follow the patient's wishes and enable him to go home
- To explore why the daughter does not agree
- To make her aware of the reasons why he should go home
- Ultimately to gain her support for his return home.

Key points in the consultation

- Introduction and establish rapport.
  Explore her knowledge and views of her father's medical and social circumstances and why she feels that he is unsafe to return home.
- Explore her reasons: social needs, guilt, eg she may not be able to look after him at home for that particular week only; under these circumstances a compromise can be sought.
- Explain his medical condition and that his condition has now returned to his preadmission state.
- Explain that he has been assessed by the multidisciplinary team (occupational therapy, physiotherapy and social worker), all of whom think that he is safe to go home.
- Explain the risks of staying in hospital (eg infections, immobility).
- Determine what can be done to get her to change her mind.
- Explain that your duty of care is to the patient who wants to go home.
- He may be eligible for additional help:
  - home help
  - meals at home services 'meals on wheels'
  - attendance at a day centre.
- Explain that he will be carefully observed with a follow-up appointment.

Directions of the consultation

Scenario A

She remains adamant that he should stay in hospital.

- Under these circumstances a form of compromise or trial period at home can be attempted.
- The daughter must be made aware that it is in the patient's best interests to go home, but if things do not work out the situation can be reassessed.
- Impress on her that he will have continuing care and follow-up in the community and that hospitals are not necessarily the safest place to be.
- Arrange a case conference of all involved parties

Scenario B

There is something specific troubling her.

- The doctor should address this point and attempt to solve it.

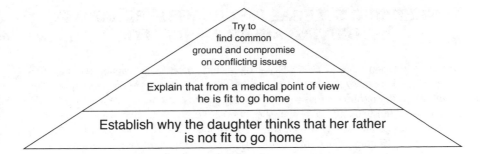

Try to
find common
ground and compromise
on conflicting issues

Explain that from a medical point of view
he is fit to go home

Establish why the daughter thinks that her father
is not fit to go home

Finishing

- Ask if she has any further questions.
- Agree a date for him returning home.
- Arrange for further discussions, if requested.
- Ensure that the nurses and team in the community are aware of the situation and your discussions.

SCENARIO 8. LEGAL ISSUES WITH REGARD TO DRIVING AFTER A FIRST FIT

You are the neurology SHO. A 24-year-old fashion model was diagnosed as having 'grand mal' epilepsy 6 months ago, but has failed to attend for follow-up appointments. In the last few weeks she has had several fits. She lives an extremely busy and social lifestyle and claims that she 'needs to drive a car' because of her work and social commitments, which she is still doing. She has a busy social life and drinks 20–30 units of alcohol a week, but also takes recreational drugs (predominantly cocaine). Although she is keen for any help to prevent her fits, she is very unwilling to take regular medication.

Please discuss the management of her epilepsy.

Preliminary thoughts

- The effects of alcohol/cocaine on epilepsy
- Which other drugs does she take?
- Legal issues about patient confidentiality vs informing the DVLA (see page 173)
- Medical treatment options.

A good candidate

- Will attempt to put the patient at ease and explain that the current situation cannot continue
- Will know the rules about driving and fits.

Goals of the consultation

- Attempt to build a rapport and maintain her trust.
- Ensure that she stops driving and informs the DVLA; if she does not, you will have to.
- She must understand that:
  - her fits will continue or get worse if she does not seek help
  - the fits may stop if she changes her lifestyle and seeks help.

Key points in the consultation

- Introduction and putting patient at ease
- Establish patient's expectations/fears – why has she turned up today?
- Establish this patient's level of understanding of her diagnosis, complications and possible treatment
- Establish her knowledge of precipitating factors, including alcohol, recreational drugs, late nights and general lifestyle
- Discuss the importance and benefits of stopping/preventing such precipitating factors

- Maintain balance between *realistic* aims and *ideal* aims. Is it likely that she will significantly change her behaviour?
- Discuss her need for possible medication, side effects, drug interactions (especially with the oral contraceptive pill or OCP)
- Impress upon her the ethical issues of continuing to drive and her responsibility to society
- Emphasise the legal requirement for her to inform the DVLA and to stop driving (possibility of re-commencing driving if fit free for 1 year), but that you have a legal duty to inform the DVLA if, in the future, you suspect that she is continuing to drive.
- Emphasise that most patients are free from medication within 5 years.

Directions of the consultation

Scenario A

The patient remains adamant that her lifestyle and fits are unrelated and/or is unwilling to stop driving.

- It is important repeatedly to stress to her the seriousness of her condition and the ethical issues associated with her continuing to drive: a firm but sympathetic approach may be required.
- All discussions should be well documented in her medical notes.
- As it is important for her to maintain faith in you, some form of compromise may be appropriate, eg stopping the recreational drugs for a week and returning to the clinic to see how things are. No compromise can be made concerning the driving.
- She should be aware that, ultimately, you will have to inform the DVLA.

Scenario B

She accepts the nature of her condition and agrees to modify her lifestyle, but is unwilling to stop driving.

- A more sympathetic nature should be pursued but stressing the legal and ethical reasons for stopping driving.
- She should be aware that, if she goes along with the medical advice and modifies her lifestyle, there is a good chance that her health will turn to normal and she will be able to lead a normal lifestyle, including driving.

Finishing

- Ask her if she has any questions.
- Ensure that she understands the nature of her condition.
- Make follow-up arrangements.

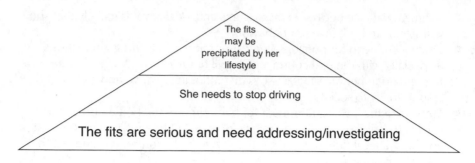

The fits
may be
precipitated by her
lifestyle

She needs to stop driving

The fits are serious and need addressing/investigating

Discussion

The GMC and DVLA Criteria for Driving (October 2001)

See also page 173.

If patients are suffering from conditions that may affect their driving, the onus lies with them to report this to the DVLA. If the patient is incapable of understanding this advice, the doctor should inform the DVLA immediately. Ultimately the DVLA is legally responsible for deciding if that patient is medically fit to drive. If patients refuse to accept their doctors' diagnosis, doctors should suggest a second opinion. If patients continue to drive when considered unfit, the doctor should report this to the medical officer at the DVLA. Before discussing legal issues it is often beneficial to discuss the ethical context in which the law arises. Individuals are more likely to comply with legislation if they understand the reasoning behind it. Candidates should be aware of the current regulations with regard to medical restrictions on driving (www.dvla.gov.uk).

Explaining a procedure and obtaining consent: Scenarios

This is the third type of scenario that occurs in communication skills exams. The most common procedures are included below.

1. Cardiac procedures – 1
2. Cardiac procedures – 2
3. Respiratory procedures
4. Consent for renal transplantation
5. Discussion about newly diagnosed diabetes
6. Genetics and HRT in breast cancer
7. Genetics: Huntington's disease
8. Breaking bad news and cancer procedures

SCENARIO 1. CARDIAC PROCEDURES – 1

As a cardiology SHO you know that there is a long waiting list of patients for coronary intervention. Your next patient is a 52-year-old man who, despite having had two previous myocardial infarctions and a coronary artery bypass graft (CABG) 5 years ago, continues to smoke 40 cigarettes per day. He is now having recurrent worsening angina, with an exercise tolerance of 50 m. An angiogram shows diffuse disease not amenable to angioplasty, but suitable for re-do CABG.

Please discuss the results of this test and further management. He is on maximal medical therapy.

Preliminary thoughts

- A re-do CABG may alleviate symptoms, but the risk vs benefits must be considered
- Effects on his overall prognosis
- Does his lifestyle affect the decision vis-à-vis smoking?
- Attitude of patient and compliance with treatment
- Any previous attempts to stop smoking (nicotine gum, acupuncture, peer pressure)?

A good candidate

- Will ensure that the patient understands the implication of continuing to smoke
- Will ensure that the patient has had the opportunity to have help to quit
- Will not appear over-judgemental – after all what he is doing is perfectly legal and at no time in the past was he told that it may have an effect on allocation of health-care resources.

Goals for consultation

- He must understand that life modification is required (ie stopping smoking).
- He must understand the morbidity and mortality associated with and without surgery.
- He must be aware that further intervention may not happen immediately (the waiting list principle associated with limited resources).

Key points

- Introduction and establish a rapport
- Establish this patient's understanding of his disease, its severity and consequences of continuing to smoke
- Avoid being judgemental about his smoking
- Explain the results of his recent angiogram

- Establish this patient's understanding and expectations of his possible treatment options
- Explain the risks and benefits of repeat CABG:
  - possible relief of symptoms
  - limited benefit in 5-year survival rate
- Ensure that other risk factors have been addressed.

Direction of consultation

The doctor can approach the consultation in one of many ways, which will be influenced by both his or her own views and the attitude of the patient. The doctor should try to avoid preaching or being judgemental. The patient should be made aware that there is a need to stop smoking. However, there are ethical issues with regard to whether his future management should depend on him agreeing to give up.

There are two extremes and most doctors' approaches tend to be somewhere in the middle.

Approach A

We will not go ahead with the surgery unless you agree to stop smoking.

Reason: the money could probably be better spent on individuals who have stopped or never smoked.

Approach B

You probably should try to give up, but we will put you on the waiting list anyway.

Reason: he has paid his national insurance (and a large amount of tax on cigarettes) and therefore deserves the same care as everyone else. After all, there is no guarantee that, once the procedure has taken place, the patient will not start smoking again, even if he promises to give up.

There is a debate about allocation of resources in this setting. Some NHS trusts advocate that, unless individuals stop smoking (or even lose weight), they will not be eligible for an operation. They argue that, unless this takes place, the chance of success is reduced, so patients are being asked to stop smoking before the procedure can take place. Whether or not this genuinely has the patient's interests at heart is open to debate that will continue.

Finishing

- Ensure that he understands the need to stop smoking and the possibility of further surgery
- Summarise the consultation
- Ask if he has any questions
- Arrange follow-up.

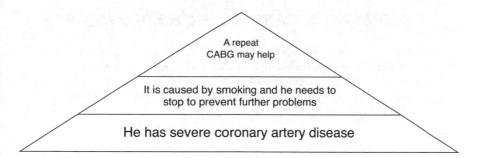

SCENARIO 2. CARDIAC PROCEDURES – 2

This 45-year-old man, who is a hypertensive smoker, has had a recent exercise tolerance test that was positive (he does not know the result). He has had his blood pressure controlled and been advised to stop smoking. He will need coronary angiography. Please discuss the result of the exercise test with him and the need for coronary angiography.

Points to consider

The exercise tolerance test (ETT) was positive which is highly suggestive of coronary artery disease (CAD). The following are benefits and consequences of angiography:

- Identification of coronary lesions
- The potential need for angioplasty or even CABG.

Possible side effects of angiography

- Death 0.05%
- Cerebrovascular accident (CVA) 0.05%
- Nephropathy 2%
- Femoral haematoma 10%
- Femoral artery pseudoaneurysm 1%

Risk factors for complications include technician's inexperience, greater catheter size and high BMI.

How successful has he been with modification of risk factors associated with CAD:

- Smoking: smoking cessation groups, nicotine replacement
- Weight gain: often temporary after cessation of smoking
- Blood pressure: is it being monitored?
- Cholesterol: has it been measured? What was the result?

A good candidate

- Will explore the patients understanding of why he had an ETT before giving him the results
- Will know the benefits and risks of angiography
- Will not forget to address the risk factors associated with smoking.

Approach to the patient

- Introduce yourself.
- Ask an open question about what he knows about why he had the ETT.
- Ask how he has been since the ETT. This is controversial in that it is not a history-taking session. It is possible that the actor will say that he has had

ongoing chest pain. This would be a mistake on the part of the examining team and suggests that the actor has not been briefed properly. However, this does need to be dealt with and these symptoms must be further investigated. The best way to deal with this is to say that initially we will discuss the results and implications of the ETT and then at the end go through the ongoing symptoms of chest pain. There are few marks in this part of the exam for history-taking skills.

- Explain that he has come today to discuss the results of the ETT.
- Give him the results.
- Explain that it is highly likely that he has CAD.
- Explain the need for further investigation (see above).
- Explain that a wire will be passed through the groin or arm, and dye will be used to look more carefully at the coronary arteries. The procedure is done as an outpatient and the main side effect is a bruise or bleeding in the site of insertion of the wire. The procedure is carried out under local anaesthetic, so patients should not drive home. The results will not be given immediately.
- Discuss the progress with modification of risk factors (see above).

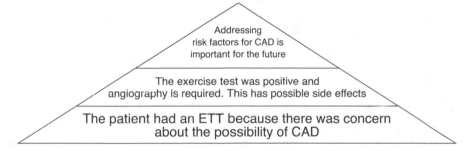

Discussion

If the candidate does not know the details of angiography it is not a necessarily irredeemable. It is, however, important to know in broad terms what it involves, ie a local anaesthetic, a day-case procedure and a wire is passed through the groin/arm. Results from previous candidates suggest that a failure to know, in broad terms, what is involved leads to failure. Making up details, when there is uncertainly, is a very efficient way of failing the exam, eg 'You will need to stay in hospital for a few days after the general anaesthetic'. If there is uncertainty candidates are advised to say that they will speak to the senior cardiologists performing the procedure to find out the details.

Coronary angioplasty and stenting (percutaneous transluminal coronary angioplasty or PTCA)

The procedure is similar to angiography, although it takes longer and is technically more difficult.

COMPLICATIONS

- Death 0.4%
- Acute coronary occlusion 1.3%
- Emergency CABG 0.6%
- Stent occlusion and re-stenosis
- Femoral haematoma 10%.

RISK FACTORS FOR COMPLICATIONS

- Older age (> 80: 3% mortality rate)
- Valve disease
- Emergency (primary) PTCA.

Radiofrequency pathway ablation

The patient needs to know that, although the procedure is similar to angiography, during the process of identification of the abnormal pathway or focus the heart rate may be increased and the patient experience chest pain and palpitations. These are expected and controllable. Greater catheter manipulation is probably responsible for increased rates of tamponade. It is worth mentioning that defibrillators can be inserted for potentially 'shockable' rhythms. The process of activation of the defibrillators is substantial in that patients feel like they have been kicked in the chest by a horse

COMPLICATIONS

- Death 0.05%
- Tamponade 1.22%
- High-grade arteriovenous (AV) block 0.79%
- Left-sided procedures:
  – CVA (0.2%)
  – transient ischaemic attack (TIA) 0.6%
  (otherwise as for diagnostic angiography)
- Pulmonary vein stenosis.

Permanent pacemaker insertion

A pacemaker is usually inserted for symptomatic or life-threatening bradycardias. There are a number of different pacemakers and candidates are advised not to go into too much detail about the advantages of one type as opposed to another, unless specifically asked. Patients need to know that the pacemaker will go under the skin on the chest wall, and that it is done under local anaesthetic as a day case. It will turn on and take over the pacing of the heart and will need to be checked on a regular basis.

COMPLICATIONS

- Pneumothorax 1.8%
- Cardiac perforation 0.98%
- Box erosion 0.5%
- Electrode displacement 1.6%
- Surgical revision required 5%.

DC cardioversion

DC cardioversion can take place either acutely or as a planned procedure. To our knowledge no candidate has been asked to discuss DC cardioversion in the acute setting. There are obviously reasons for this, in that the exam lasts for 15 min and acute DC cardioversion is a medical emergency. Therefore we focus on planned CD cardioversion, which is usually performed for atrial fibrillation. The procedure is carried out in an intensive care setting. Patients are given an anaesthetic and should not remember the procedure. Recurrence of the arrhythmia is the most common problem encountered. Repeated attempts are a story of diminishing returns.

COMPLICATIONS

- Thromboembolic event: < 48 h – 0.8% irrespective of anticoagulation
- Thromboembolic event: > 48 h – 0.93% if INR (international normalised ratio) < 2.5; 0–0.48% if INR > 2.5
- Superficial burns/pain: 84% mild-to-moderate pain, 23% moderate-to-severe pain on visual analogue scale
- Generation of more serious arrhythmia/asystole: rare enough for case reports to be submitted
- Anaesthesia-associated risk.

SCENARIO 3. RESPIRATORY PROCEDURES

A 56-year-old man who is a smoker has coughed up blood on three separate occasions over the last month. His GP has had a radiograph taken which shows a 3 cm coin-shaped lesion in the left upper lobe. Five days earlier his GP told him that the abnormality was present and has discussed the fact it may be a cancer. He has been referred to you for a bronchoscopy.

Points to consider

- Do not assume that the patient knows that he may have cancer, despite the letter from the GP.
- It is essential to ask open questions at the start of the consultation. 'Your GP has asked you to come and see me. Did he say what he thought was wrong?'
- Although it is likely that he has lung cancer, there is no histology and uncertainty exists. Therefore it must be stressed that it is not possible to be sure of the diagnosis without the biopsy. Use phrases such as 'We do not know the cause of this X-ray abnormality without histology, so anything we discuss about the cause is speculation'.
- Other phrases that are helpful include: 'Some of the causes are quite serious and that's why we are keen to do this soon.' If this phrase is used patients must be given an opportunity to ask questions. We are not convinced that there is any need to discuss lung cancer specifically to pass this communication skills scenario. This is especially true if the patient does not pick up on the warning shot (see Breaking Bad News, page 379). However, if the candidate is keen to raise cancer as a possibility as part of a differential diagnosis, this can be successful but should be approached with caution.
- After the initial open question, it may become apparent that the patient has gone through a long discussion about cancer with his GP and may not want to go through it all again. You therefore need to gain consent for the procedure and to explain why it is necessary.

During a bronchoscopy, patients have a local lidocaine throat spray and a sedative, which is usually a drug such as midazolam. The procedure is quick and done as a day case.

COMPLICATIONS
- Death 0.01%
- Pneumothorax 5%
- Risks of sedation increased with airway disease
- Major haemorrhage 0.9%.

A good candidate

- Will attempt to discover how much information the GP has told the patient
- Will explain that without a tissue diagnosis no definitive diagnosis can be made
- Will give the patients a chance to ask questions
- Will not necessarily discuss the possibility of cancer if it is clear that the patient does not want to talk about it.

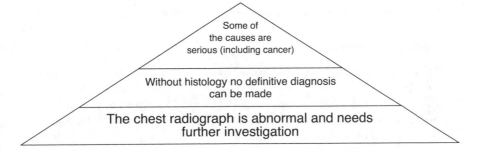

SCENARIO 4. CONSENT FOR RENAL TRANSPLANTATION

You are the SHO in the renal clinic. A 54-year-old man has had poorly controlled type 2 diabetes for the last 15 years. He also has hypertension and has been on continuous ambulatory peritoneal dialysis (CAPD) for the last 2 years. Previous haemodialysis has failed. He is not coping with CAPD. The renal MDT has decided that he should be placed on the renal transplant list.

Discuss with him the possibility of a renal transplantation.

Preliminary thoughts

- Why is he not coping (eg false expectations, social, compliance, recurrent infections)?
- Advantages and disadvantages of CAPD vs renal transplantation
- Short-, medium- and long-term complications of renal transplantation
- Practicalities of obtaining a transplant
- Legal and ethical issues
- Do patients with diabetes benefit from transplantation? Is it a good use of a limited resource? The answer to both is yes
- It is illegal to buy and sell kidneys for transplantation in the UK
- Should transplanted kidneys be allocated on a waiting list or where doctors perceive the greatest utility?

A good candidate

- Will not be over-critical of his poor diabetic control (after all it is not the goal of the consultation)
- Will allow the patient to express where he thinks diagnosis is going
- Will explore kidney transplantation and his views of it
- Will not put pressure on the patients to make a decision
- Will put the patient in touch with information about transplantation.

Goals for the consultation

- He must understand the benefits of changing from CAPD.
- He must understand the implications of transplantation.
- By the end of the consultation he should be in a position to make an informed decision about his future management.

Key points in the consultation

- Introduction and establish rapport
- Explore patient's understanding of his condition

Discuss reasons for non-coping with CAPD
- Explore patient's expectations of CAPD and transplantation
- Explain that he has end-stage renal failure and requires support. If he is not managing CAPD, renal transplantation is the only alternative, because haemodialysis has previously failed
- Practicalities of obtaining a transplant:
  - cadaveric vs live donor
  - the principle of waiting list – cannot guarantee that he will get one
  - the duration to transplantation depends upon an acceptable HLA match
- Complications of transplantation:
  - short term: surgical risks – will need to see surgeons
  - medium term:
    - immunosuppression: infection and side effects
    - risk of rejection
  - long term:
    - immunosuppression – secondary malignancy and infection
    - recurrent renal failure – 5-year graft survival (see Transplantation, page 19).

Finishing

- Ensure that the patient understands what has been said
- Ask if he has any questions
- Arrange follow-up appointment.

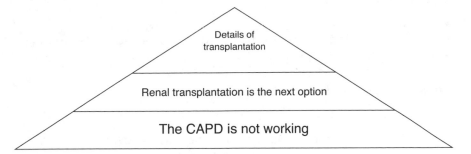

SCENARIO 5. DISCUSSION ABOUT NEWLY DIAGNOSED DIABETES

A 48-year-old man who is a company director has recently undergone a routine employment medical that has revealed glycosuria (no ketones). A subsequent fasting glucose is 12 mmol/l. He smokes 20 cigarettes/day, watches a lot of football and is obese. He has been referred to a new patient diabetes clinic for further advice and management.

Please discuss the results with him.

Preliminary thoughts

This scenario requires the candidate to impart knowledge of diabetes to the patient. It is commonly seen in exams:

- Does the patients have any idea about his diagnosis (probably not because of the routine nature of the medical)?
- Lifestyle influences may have a large part to play in the process and modification will help in the future
- Lifelong management
- Complications of diabetes
- Treatment options
- UKPDS (UK Prospective Diabetes Study) data.

A good candidate

- Will discuss risk factors
- Will emphasise the need for the patient to be in control of his health care
- Will know the treatment plan.

Goals for consultation

For him to understand:

- The importance of the patient and doctor (as part of the MDT) working together to control the disease (his input is vital).
- The lifelong nature of the disease, its complications and the need for treatment and lifestyle modification to prevent these complications.

Starting the consultation (after introductions, etc)

'We performed a series of tests when we saw you last time. Did someone explain which tests we were measuring and why?'

'No.'

'One of these was a measurement of your blood glucose. Have you had raised blood sugars in the past?'

'No.'

'The results performed last time show a raised blood sugar, you see.'

Key points in the consultation

- Introduction and establish rapport
- Establish patient's understanding of diabetes and its implications
- Establish patient's expectations
- Explain to the patient the basic mechanisms underlying his diabetes.
- Explain the aims of treatment: to reduce the risk of complications:
  - macrovascular: IHD (ischaemic heart disease), cerebrovascular and peripheral vascular disease
  - microvascular:
  - nephropathy
  - retinopathy
  - neuropathy
- All of these can be reduced with optimal glycaemic control
- Explain UKPDS data
- Emphasise need for lifelong treatment
- Emphasise the multidisciplinary approach:
  - diabetic specialist nurse
  - dietician
  - chiropodist/podiatrist
  - ophthalmologist
  - need for team work, but 'patient is the driver of the train'
- Outline possible treatments:
  - emphasise that dietary modification is the most important aspect of treatment combined with exercise
  - discuss oral medication if this is unsuccessful
  - discuss the possibility of insulin therapy in the future
- Address other risk factors, ie hypertension, hyperlipidaemia, smoking
- Emphasise the need for compliance and regular review.

Finishing

- Introduce him to the diabetic team
- Give him information about diabetes
- Arrange patient education sessions
- Arrange follow-up with MDT.

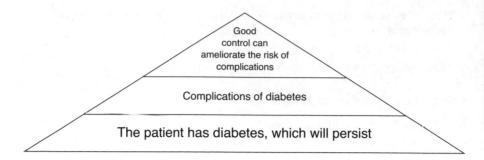

SCENARIO 6. GENETICS AND HRT IN BREAST CANCER

A 55-year-old woman has recently entered the menopause. She has very sympto-matic and troublesome hot flushes and some vaginal dryness. She has read about hormone replacement therapy (HRT) and wishes to discuss this with you. Her younger sister died 2 years ago of breast carcinoma (the only member of her family with the disease).

Please discuss HRT with her.

Preliminary thoughts

- Pros and cons of HRT
- Risk vs benefit: cancer, osteoporosis, symptoms, cardiovascular status
- Alternatives to HRT for symptoms
- Mammography screening for breast cancer and its reduced efficacy with HRT
- Legal and ethical issues about informed consent.

A good candidate

- Will make it clear that she is increasing her risk of breast cancer
- Will ask if her sister had genetic testing (the patient cannot be tested now, see below)
- Will discuss the alternatives
- Will ultimately let the patient make an informed decision
- Will encourage the patient to seek other advice before starting HRT.

Goals for consultation

- She must be in a position to make an informed decision.
- She must be aware of the increased risks in her particular case.
- A discussion about alternative treatments (eg clonidine for hot flushes).

Key points in the consultation

- Introduction and establish rapport.
- Establish patient's knowledge of HRT and concerns about it.
- Establish patient's expectations.
- Explain the risks/benefits of HRT.
- Benefits:
  - relieves symptoms of oestrogen deficiency
  - prevents osteoporosis,
  - possible decrease in risk of IHD, but evidence is unclear
  - decreases risk of uterine carcinoma and possibly colonic carcinoma.

- Risks: contraindications revolve predominantly around an increased risk of breast carcinoma. This is increased as a result of a family history. Oestrogens increase the risk of breast cancer by approximately twofold, but by sixfold with a family history. You should remember that taking a detailed family history is not part of the communications skills section and candidates will not be rewarded for this. However, it is worth asking if the sister was tested for genetic mutation (BRCA-1 or -2).
- Discuss alternatives to HRT, eg clonidine for hot flushes, evening primrose oil, topical oestrogens.
- Need for mammograms and self-examination.
- Explain that mostly HRT will result in her continuing to have regular withdrawal bleeds that may be troublesome to her. Tibolone can be taken continuously, however, avoiding withdrawal bleeds.
- Ultimately the decision is the patient's and she needs to weigh up the theoretical risks and inconvenience against her troublesome symptoms.

Direction of the consultation

Scenario A

She has made her mind up and ultimately wants treatment

- Under these circumstances the patient should be aware of the possible risks and these should be carefully documented in her notes.
- As a result of the great increase in potential risk of cancer, it is advisable to arrange a further consultation to discuss this more.
  If the doctor feels that he or she is ethically unable to prescribe the drug, she should seek a second opinion.
- She may feel that she wants to have genetic testing for breast cancer. This is not possible (see below).

Scenario B

She remains unsure what to do and is looking for advice.

- Under these circumstances she should be made aware of the increased risks and encouraged initially to try alternatives with a regular follow-up arrangement.

Finishing

- Ensure that she understands all the issues.
- Ask if she has any questions.
- Everything should be carefully documented in the notes.
- If she has decided to try HRT, she must be aware of the gravity of her decision.
- Follow-up arrangements should be made in both cases.

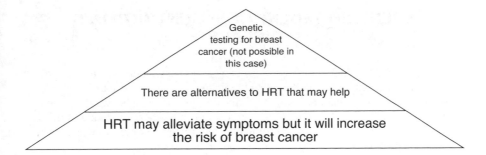

Genetic
testing for breast
cancer (not possible in
this case)

There are alternatives to HRT that may help

HRT may alleviate symptoms but it will increase
the risk of breast cancer

Genetic risk of breast cancer

BRCA-1 and -2 genetic abnormalities predispose women to develop breast cancer (life-time risk > 80%). The mutations are inherited in an autosomal dominant manner.

The exact mutations within the gene must be identified in an individual (family member) with cancer (case). That specific mutation can then be tested in the rest of the family (according to autosomal dominant inheritance). Those with the mutation within the gene, which has already been identified in family member with cancer, are at increased risk of cancer. The reason that the mutation has to be identified in a case is that a number of other mutations/poly-morphisms can occur within the gene, which may not be responsible for the development of cancer. There are screening issues and treatment issues surrounding this (including bilateral mastectomies!).

If a candidate is asked to screen a woman genetically for *BRCA*-1/-2 the first thing to do is take a family history, and then identify a family member who is alive with cancer and willing to be tested. Once the genetic abnormality within the gene has been identified, we can test the individual who wants to be screened.

Remember to discuss the issues and implications for siblings and children.

Currently we do not have to answer 'genetic test' questions on life insurance. This may change in 2011.

BRCA-1 and -2 mutations account for a small minority of breast cancers, so the majority are considered to result from other causes (currently unknown at a genetic level). If an individual does not have a *BRCA*-1 or -2 mutation and a first-degree relative with breast cancer, the hazard ratio for that individual is increased (relative risk or RR 2–5).

SCENARIO 7. GENETICS: HUNTINGTON'S DISEASE

You are a medical SHO in the neurology clinic. The next patient is a 46-year-old woman who wants a genetic test for Huntington's disease. She had previously found out that her father had committed suicide aged 50 when he was diagnosed as having the disorder, but none of her three younger brothers knows about their father's condition. She has noticed some early neurological symptoms with ataxia and forgetfulness. She has two daughters aged 4 and 7 years.

Please counsel the patient with a view to discussing screening for the rest of her family.

Preliminary thoughts

- She needs to be consented appropriately for the genetic test and thus understand the nature of the disease and implications of the result (progressive untreatable dementia, ataxia, etc).
- She must be mentally fit enough to give consent (there is no reason in the text to indicate that this should not be the case and it is very unlikely that this would happen in an exam setting).
- The patient must consider children and siblings and may want to reconsider testing until she has discussed the situation with them. She is entitled to do the test in complete isolation and confidentiality must be respected.
- The median onset of symptoms of the disease is between 30 and 45 years. Life expectancy is only 10 years after onset of the symptoms. Chorea tends to occur first and dementia a few years after.
- The disease is autosomal dominant and shows anticipation, where symptoms occur earlier and are more severe from one generation to the next.
- Support groups for Huntington's disease and information for the patient about it.
- The Huntington Disease Association guidelines suggest that the same doctor should take the consent and give results.
- Patients are always asked what they would like to happen to the results if they were not able to receive them themselves.
- Although individuals do not currently have to answer questions about genetic testing on life insurance forms, this may change in the future (2011).

A good candidate

- Will ensure that she understands the disease
- Will discuss the implications of being positive: 'Who will you tell?'
- Will discuss details about how her family will react and whom she has told

- Will encourage her to discuss the situation with her family before having the test
- Will respect her rights to confidentiality.

Key points in the consultation

- Introduction and establish rapport.
- Ensure that she is fit to give consent.
- Ask if she would like someone with her, ie family member.
- Establish patient's understanding of Huntington's disease and its inheritance.
- Explore why she has had the test now.
- At this point the patient must understand the nature of the disease for which she is being tested. She must be aware of the seriousness of the condition and its untreatable nature. If she is not fully aware, the doctor should discuss the nature of the disease at length with her before moving on.
- It is essential to ask her what she would do if the test was positive, who she will tell, etc.
- She should be encouraged to inform her support structure that she is having the test (this may be her family).
- She should consider bringing someone with her to the next consultation.
- She must be offered more time to discuss the situation with her family if she wishes.
- Make provisions for what she would like to happen if she was unable to receive the result herself.
- Ask if she has any questions.

Finishing

- Summarise the discussion
- Ask if she has any further questions
- Arrange follow-up for the test result (weeks).

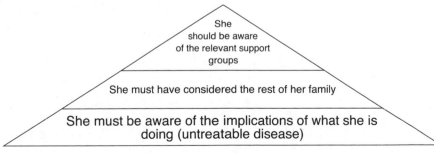

She should be aware of the relevant support groups

She must have considered the rest of her family

She must be aware of the implications of what she is doing (untreatable disease)

Discussion

Antenatal diagnosis from amniocentesis can be offered as appropriate and pre-implantation in vitro diagnosis is a possibility. These are clearly good reasons for having the test. Other autosomal dominant genetic conditions, which have appeared in communications exams, include spinal cerebellar ataxia, myotonic dystrophies, BRCA-1 and -2 mutations in breast cancer, familial adenomatous polyposis (FAP) and hereditary non-polyposis colon cancer (HNPCC). Currently there are no questions about genetic testing on life insurance policies; however, this may change in the future.

Autosomal recessive conditions occur less frequently in communication skills exams. Cystic fibrosis is perhaps the best example; however, it needs to present in adulthood for this exam. An example is a man presenting who is being investigated for fertility problems, although this is rare.

SCENARIO 8. BREAKING BAD NEWS AND CANCER PROCEDURES

A 22-year-old man has recently noticed a lump in his left testicle. Ultrasonography was highly suspicious of malignancy, which was confirmed histologically (germ-cell tumour) after unilateral orchidectomy. CT staging has shown local lymph node involvement, which will require cytotoxic chemotherapy; with the correct treatment his long-term survival rate is > 90%.

Please discuss with the patient his diagnosis and the need for chemotherapy.

Preliminary thoughts

- Underlying diagnosis is cancer
- What does he know or suspect?
- Good prognosis
- Treatment
- Fertility issues: reduced with chemotherapy.

A good candidate

- Will discover if the patient is prepared and wants to talk about a diagnosis of cancer before progressing
- Will know some information about chemotherapy in broad terms and will explain that the patient will need to see an oncologist
- Will allow time for questions at the end of the consultation
- Will put the patient in contact with support from the cancer centre.

Goals for consultation

- Establish his current understanding of his condition
- Explain his diagnosis to him
- Ensure that he understands the need for chemotherapy and the good prognosis
- Ensure follow-up and support.

Key points in the consultation

- Introduction and establish rapport
- Ask if he wants anyone else present
- Establish patient's views on what he thinks might be the diagnosis and what he knows
- Determine which category he falls into (he wants all information at once, or a 'nugget' type – see Breaking Bad News, page 379)
- Once the patient's understanding of the condition has been established, it is possible to predict if he is expecting a diagnosis of cancer.

Direction of the consultation

Scenario A

He is aware that testicular cancer is a possibility

- The patient should be informed of the diagnosis in a clear and sympathetic manner. He may wish to see his CT scans or the histology report, which is sometimes helpful.
- Explain the nature of the disease, and the need for cyclical combination chemotherapy over a period of several weeks and its side effects.
- Explain that with treatment he has a very good outcome.

Scenario B

The patient has not considered cancer as a possible diagnosis.

- The patient should be given small pieces of information at a time, working towards the diagnosis.
- The doctor should be relatively positive, because the outcome is usually good with chemotherapy.
- Remember that, once the patient has been told his diagnosis, he should be allowed time to react.
- The doctor should pause before moving on.
- Explain the need for subsequent cytotoxic chemotherapy
  - logistics – when, where, frequency (he should start very soon)
  - side effects, eg infection, alopecia, nausea, infertility.
- Discuss the squelae of his condition:
  - cosmetic – testicular prosthesis can be inserted
  - fertility – unaffected by previous surgery, likely to be infertile after chemotherapy; semen can be frozen and stored.
- Need for future monitoring of response to treatment:
  - CT of body
  - blood tests – human chorionic gonadotrophin (hCG)/α-fetoprotein (AFP)/lactate dehydrogenase (LDH).
- Emphasise the very good prognosis for testicular cancer: > 90% cure.

Finishing

- Ask the patient if he understands what has been said
- Summarise the consultation
- Ask if he has any questions
- Arrange medical follow-up
- Arrange point of contact (eg telephone no.) with oncology nurse specialist
- Make sure that there is someone he can talk to or someone at home with him.

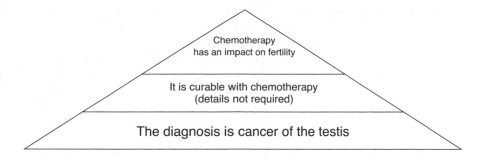

Chemotherapy
has an impact on fertility

It is curable with chemotherapy
(details not required)

The diagnosis is cancer of the testis

Cancer procedures

When patients are told of a cancer diagnosis, they do not tend to remember too many details of the consultation. The type of cancer, whether or not it is treatable/curable, is usually about as far as it goes. Candidates should try to avoid life expectancy issues, because it is very unreliable and often unhelpful at this stage (see Breaking Bad News, page 379). This also applies to details of treatment, which is why it is often possible to talk about chemotherapy and radiotherapy in broad terms. To our knowledge no communication skills station has specifically named a regimen and asked the candidate to obtain consent – which is good news.

Chemotherapy and targeted therapy

Many communication skills scenarios mention that patients will need chemotherapy, so candidates should know in broad terms what chemotherapy is about. It is important to stress to the patient that the detailed information needs to be given by an oncologist, because there are an enormous number of permutations for treatment and staging may not be complete.

However, in broad terms chemotherapy is usually given in 3- or 4-weekly cycles. The number of cycles depends on the cancer and the drugs, but is usually between four and six. It is traditional to do a radiological scan before and after chemotherapy.

The drugs are usually given in combination, over a few hours as an intravenous infusion. Very few regimens are given as an inpatient. Recently oral chemotherapy has become widely used, especially in colorectal cancer. The side effects vary according to the drug regimen, but the most important side effect is neutropenic sepsis, which can occur with almost all regimens. Hair loss is not universal.

Common side effects for chemotherapy

- Short term: nausea and vomiting, change in bowel habit, stomatitis
- Medium term: neutropenic sepsis, anaemia, bleeding, lethargy
- Long term: lethargy, second cancers (with topoisomerase II inhibitors).

New classes of drugs such as monoclonal antibodies and tyrosine kinase inhibitors have increased treatment options further. These drugs have specific side effects, the most commonly encountered including: allergic reactions, rash, hypertension, hand and foot syndrome, and cardiac toxicity. Neutropenic sepsis does not tend to occur with these agents.

Radiotherapy

Palliative

This type of radiotherapy is given to alleviate symptoms, especially bone pain, and involves only a small number of fractions (often as few as one). It can be given to the soft tissues and the brain. It is rarely associated with major side effects and, because it is palliative in nature, is rarely associated with significant long-term side effects.

Curative

Radiotherapy with curative intent is given for many cancers. A large number of cycles are given, eg 25 daily fractions. It requires planning, which is done in conjunction with CT.

Side effects include local skin irritation and toxicity to local structures (eg urinary symptoms for prostate or bladder cancer). It can cause long-term changes to the skin or local structures and is associated with second cancers.

STATION 5

The Skin, Locomotor, Eye and Endocrine Examinations

EXAMINATION OF THE SKIN

Examination of the skin as a whole

- Examine in good (ideally natural) light.
- Expose the patient as much as the situation will allow.
- Inspect the patient as a whole and consider:
    - Is there a rash and what is its distribution?
    - Is there any hair growth or loss?
    - Are there any features of systemic disease?
- And more specifically:
    - If there is a rash – is it red or not?
    - Is the rash macular, papular, in patches or plaques?
    - Are there scales or evidence of excoriation?
    - Are there fluid-filled lesions? Are these vesicles, pustules or blisters?

If pointed to a particular area examine this first, but be aware that you may need to examine the skin as a whole as follows (where a specific condition is important it is mentioned):

- Are there signs of systemic disease giving clues as to the aetiology of the skin lesion, eg a colostomy bag suggesting ulcerative colitis?

You will see from the following that there are numerous 'dermatological diagnoses' and numerous dermatological manifestations of systemic disease. The list is not exhaustive – consider yourself what you might see as you examine a patient's skin and the associations of these cutaneous signs.

Nails and hands

- Pitting: psoriasis or fungal infection
- Onycholysis: psoriasis or thyrotoxicosis
- Paronychia: Cushing's disease or diabetes mellitus
- Pigmentation under the nail: possible subungual melanoma
- Splinter haemorrhages: vasculitis, infective endocarditis
- Telangiectasias: systemic lupus erythematosus (SLE), systemic sclerosis
- Gottren's papules: purplish discoloration seen over the knuckles – dermatomyositis
- Blisters: seen in pemphigus and pemphigoid:
    - in pemphigus (S – superficial) they are fragile and may be open
    - in pemphigoid (D – deep) they are tense
    - if the blisters are only on the hands consider photosensitivity, eg porphyria cutanea tarda
- Papules, scratch marks and tracks between the knuckles: scabies
- Viral warts: common on the fingers or hands

- Dupuytren's contracture: may be familial, associated with alcohol excess and in those who operate vibrating machinery
- Xanthomas: palmar creases and/or tendons
- Pigmentation: Addison's disease, particularly in the skin creases and knuckles; haemochromatosis; amiodarone therapy (slate-grey skin)
- Thin skin: Cushing syndrome, with bruises or purpura.

Forearms and arms

- Lichen planus: on the flexor surfaces, small, shiny purplish papules; if they are itchy Koebner's phenomenon (scarring in scratchmarks) may be seen.
- Psoriasis: usually on extensor surfaces in silvery plaques
- Eczema: flexural surfaces, with prominent excoriations
- Acanthosis nigricans: raised, dark, velvety areas of skin frequently in the axillae and on the neck, occurring in:
  - insulin-resistant states, eg polycystic ovarian syndrome (PCOS), diabetes mellitus
  - solid malignancy

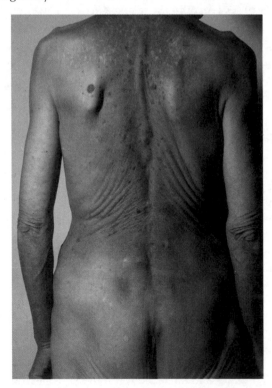

Figure 5.1   Acanthosis nigricans.

- Eruptive xanthomas: hypertriglyceridaemia (are there scars from operative management of acute pancreatitis?)
- Dermatitis herpetiformis: blistering, extensor, itchy rash on extensor surfaces, seen in inflammatory bowel disease.

Hair and scalp

What is the distribution of hair on the scalp?

- Alopecia:
  With normal skin:
  - traction alopecia in nervous children
  - ringworm – tinea capitis
  - autoimmune alopecia areata – patchy hair loss
  Scarring alopecia:
  - discoid lupus
  - trigeminal zoster
  - burns
  Diffuse, temporary, hair loss is seen with chemotherapy
  Male pattern hair loss with growth of body hair in women may point to virilising conditions, eg congenital adrenal hyperplasia or androgen-secreting tumours
- Exclamation mark hairs: short hairs at the temples seen in SLE
- Dry, brittle hair: hypothyroidism
- Scaling: psoriasis, psoriatic scaling often also present in the navel
- Sebaceous cysts in the scalp are common.

Eyebrows and eyelids

- Greasy and scaling skin: seborrhoeic dermatitis
- Heliotrope rash: seen in dermatomyositis on the eyelids, very easily missed
- Xanthelasma: in types IIa and IIb hyperlipidaemia, familial and not necessarily associated with dyslipidaemia.

Face

- Capillary haemangiomas: Sturge–Weber syndrome, in the division of cranial nerve V usually ophthalmic (see page 529); may be associated with intracerebral arteriovenous malformations (AVMs)
- Rosacea: bright erythema on the nose, cheeks, forehead and chin
- Rhinophyma: disfiguring swelling of the nose
- Acne vulgaris: papules, pustules and scarring on the face, neck and upper trunk

- Butterfly rash: SLE, look closely for fine scales which plug the follicles as these are pathognomic of SLE
- Lupus pernio: dark-red discoloration of the nose in sarcoidosis
- Ulceration:
  - basal cell carcinoma
  - squamous cell carcinoma
  - lupus vulgaris – tuberculosis (looks like apple jelly if a glass slide is pressed against the lesion)
- Keratoacanthoma: benign; volcano-like lesion arising out of a sebaceous gland
- Vesicles in the division of the trigeminal nerve: herpes zoster
- Lipodystrophy: with antiretroviral therapy in HIV.

Lips/mouth

- Osler–Weber–Rendu (hereditary haemorrhagic telangiectasia)
- Peutz–Jeughers syndrome
- Addison's disease: diffuse pigmentation next to the teeth (check the postural blood pressure) (see page 629)
- Fissured lips with ulceration: Crohn's disease
- Herpes simplex.

Neck/trunk

- Loose folds of redundant 'chicken skin': pseudoxanthoma elasticum
- Lymphadenopathy: where is it draining – infection or primary malignancy? Look closely at the scalp/face (and in the mouth)
- Depigmentation:
  - vitiligo – consider other autoimmune disease
  - pityriasis versicolor – loss of pigmentation, like raindrops on the skin; surrounding increase in pigmentation
  - leprosy – anaesthetic patches, asymmetrical
- Spider naevi: in the distribution of the drainage of the superior vena cava (SVC) – liver disease, pregnancy
- Campbell de Morgan spots: of no significance; to mistake them for telangiectasia is shameful
- Gynaecomastia: implies an imbalance between oestrogen and testosterone, eg hypogonadism, spironolactone
- Neurofibromas: NF type I
- Café-au-lait patches: if more than five associated with NF type I, as is axillary freckling

- Morphoea: faintly yellow/ivory, thickened skin, either plaques, generalised or linear lesions. It does not progress to systemic sclerosis. In children and adolescents the 'en coup en sabre' form of linear morphoea may be associated with seizures or headache.
- Livid striae: broad and purple in active Cushing's syndrome; they become silvery on removal of the excess steroid
- Striae gravidarum: previous pregnancy, obesity; more rarely previous Cushing's syndrome
- Mycosis fungoides: scaly, erythematous lesions, a cutaneous T-cell lymphoma.

Pattern of hair

- Axillary loss in hypogonadism
- Hirsutism in androgenisation, eg PCOS

Lower limbs

- Moles:
  - the leg is the most common site for a malignant melanoma in females, the forearm in males
  - irregular shape and colour, bleeding, itchy, with satellite lesions and regional lymphadenopathy
- Vasculitis: commonly first appears on the legs
- Erythema nodosum: tender, raised, red lesions, associated fever
- Erythema multifome: associated mucosal ulceration in Stevens–Johnson syndrome
- Graves' dermopathy, classically on the shins or round the ankle
- Granuloma annulare: diabetes mellitus
- Necrobiosis lipoidica diabeticorum
- Ulcers: venous, arterial, neuropathic or malignant
- Pyoderma gangrenosum: inflammatory bowel disease.

Feet

- Keratoderma blenorrhagica: Reiter syndrome
- Ischaemia
- Neuropathic ulcers: diabetes mellitus.

Skin Scenarios

1. Systemic lupus erythematosus
2. Necrobiosis lipoidica
3. Leukoplakia
4. Granuloma annulare
5. Xanthomas
6. Psoriasis
7. Eczema
8. Rosacea
9. Hereditary haemorrhagic telangiectasia – Osler–Weber–Rendu syndrome
10. Ulcer
11. Lichen planus
12. Dermatitis herpetiformis
13. Dermatomyositis
14. Sarcoidosis
15. Erythema nodosum
16. Kaposi's sarcoma
17. Vitiligo
18. Pigmentation
19. Vasculitis/purpura
20. Neurofibromatosis
21. Palmar erythema
22. Dupuytren's contracture
23. Cheilosis
24. Herpes zoster
25. Peutz–Jeghers syndrome

26. Lipodystrophy
27. Capillary haemangioma
28. Pseudoxanthoma elasticum
29. Erythema multiforme
30. Scleroderma
31. Leukonychia
32. Pemphigoid
33. Pemphigus

SCENARIO 1. SYSTEMIC LUPUS ERYTHEMATOSUS

Face

There is a classic butterfly rash – a symmetrical patchy erythematous rash on the cheeks and the bridge of the nose (malar), tending to spare the nasolabial folds; it may also be present on other sun-exposed areas.

On close inspection this may simply be nothing more than non-specific patchy erythema or a more discrete maculopapular eruption; the (almost) pathognomic feature is raised keratotic 'scaling' with follicular plugging (discoid rash) and telangiectasia; atrophic scaring may occur in older lesions.

The scarring may lead to scarring alopecia with exclamation mark hairs, and the scarring can give the appearance of vitiligo.

Oral or nasal ulceration (usually painless) is present.

Hands

The appearance of the skin of the hands may include:

- Photosensitivity
- Raynaud's phenomenon
- Vasculitis, nailfold infarcts or splinter haemorrhages
- Palmar erythema.

There is a symmetrical non-deforming arthritis (compare deforming in rheumatoid), characterised by tenderness, swelling or effusions.

The important discriminating, diagnostic signs are:

- Malar flush
- Photosensitivity
- Discoid rash
- Oral or nasal ulceration
- Symmetrical, non-deforming arthritis

A good candidate

Will note the following:

- Jaccoud's arthropathy: the hands may be deformed, suggesting a deforming arthropathy, but in SLE this is the result of tenosynovitis and tendon dysfunction, causing reversible subluxation of the joints, rather than destruction

- Livido reticularis: a pattern of the skin of trunk, arms or legs that is persistent, not reversible with re-warming, violaceous, red or blue, reticular or mottled
- Cushing syndrome: from exogenous steroids
- Fever
- Pallor, splenomegaly ± lymphadenopathy
- Haematuria/proteinuria
- Oedema: associated with the nephritic syndrome
- Thrombosis associated with the antiphospholipid syndrome or the nephritic syndrome
- Mononeuritis multiplex
- Peripheral neuropathy.

The American College of Rheumatology Criteria for Classification of Systemic Lupus Erythematosus were last revised in 1997.

Criterion	Definition
Malar rash	Fixed erythema, flat or raised, over the malar eminences, tending to spare the nasolabial folds
Discoid rash	Erythematous raised patches with adherent keratotic scaling and follicular plugging; atrophic scarring may occur in older lesions
Photosensitivity	Rash as a result of unusual reaction to sunlight, by patient history or physician observation
Oral ulcers	Oral or nasopharyngeal ulceration, usually painless; observed by physician
Arthritis	Non-erosive arthritis involving two or more peripheral joints, characterised by tenderness, swelling or effusion
Serositis	Pleuritis: convincing history of pleuritic pain or rubbing heard by a physician or evidence of pleural effusion Pericarditis: documented by ECG or rub or evidence of pericardial effusion
Renal disorder	Persistent proteinuria > 0.5 g/day or > 3+ if quantitation not performed Cellular casts: may be red cell, haemoglobin, granular, tubular or mixed
Neurological disorder	Seizures: in the absence of offending drugs or known metabolic derangements, eg uraemia, ketoacidosis or electrolyte imbalance Psychosis: in the absence of offending drugs or known metabolic derangements, eg uraemia, ketoacidosis or electrolyte imbalance

Haematological disorder	Haemolytic anaemia: with reticulocytosis
	Leukopenia: < 4000/mm³ total on two or more occasions
	Lypmhopenia: < 1500/mm³ on two or more occasions
	Thrombocytopenia: 100 000/mm³ in the absence of offending drugs
Immunological disorder	Anti-DNA: antibody to native DNA in abnormal titre
	Anti-Sm: presence of antibody to Sm nuclear antigen
	Positive finding of antiphospholipid antibodies, including IgG or IgM anticardiolipin antibodies and lupus anticoagulant
Antinuclear antibody (ANA)	An abnormal titre of ANA by immunofluorescence or an equivalent assay at any point in time and in the absence of drugs known to be associated with 'drug-induced lupus' syndrome

Formally, 4 of the 11 criteria should be present (though not necessarily at the same time) for a secure diagnosis; these are research classification criteria and may be too stringent for everyday practice, and SLE can be diagnosed on the basis of typical clinical findings in one organ or tissue, combined with the presence of appropriate autoantibodies.

Questions

1. How might the patient with SLE present?

The diverse clinical features of the disease mean that it may present to various clinicians including dermatologists, rheumatologists, nephrologists and general physicians.

It is between 10 and 20 times more common in women than men and six times more common in African–Caribbean individuals and three times more common in British Asians, respectively, than in white individuals. It is an important diagnostic consideration in any woman, between the ages of 15 and 50, who presents with symptoms or signs in different organs, either simultaneously or in sequence.

The approximate frequency of the clinical features is shown.

Clinical feature	Approximate cumulative prevalence (%)	Clinical feature	Approximate cumulative prevalence (%)
Musculoskeletal		Serum creatinine > 125 mmol/l	30
Arthralgia/arthritis	90	Haematuria	10
Myalgia	50		
Tenosynovitis	20	**Cerebral**	
Myositis	5	Migraine	40
		Seizures	20
Cardiopulmonary		Depression	15
Pulmonary function abnormalities	85	Psychosis	15
Dyspnoea	40	Hemiplegia	10
Pleurisy	35	Cranial nerve lesions	10
Pleural effusion	25	Cerebellar signs	5
Cardiomegaly	20	Meningitis	1
Pericarditis	15		
Cardiomyopathy	10	**Haematological**	
Lupus pneumonitis	5	Anaemia (of chronic disease)	75
Interstitial fibrosis	5	Leukopenia	60
Myocardial infarction	5	Lymphopenia	60
		Anaemia (iron deficiency)	30
Gastrointestinal		Thrombocytopenia	25
Anorexia	40	Circulating anticoagulants	15
Abdominal pain	30	Autoimmune haemolytic anaemia	75
Hepatomegaly	25		
Splenomegaly	10	**Dermatological**	
Nausea	15	Alopecia	70
Vomiting and diarrhoea	10	Butterfly rash	40
Ascites	10	Vasculitis/purpura	40
		Erythematous maculopapular eruption	35
Renal		Livedo reticularis	20
Proteinuria	60	Discoid lupus	20
Casts	30	Relapsing, nodular, non-suppurative	
Serum albumin < 35 g/l	30	paniculitis	5

SLE is a chronic condition with a low level of background activity and a tendency to flares of activity – it is the flares that dictate the severity to an individual patient; alongside these, weight loss and fevers may reflect overall disease activity.

Lymphadenopathy may be large and necessitate biopsy to exclude other conditions, eg lymphoma.

2. *How might you manage lupus?*

- Avoid sunlight: hats, sunscreen and long sleeves
- Topical steroids: for rashes
- Antimalarials: hydroxychloroquine and chloroquine
- Arthritis: non-steroidal anti-inflammatory drugs (NSAIDs) or steroids
- Severe rheumatological or haematological problems require steroids
- Immunosuppressants: oral cyclophoshamide, azathioprine
- Biologic agents, eg rituximab, epratuzumab and mycophenolate mofetil
- Intravenous immunoglobulin is used in resistant lupus, especially where concomitant infection makes immunosuppression risky
- Autologous stem-cell transplantation is an option in severe lupus; the treatment-related mortality rate has fallen to < 5% with a 5-year survival rate of > 80%
- Disease activity is monitored by levels of C3 or C4, dsDNA (double-stranded DNA) titres, ESR (erythrocyte sedimentation rate) and urinalysis.

3. *Tell me about the antiphospholipid syndrome*

This is a disorder characterised by recurrent venous and/or arterial thromboses and/or fetal losses, associated with characteristic laboratory abnormalities. Antiphospholipid syndrome (APS) not in association with SLE rarely progresses to SLE; the term 'secondary APS' is no longer advised because most of these patients have lupus.

Valvular regurgitation, pulmonary hypertension, migraine and livido reticularis are associated with the condition.

The patient should be risk stratified and receive either prophylaxis against thrombosis with aspirin or treatment with low-molecular-weight heparin or warfarin to a target INR (international normalised ratio) of between 2.6 and 3 depending on the clinical situation.

Catastrophic APS may require plasmapheresis alongside intensive anticoagulation with corticosteroids, cyclophosphamide and intravenous immunoglobulin.

Clinical guideline

Diagnostic criteria for APS

APS is present if at least one of the clinical criteria and one of the laboratory criteria that follow are met.

CLINICAL CRITERIA

- Vascular thrombosis: one or more clinical episodes of arterial, venous or small vessel thrombosis, in any tissue or organ. Thrombosis must be confirmed by objective validated criteria (ie unequivocal findings of appropriate imaging studies or histopathology). For histopathological confirmation, thrombosis should be present without significant evidence of inflammation in the vessel wall. Coexisting inherited or acquired factors for thrombosis are not reasons for excluding patients from APS trials.*

- Pregnancy morbidity:
  - one or more unexplained deaths of a morphologically normal fetus at or beyond week 10 of gestation, with normal fetal morphology documented by ultrasonography or direct examination of the fetus
  - one or more premature births of a morphologically normal neonate before week 34 of gestation because of:
    - eclampsia or severe pre-eclampsia defined according to standard definitions
    - recognised features of placental insufficiency
  - three or more unexplained consecutive spontaneous abortions before week 10 of gestation, with maternal anatomical or hormonal abnormalities and paternal and maternal chromosomal causes excluded.

In studies of populations of patients who have more than one type of pregnancy morbidity, investigators are strongly encouraged to stratify groups of individuals according to these criteria.

LABORATORY CRITERIA

- Lupus anticoagulant (LA) present in plasma, on two or more occasions at least 12 weeks apart, detected according to the guidelines of the International Society on Thrombosis and Haemostasis (Scientific Subcommittee on LAs/phospholipid-dependent antibodies)
- Anticardiolipin (aCL) antibody of IgG and/or IgM isotype in serum or plasma, present in medium or high titres, on two or more occasions, at least 12 weeks apart, measured by a standardised ELISA (enzyme-linked immunosorbent assay)

---

*However, two subgroups of APS patients should be recognized, according to: (a) the presence, and (b) the absence of additional risk factors for thrombosis. Indicative (but not exhaustive) cases include: age (>55 in men, and >65 in women), and the presence of any of the established risk factors for cardiovascular disease (hypertension, diabetes mellitus, elevated LDL or low HDL cholesterol, cigarette smoking, family history of premature cardiovascular disease, body mass index ≥30 kg/m², microalbuminuria, estimated GFR <60 ml/min), inherited thrombophilias, oral contraceptives, nephrotic syndrome, malignancy, immobilization and surgery. Thus, patients who fulfil criteria should be stratified according to contributing causes of thrombosis.

- Anti-f_2-glycoprotein-I antibody of IgG and/or IgM isotype in serum or plasma (in titre > 99th percentile), present on two or more occasions, at least 12 weeks apart, measured by a standardised ELISA, according to recommended procedures.

SCENARIO 2. NECROBIOSIS LIPOIDICA

There is a reddish-brown plaque on the shin of this patient (it commonly occurs on both shins in patients with diabetes); the centre is yellowish and atrophic and can sometimes ulcerate. There are often telangiectasias within the lesion (see figure below).

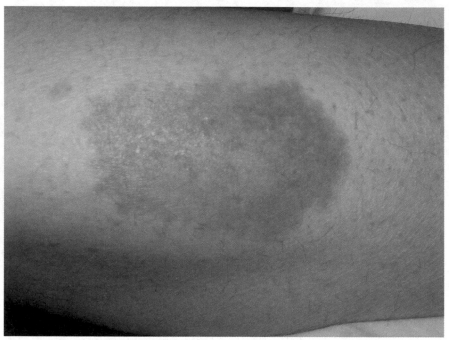

Figure 5.2   Necrobiois lipoidica.

It is a chronic condition, associated with diabetes mellitus in over two-thirds of cases; glycaemic control has no effect on its progression, and it may predate diabetes in a third of cases; it is also an occasional cutaneous manifestation of AIDS.

The advancing edge may respond to potent topical or intralesional cortico-steroids but these both have a tendency to aggravate the atrophy in the centre.

The histology is of partial necrosis of collagen and connective tissue with surrounding immunoglobulin and complement deposition and macrophages, giving a 'palisading granuloma'. Healing may result in scarring (see also Granuloma annulare see next page).

The main differential diagnosis is with granuloma annulare and basal cell carcinoma.

SCENARIO 3. LEUKOPLAKIA

There are small, discrete, white patches on an erythematous base in the oral mucosa. It is predisposed by tobacco smoking and local trauma.

Of precancerous lesions in the mouth 85% are leukoplakic, but the risk of malignant transformation of leukoplakia cannot be determined.

In AIDS it is characteristically seen as vertically ribbed keratinised plaques on the lateral border of the tongue, though it can involve other oral sites; it is usually asymptomatic.

It is associated with Epstein–Barr virus.

The occurrence of hairy leukoplakia is not clearly related to CD4 count but suggests the progression to AIDS; the mean CD4 count of those with leuko-plakia is 340/mm³ (Jung and Paauw [1998] provides a useful overview of the common infections in HIV related to the CD4 count).

It usually responds to treatment of the HIV infection, eg HAART.

SCENARIO 4. GRANULOMA ANNULARE

This young patient has rings of smooth, skin-coloured (or slightly violaceous) papules on the dorsum of the hands/feet, or fingers, ankles, elbows or elsewhere.

It can occur as a solitary lesion.

More widespread granuloma is often associated with diabetes mellitus.

The smooth surface is an important feature and helps to distinguish it from the most common misdiagnoses – warts and fungal infection.

A potent corticosteroid, either topically or more rarely by injection, can be used for symptomatic lesions, but, as it is asymptomatic and self-limiting – resolving within 1–2 years – it usually needs no treatment.

The histology is of partial necrosis of collagen and connective tissue with surrounding immunoglobulin and complement deposition, and macrophages giving a 'palisading granuloma'. It is entirely reversible, and usually does not result in scarring (see also Necrobiosis, previous page).

SCENARIO 5. XANTHOMAS

Extensor tendon xanthomas

Classically these occur on the back of the hands and Achilles' tendon. Associated xanthelasma (skin lipid deposit around the eyelids, 495) and arcus occur.

A good candidate

- Will look for the signs of associated ischaemic heart disease – bradycardia (from β blocker or ivabradine), sternotomy or vein harvest scars.

What is the aetiology?

- Raised LDL-cholesterol
- Type IIA familial hypercholesterolaemia
- Autosomal dominant disease caused by a defect in the LDL receptor (chromosome 19). This occurs in 0.2% of white, western European populations.

Eruptive xanthomas

Multiple small yellow vesicles are present on the extensor surfaces.

A good candidate

- Will perform fundoscopy – this often reveals lipaemia retinalis
- Will examine the abdomen for hepatosplenomegaly caused by accumulation of fat-laden macrophages
- Will consider the factors associated with recurrent pancreatitis.

What is the aetiology?

- Raised triglycerides
- Very-low-density lipoproteins (VLDLs): familial hypertriglyceridaemia
- Chylomicrons: lipoprotein lipase deficiency
- Primary: type IV familial hypertriglyceridaemia and lipoprotein lipase deficiency (autosomal recessive diseases)
- Secondary: associated with poorly controlled diabetes mellitus.

Palmar xanthomas

There is yellow (often) raised discoloration of the creases of the palms.

A good candidate

- Will look at knees for tubero-eruptive xanthomas
- Will look for:
  - associated xanthelasma
  - signs of associated ischaemic heart disease
  - secondary causes, eg hypothyroidism.

What is the aetiology?

- Raised cholesterol and triglycerides
- Primary: remnant particle disease (type III); *synonym*: broad β disease
- Secondary: diabetes, hypothyroidism, renal disease.

Xanthelasma

There are symmetrical yellow plaques around the inner canthus of the eyelids (upper more commonly than lower but all four can be involved); this is xanthoma (plural xanthelasma).

Over half of these patients with xanthelasma will have an elevated cholesterol. They are common in familial hypercholesterolaemia (type IIa and IIb) and familial hypertriglyceridaemia (type IV) in lipoprotein lipase deficiency (type IV).

SCENARIO 6. PSORIASIS

Plaque psoriasis

There is a symmetrical rash characterised by sharply demarcated, erythematous areas covered with thick, silvery scales; these (commonly) affect the extensor surfaces, especially of the elbows and knees as well as the scalp (particularly behind the ears and the hairline) and the navel. Often a resistant plaque at the sacrum is common.

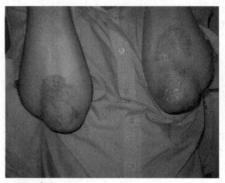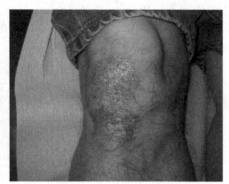

Figure 5.3   Plaque psoriasis.

On removal of a scale you might see pinpoint bleeding.

A good candidate (for all types of psoriasis)

- Will know that lesions can occur at sites of minor trauma – Koebner's phenomenon.
- Will know that the other lesions seen displaying Koebner's phenomenon are warts and lichen planus (see page 509)
- Will examine for:
  - Nail pitting
  - Psoriatic arthritis:
    - pitting occurs on the fingers in 50% and the toes in 35% of patients; occurs in most patients with psoriatic arthritis
    - psoriatic arthritis occurs in at least 5% to as many as 20% of patients with psoriasis
  - Onychodystrophy.

Flexoral psoriasis

Plaques of psoriasis occurring in flexoral or intertriginous areas that usually show only scant scaling.

Guttate psoriasis

History of abrupt onset of a rash, usually in a young adult or child, characterised by 'droplet'-shaped, erythematous, scaly lesions distributed widely on the trunk and limbs with no predilection for extensor surfaces.

A good candidate

- Will know that it is often precipitated by a streptococcal sore throat 2–3 weeks earlier
- Will know that, although it usually resolves completely, individual plaques may enlarge and turn into plaque psoriasis, or plaque psoriasis may appear later in life.

Pustular psoriasis (psoriasis vulgaris)

Localised chronic pustular psoriasis most commonly occurs on the palms and soles (palmoplantar pustulosis). It is characterised by small sterile pustules; the hands and soles are not tender or oedematous.

Rarely these may coalesce into disseminated 'lakes' of pus on deeply erythematous skin, fever and systemic upset coexist and it can be rapidly fatal – generalised pustular psoriasis.

It can be precipitated by topical or systemic steroids, drug reactions or infections.

Questions

1. What drugs are known to worsen psoriasis?

- Alcohol
- Lithium
- Chloroquine
- Mepacrine
- NSAIDs
- Possibly β blockers
- Possibly angiotensin-converting enzyme (ACE) inhibitors.

2. How would you manage psoriasis?

Clinical guidelines from the British Association of Dermatologists

Assessment of severity should include the patient's own perception of disability, the need for treatment, and an objective assessment of the extent and severity of the disease. A quality-of-life assessment, such as the Dermatology Life Quality Index or Children's Dermatology Life Quality Index, is a useful tool to monitor treatment with.

TREATMENT OF CHRONIC PLAQUE PSORIASIS

Emollients should be used to soften scaling and reduce any irritation.

For **localised plaque psoriasis**, eg on the elbows or knees, one of more of the following can be tried:

- A tar-based cream or a tar/corticosteroid mix.
- A moderate potency topical corticosteroid (eg 0.05% clobetasone butyrate) – use of topical corticosteroids may lead to rebound exacerbation when discontinued and thus should be given only under specialist supervision.
- A vitamin D analogue, with caution:
  - calcipotriol is effective for mild-to-moderate chronic plaque psoriasis, more so than calcitriol, tacalcitol, coal tar or short-contact dithranol. Only potent topical corticosteroids have comparable efficacy at 8 weeks
  - calcipotriol is useful in addition to PUVA (psoralen and UVA), ciclosporin and ultraviolet B light (UVB)
  - calcitriol is less irritant and may thus be suitable for the face and flexures
  - none has data to support use in pregnancy.
- Calcipotriol with betamethasone dipropionate in combination: not recommended in those under age 18, or on the face or flexures.
- A vitamin A analogue – tazarotene:
  - suitable for moderate plaque psoriasis affecting up to 10% of the skin area
  - not licensed in pregnancy, adequate contraception mandatory, not recommended if breastfeeding or under age 18.
- A dithranol preparation: usually as a short-contact treatment; effective but difficult to use especially on small lesions. It is irritant to normal skin and should be used only under expert guidance on the face and flexures:
  - once lesions are palpably flat dithranol should be discontinued
  - it is frequently combined with UVB phototherapy and a tar bath (the Ingram regimen); the addition of UVB phototherapy prolongs remission.

For more **widespread plaque psoriasis**, eg on the trunk or the limbs, the same treatments as above may be appropriate but:

- Dithranol may be impractical (as mentioned above) and will irritate flexures; application or treatment by trained nurses may alleviate some of these problems.
- Topical corticosteroids may be inappropriate for use in widespread psoriasis, particularly more potent agents if used on a long-term basis.

For **scalp psoriasis** a tar-based shampoo should be tried first; this can be combined with the use of:

- A 2–5% salicylic acid preparation
- A coconut oil/tar/salicylic acid combination ointment

- A potent topical corticosteroid preparation (eg 0.1% betamethasone valerate)
- Calcipotriol scalp application
- More than one of these.

Use a keratolytic agent (eg 5% salicylic acid in emulsifying ointment) first when there is significant scaling, or other treatments will fail.

Use milder agents for flexures and mild agents in facial psoriasis.

Treatment of resistant disease

Phototherapy

UVB PHOTOTHERAPY

- Effective treatment for guttate or plaque psoriasis resistant to topical therapy but must be started under guidance of an experienced dermatologist and supervised by trained staff.
- Patients with previous skin malignancy, SLE or xeroderma pigmentosum are excluded.
- It has the advantages of PUVA in that it can be used in pregnancy and in children.
- It can be used in combination with tars, topical calcipotriol and oral retinoids, and increases the rate of total clearance with reduced total UVB exposure to clearance.
- As most patients enjoy the freedom from topical therapies and the accompanying adverse effects, adjunctive treatment is reserved for resistant cases.

PHOTOCHEMOTHERAPY (PUVA)

- Oral or topical psoralens are administered followed by irradiation with UVA; it is effective and widely used but unlicensed in the UK. It is used to clear psoriasis resistant to topical preparations and UVB.
- Adjunctive therapy with vitamin D analogues and retinoids has been shown to be effective.

METHOTREXATE

- It is especially effective in acute, generalised, pustular psoriasis, psoriatic erythroderma, psoriatic arthritis and for extensive chronic plaque psoriasis in patients who are inadequately controlled by topical therapy alone.
- It can be used as a short-term measure to gain control of unstable psoriasis, such as pustular psoriasis or erythroderma, before returning to the other modes of treatment.
- Acute marrow suppression is the most important side effect. Long-term therapy carries a risk of hepatic fibrosis and cirrhosis.

ORAL RETINOIDS

- **Acitretin**:
  - effective as monotherapy or in combination with PUVA – with a reduction in the dose of UVA and acitretin
  - mucocutaneous side effects troublesome in virtually all patients
  - teratogenic and, because of the long half-life of its reverse metabolite – etretinate – pregnancy should be avoided for 2 years after stopping it; secure contraception is mandatory.
- **Ciclosporin** is highly effective and rapidly acting:
  - main side effects are renal impairment and hypertension, both of which are largely reversible if the dose is reduced or stopped
  - all forms of psoriasis respond; it has a licence for the treatment of severe psoriasis
  - certain amounts of dose sparing can be achieved by using topical treatment together with ciclosporin.
- **Mycophenolate** has shown beneficial effects in several reports but no randomised trials have been conducted. Effective contraception is required and patients should not breastfeed.
- **Azathioprine** and biologic agents, eg anti-TNF (tumour necrosis factor) agents or efalizumab, should be considered only in severe, recalcitrant disease in very specific circumstances and under close supervision.

SCENARIO 7. ECZEMA

Atopic eczema

The skin is dry and lichenified, symmetrically in the flexural aspects of this patient's elbow and knee flexures, wrists and ankles – there is often evidence of excoriation from scratching; this is eczema, it is intensely itchy.

A good candidate

- Will ask for a personal and family history of asthma, hay fever and infantile eczema
- Will know that:
  - atopic eczema most commonly develops in childhood and usually clears up by adulthood
  - commonly involves the face of babies
- Will consider the patient's occupation in the context of the distribution of the rash, eg:
  - hairdressers: may have atopic eczema on the back of the hands or in the webspaces of the fingers from contact with chemicals
  - nurses and doctors: atopic eczema caused by contact latex allergy from gloves. This is alleviated by using latex-free gloves in many clinical areas.

Question

1. What treatment might you give?

Avoid irritants such as bubble bath and soap; the following are all useful: mild topical steroids and plentiful emollients when the skin is dry, antibiotics for secondary infection where necessary, tar preparations for more chronic and less inflamed lesions, and a sedative antihistamine at night. Cotton clothes can be helpful as can the use of emollient soap substitutes. Children of atopic families should (perhaps) be breastfed for at least up to 3 months.

Seborrhoeic eczema

This young man (usually) has greasy scales on a background of erythema involving the scalp, ears, eyebrows, eyelids, nasolabial folds, central chest and pubis.

In elderly people it is commonly intertriginous; these moist erythematous areas are often the sites of bacterial/candidal infection.

Treatment consists of soap substitutes, weak topical steroids, with the addition of a mild tar, salicylic acid, imidazole. Shampoos containing ketoconazole, selenium sulphide or zinc pyrithione are useful for scalp involvement.

Gravitational eczema

There is haemosiderin staining, patchy atrophy, sclerosis and (perhaps) ulceration of this elderly woman's legs, particularly evident near the medial malleolus – this is gravitational, or venous, eczema (see also Ulcer, page 505).

This is a frequent long-term complication of previous deep vein thrombosis but may also be seen in relation to varicose veins and incompetent perforating veins. It is caused by long-term venous stasis in the area in question. Increasing intracapillary pressure leads to diapedesis of red cells; having passed through the walls of the anoxic capillaries the corpuscles disintegrate, and the contained haemoglobin is converted into haemosiderin, which stains tissues brown. It is not truly eczema.

SCENARIO 8. ROSACEA

The patient has facial erythema with pustules and papules (acne rosacea) and telangiectasia involving the nose, chin, glabella and cheeks.

You may see conjunctival suffusion, conjunctivitis and blepharitis; rarely keratitis may be seen. Oral tetracyclines or metronidazole gel and lotion are effective treatments. Some clinicians recommend eradication therapy for *Helicobacter pylori* but the link is controversial.

The condition starts as facial flushing before becoming permanent – this flushing might respond to clonidine. The clinical picture in an individual patient tends to be dominated by a particular manifestation:

- Erythema telangiectatic
- Papulopustular
- Phymatous
- Ocular.

It can be exacerbated by sun, heat, alcohol and spicy/hot foods. The onset is most common between the ages of 30 and 50 and it is more common in women, particularly of those of Celtic origin. Rosacea is uncommon on black skin. Up to 30% of patients report a family history. The common misconception that the facial redness and the phymatous change are caused by excessive alcohol consumption can make rosacea a socially stigmatising condition.

An erythematous rash and telangiectasia may be seen in lupus but in this there is follicular plugging, destruction of the skin and scarring, and the margin is often more abruptly demarcated.

Sarcoid (see page 513) can give a similar appearance, particularly lupus pernio, and mitral and pulmonary stenosis can have a persistent malar flush.

Rhinophyma

There is erythema and swelling of the nose of this (usually) male patient. The pores are very prominent and can give the nose a strawberry-like appearance. It is caused by adenomatous enlargement of the sebaceous glands. It is a consequence of long-term rosacea. Plastic surgery is the treatment, if the patient requires treatment.

SCENARIO 9. HEREDITARY HAEMORRHAGIC TELANGIECTASIA – OSLER–WEBER–RENDU SYNDROME

There are dilated post-capillary venules on the surface of the skin, particularly around the mouth and on the tongue, gums and mucous membranes. They blanch on pressure. This distribution is suggestive of hereditary haemorrhagic telangiectasia (HHT) – Osler–Weber–Rendu (OWR) syndrome.

A good candidate

Will have a detailed knowledge of this diagnosis. HHT is an autosomal dominant condition characterised by epistaxis, cutaneous telangiectasia and visceral arteriovenous malformations (AVMs). The cutaneous telangiectasias are fragile and prone to bleeding – the patient may have had episodes of epistaxis in childhood that were heavier or more troublesome than for other children; epistaxis is the presenting feature in 90% of patients. The condition has high penetrance of over 95% by 40 years of age. Half to two-thirds present before 21 years of age.

The diagnosis of HHT is based on the Curaçao criteria (Shovlin et al. 2000):

- Epistaxis: spontaneous, recurrent nosebleeds
- Telangiectasias: multiple, at characteristic sites (lips, oral cavity, fingers, nose)
- Visceral lesions: GI telangiectasia (with or without bleeding), pulmonary AVMs, hepatic AVMs, cerebral AVMs, spinal AVMs
- Family history: a first-degree relative with HHT.

Three criteria indicate a definite diagnosis of HHT; two mean possible or suspected.

Visceral AVMs can cause significant morbidity and mortality if overlooked and untreated. The patient should receive close follow-up because telangiectasias can develop, and increase in size and number with age.

SCENARIO 10. ULCER

The most common site of an ulcer is on the lower leg.

Venous/varicose ulcer

On the lower, medial leg there is a shallow, irregularly shaped ulcer with a shelved edge, often with a characteristic blue line of growing epithelium. The base will contain pink granulation tissue, pale granulations or slough. This may be large and encircle the limb. There is (often) a feeding vein that proceeds towards the edge of the ulcer; if there is scarring this feeding vein is often not visible but can be palpable.

They are more common on the medial side (long saphenous vein), rather than the lateral side (short saphenous vein). A considerable proportion lies above and behind the medial malleolus.

A venous ulcer is a consequence of the long-term presence of incompetent superficial varicose veins or incompetent perforating veins.

If the ulcer does not lie in the illustrated area, it is improbable that it is venous in origin. They tend to be painless.

Very occasionally an equinus deformity can be seen at the ankle after years of persistent venous ulceration, as a consequence of long-continued walking on the ball of the foot to relieve the pain (unusually) caused by an ulcer, by full dorsiflexion of the ankle joint.

Post-thrombotic ulcer

Little different from a venous/varicose ulcer except pain is frequently a fairly constant accompaniment of a post-thrombotic ulcer. There is often a clear antecedent history of venous thromboembolism from childbirth, abdominal surgery or an accident involving the leg. It is seen less in younger patients from the UK because of effective thromboprophylaxis and prompt treatment of recognised venous thromboembolism. Varicose veins are lacking. The leg is often extensively indurated half-way up the calf, producing a peculiar, but characteristic, shape of the leg, akin to an inverted beer bottle. The skin is firm and tends to be tethered to the underlying structures.

Arterial ulcer

These are extremely painful ulcers, often at sites of trauma, such as the shin or lateral malleolus. They are deep, penetrating the deep fascia and not uncommonly exposing tendons in the base. The pedal pulses are absent; the foot is usually pale and cool. There may be an antecedent history of intermittent claudication; the toes may be discoloured, suggesting that the onset of gangrene is imminent.

You should expect the patient to be a current or past smoker, and enquire whether he or she has diabetes.

Ulcers can have a mixed venous and arterial aetiology. As the treatment of venous ulcers is compression bandaging, any suspicion of an arterial component must be investigated by an arterial assessment; this may be satisfactorily accomplished in many with an ankle/brachial pressure index or arterial Doppler ultrasonography.

Pyoderma gangrenosum

There is an ulcer on the lower limb, most commonly the pretibial area (although it can be found all over the body, including the breast, upper limbs, head and neck); it has a ragged, purplish, overhanging edge with infiltration and oedema of the surrounding skin. It has a mucopurulent or haemorrhagic exudate and secondary infection can make it malodorous and markedly painful. It can be huge and lesions can be multiple.

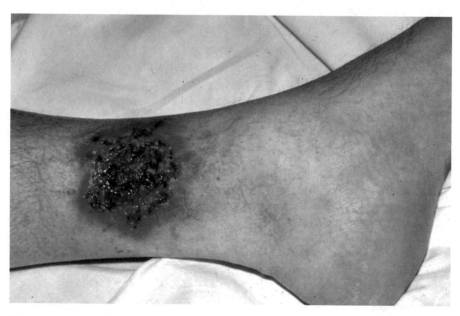

Figure 5.4   Pyoderma gangrenosum.

Questions

1. What is the natural history?

It starts as a sterile pustule that rapidly grows before breaking down and spreading to form the sterile ulcer. Minor trauma (pathergy) may precede the ulcer.

The incidence is higher in women and the onset is between 20 and 50 years of age.

2. What conditions is pyoderma associated with?

About 50% of the diagnosed cases are associated with other diseases:
- Ulcerative colitis: 10–15%
- Crohn's disease: 10–15%
- Other diagnoses:
  - hepatitis C
  - seronegative or seropositive polyarticular arthritis
  - malignant lymphatic disorders, eg leukaemia and lymphoma, paraproteinaemia.

3. How is it diagnosed and treated?

It is primarily a clinical diagnosis but of exclusion. Particular conditions that simulate pyoderma are venous ulcers, vasculitis, cancer, infection, exogenous tissue injury and other inflammatory disorders. There are no diagnostic features on biopsy, and if one is necessary it is to exclude other diagnoses.

The mainstay of treatment is prednisolone 1–2 mg/kg per day.
Other immunosuppressants can be combined with the corticosteroid such as ciclosporin or mycophenolate. Sulfa drugs (eg dapsone up to 200 mg/day) can be used with less aggressive ulcers.

Azathioprine is a useful steroid-sparing agent but its effects are delayed for 2–4 weeks; blood counts and transaminases must be monitored closely. Azathioprine and sulfasalazine can be used in case inflammatory bowel disease (IBD) is the underlying condition.

TNF-α antibody has been used in IBD combined with specific therapy for the bowel disease.

The patient must receive close, continuous follow-up from a specialist to monitor the response to therapy; if there is no response to therapy reconsider the diagnosis and repeat a biopsy.

Topical wound treatment should be performed in all cases; local, potent steroids, in particular, may reduce the pain.

Vasculitic ulcers

These are comparatively rare. You might consider the diagnosis if the site of the ulcer is atypical for a venous or arterial ulcer.

Vasculitic skin lesions are polymorphic, palpable purpura (see also Vasculitis, page 520) is classic, but macules, papules, urticaria, pustules, vesicles, necrosis and livido reticularis may also be present. Subcutaneous oedema below the ulcer may occasionally be seen. The legs are a common site, as are other dependent areas, such as the back and gluteal region. They are uncommon on the face, palms, soles and mucous membranes. The oedema and inflammatory reaction mean that they are often painful. One should consider the presence of fever, arthralgia or myalgia – irrespective of an associated disease – together with the cutaneous lesions, alongside looking for other small vessel involvement in the gastrointestinal tract, peripheral nerves and kidneys.

Consider also the presence of associated disease such as:

- Rheumatoid arthritis (RA): the development of vascular lesions is related to the severity of the disease, which is usually, not always, seropositive (see Rheumatoid Arthritis, page 543). Subcutaneous nodules may also be present. Patients with RA often have involvement of larger vessels with associated peripheral neuropathy, nailfold infarcts and digital gangrene.
- SLE: vasculitis is usually associated with an exacerbation of the underlying disease (see SLE, page 485).
- Sjögren syndrome: these are located on the lower extremities and appear after exercise.
- Paraneoplastic vasculitis: associated with malignant conditions including Hodgkin's lymphoma, lymphosarcoma, T-cell leukaemia, mycosis fungoides, myelofibrosis, acute and chronic myeloid leukaemia, and bronchogenic, prostatic, renal or colonic carcinoma. The association is, however, rare and you would not necessarily evaluate all patients for an associated malignant condition.

Consider also the presence of precipitating drugs and infections:

- Group A haemolytic streptococci
- *Staphylococcus aureus*
- Mycobacteria
- Hepatitis B and C
- Penicillin
- Sulphonamide
- Thiazides.

SCENARIO 11. LICHEN PLANUS

The patient has a rash with small, shiny, flat-topped, polygonal, purplish papules with an overlying network of fine white lines (Wickham's striae).

It (characteristically) affects the flexor aspect of the wrists, the forearms, shins, trunk and lower back; larger more warty areas may be seen on the legs.

The lesions are very itchy.

Koebner's phenomenon is seen with the induction of new lesions at sites of skin trauma.

Lesions that are healing do so (often) with hyperpigmentation.

A good candidate

- Will look in the mouth: a network of fine white lines on the buccal mucosa and white patches on the tongue are often seen.
- Will examine the nails: these can be affected and show longitudinal areas of thinning or more rarely permanent loss.

The scalp can be involved with patches of inflammation and scarring alopecia. Lichen planus tends to last for a year or more.

Topical steroids may help the inflammation alongside sedative antihistamines for symptomatic relief, although in mild cases no treatment is required.

In more widespread symptomatic lichen planus, prednisolone 20–30 mg daily for 4–6 weeks before tapering often shortens the course of the disease.

Hypertrophic plaques can be treated with potent topical steroids or injected with intralesional steroids.

What is the differential diagnosis of mucosal lichen planus?

- Candidiasis
- Secondary syphilis
- Leukoplakia.

SCENARIO 12. DERMATITIS HERPETIFORMIS

There are grouped papules, weals and vesicles, with surrounding excoriation and urticaria, involving the elbows, knees, buttocks, scalp and scapular areas.

It can be very widespread or, alternatively, it can be localised to the elbows.

Although it is a condition of subepidermal blistering, the intense itch with excoriation often dominates the clinical picture.

It is an autoimmune disease associated with gluten-sensitive enteropathy (coeliac disease) with deposition of IgA in the dermal papillae throughout the skin. The enteropathy may not be symptomatic.

The diagnosis is best made by demonstrating the typical histology in early lesions with surrounding IgA deposition; tissue transglutaminase antibodies and a jejunal biopsy may complete the picture alongside the consideration of other autoimmune diseases (that are more common in these patients).
Dapsone and a gluten-free diet are the treatment.

SCENARIO 13. DERMATOMYOSITIS

There is a heliotrope (faint lavender or purplish tint) rash around the eyes (this can be difficult to see and must be looked for), often accompanied by eyelid oedema.

- Cutaneous erythema is common; this may involve several sites:
  - shoulders and upper back: 'shawl' sign
  - upper chest, in a 'V' distribution
  - face and hands
- Gottren's papules are present on the metocarpophalangeal (MCP) joints (these can also affect other extensor surfaces)
- Diffuse subcutaneous calcification within the muscles
- Proximal muscle weakness (see Proximal Myopathy, page 362 and 366) with wasting and muscle tenderness.

A good candidate

- Will examine for features of systemic malignancy (especially carcinoma) in an elderly patient: lung, oesophageal, breast, colon and ovarian tumours are all reported: consider clubbing, Horner syndrome, ascites, lymphadenopathy or hepatomegaly.
- Will know the extramuscular/extracutaneous features:
  - interstitial lung disease: basal fibrosis (the typical pattern of connective tissue disorders), occurring in 30%, although it may be asymptomatic
  - cardiac involvement: usually asymptomatic but clinically evident myocarditis may occur leading to cardiac failure or intractable, life-threatening arrhythmias: the ECG usually shows no specific ST–T wave changes and the creatine kinase CK-MB isoenzyme is frequently elevated even in the absence of symptoms.

Question

1. How might the patient present?

The clinical presentation is divided into five subgroups of patients:

1. Primary idiopathic polymyositis, with voluntary muscle weakness mainly affecting the proximal limb and girdle muscles
2. Primary idiopathic dermatomyositis
3. Either disorder associated with a malignancy
4. Childhood dermatomyositis, or more rarely polymyositis
5. Overlap syndromes: mixed connective tissue disease, eg polymyositis, SLE and systemic sclerosis.

Symmetrical muscle weakness develops slowly, usually over weeks to months; routine tasks become increasingly difficult. Weakness of the extremities, skeletal muscles at other sites, the upper third of the oesophagus, the muscles of neck flexion, intercostal muscles and diaphragm are susceptible to inflammation.

Neck flexion can be so weak that the patient cannot lift the head off the pillow.

Hypercapnic respiratory failure can occur.

It usually spares facial expression and the extraocular muscles even if there is profound weakness elsewhere.

Handgrip strength and fine motor movements remain preserved until advanced stages of the disease.

Prominent muscle pain and tenderness are atypical.

Deep tendon reflexes and muscle bulk are preserved except in severe, advanced disease.

Fasciculations are absent in polymyositis and sensory function remains normal.

Muscles enzymes are released into the blood: CK, AST (aspartate transaminase), ALT (alanine transaminase), LDH (lactate dehydrogenase).

Gottren's papules in a patient with proximal weakness and elevated muscle enzymes obviate the need for a muscle biopsy, otherwise confirmation of the diagnosis with a biopsy is essential.

SCENARIO 14. SARCOIDOSIS

Lupus pernio

There are soft, waxy, blue–red, indurated plaques/maculopapular lesions over the nose, ears, cheeks, fingers and back.

The term 'lupus pernio' is particularly used when the lesions occur on the face.

Erythema nodosum (see next page)

There are tender red nodules with a diffuse margin on the extensor surface of the legs and occasionally the forearms.

The patient may have a light fever and malaise.

The constellation of erythema nodosum, arthritis (in the ankles), uveitis and hilar lymphadenopathy is called Löfgren syndrome and is diagnostic of sarcoidosis.

A good candidate will know that the histology is not of granulomas but a paniculitis, ie inflammation of the subcutaneous fat, thought to result from circulating immune complexes.

The other manifestations of sarcoid are hyperpigmentation, hypopigmentation and keloid reaction (with granuloma formation on biopsy).

SCENARIO 15. ERYTHEMA NODOSUM

There are tender red nodules on the extensor surface of the legs and occasionally the forearms.

The patient may have a light fever and malaise.

It is most commonly idiopathic; streptococcal pharygnitis is the most commonly identified precipitant.

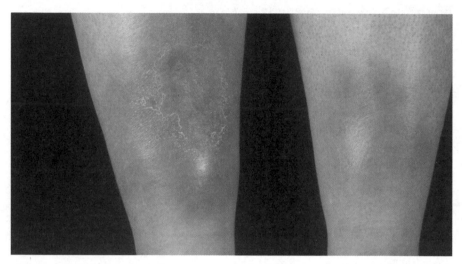

Figure 5.5   Erythema nodosum.

Causes of erythema nodosum

Common

- Infections:
  - streptococcal pharyngitis 25–50%
  - *Yersinia* spp.
  - mycoplasma
  - *Chlamydia* spp.
  - histoplasmosis
  - coccidioidomycosis
  - mycobacteria
- Sarcoidosis, with bilateral hilar adenopathy (see Löfgren syndrome, page 513): 10–25%
- Drugs: antibiotics (sulphonamides, amoxicillin), oral contraceptives – 3–10%
- Pregnancy: 2–5%
- Inflammatory bowel disease: Crohn's disease, ulcerative colitis – 1–4%.

Rare < 1%

- Infections
  - viral – herpes simplex, Epstein–Barr virus, hepatitis B and C viruses, HIV
  - bacterial – *Campylobacter* spp., rickettsiae, *Salmonella* spp., psittacosis, *Bartonella* spp., syphilis
  - parasitic – amoebiasis, giardiasis
- Miscellaneous: lymphoma, other malignancies.

Questions

1. How would you investigate a patient presenting with erythema nodosum?

- FBC, ESR, CRP
- Throat examination and swab looking for group A streptococci, anti-streptolysin O titre (ASOT)
- Chest radiograph

Depending on the clinical suspicion:

- Serum ACE, Mantoux test
- Stool culture and evaluation for ova, cysts and parasites
- Evaluation for IBD.

2. How could you treat it?

Treat the underlying condition; if it is painful and needs specific therapy then NSAIDs are useful (except in Crohn's disease where NSAIDs can cause a flare-up). If there is underlying infection, risk of bacterial dissemination or sepsis and malignancy will have been excluded by a thorough evaluation; prednisolone 1 mg/kg is useful if needed.

SCENARIO 16. KAPOSI'S SARCOMA

There are multiple raised, purplish to brown-black violaceous, well-demarcated, vascular lesions of varying size; they can be macules, patches, nodules or papules. These may also be found on other mucosal surfaces, most commonly the hard palate. Local and regional lymphadenopathy may be found.

The lesions are not painful or itchy.

Visceral disease – most commonly affecting the lung and gastrointestinal tract (anywhere from the mouth to the anus) – is an important cause of morbidity and mortality.

- Lung lesions can cause dyspnoea, cough, haemoptysis and crepitations.
- Gastrointestinal lesions may cause abdominal pain, bleeding and, rarely, a protein-losing enteropathy.
- Extensive visceral disease can cause constitutional upset with fevers, night sweats and weight loss.
- Treated lesions become browner and flatter.

A good candidate

- Will consider the matter further: Kaposi's sarcoma is associated with the following groups of patients:
  - AIDS-related Kaposi's sarcoma – suggests severe immunosuppression
  - immunocompromised Kaposi's sarcoma – post-transplantation
  - classic Kaposi's sarcoma – elderly Mediterranean men, usually on the legs
  - endemic Kaposi's sarcoma – an endemic form in Africa.
- Will be aware that Kaposi's sarcoma is caused by human herpesvirus 8 (HHV8).

Diagnosis

- Biopsy and PCR (polymerase chain reaction) for human HHV8 (strongly implicated in HIV-related Kaposi's sarcoma)
- CD4 count and viral load
- Endoscopy and bronchoscopy are required only if the patient is symptomatic.

Questions

1. *What is the treatment?*

- Antiretroviral therapy (**h**ighly **a**ctive **a**nti**r**etroviral **t**herapy – HAART) alone is often adequate.
- Intralesional chemotherapy with vinblastine for local disease – impractical in widespread disease.

- Chemotherapy with liposomal anthracyclines or taxanes has a role in more severe disease with a good side-effect profile.

Differential diagnosis

This includes:

- Cutaneous bacillary angiomatosis: lesions are often papular and red with a smooth or eroded surface; the papules may enlarge to form large pedunculated lesions, and may be solitary or multiple; subcutaneous nodules can also occur.
- Pyogenic granulomas (*synonym* granuloma telangiectaticum, pregnancy tumour): common benign vascular lesion of the skin and mucosa of unknown aetiology occurring most commonly in children, pregnant women and those taking the combined oral contraceptive, indinavir or retinoic acid derivatives.

SCENARIO 17. VITILIGO

There are patches of complete depigmentation, arranged roughly symmetrically on the body; these are sharply demarcated.

Differential diagnosis

The differential diagnosis of depigmentation includes:

- Pityriasis versicolor: irregular patches on the trunk with a fine scale – it is pale on dark skin and slightly dark on pale skin
- Tinea corporis: usually an overlying fine scale with an indistinct border
- Leprosy: anaesthetic patches
- Hypopigmented mycosis fungoides: usually multiple patches on the trunk.

A good candidate

Will consider the presence of other autoimmune conditions on history or examination:

- Graves' disease (see page 617); note that the patient should, almost certainly, be euthyroid!
- Type 1 diabetes mellitus: injection marks, lipohypertrophy or lipoatrophy, white stick, nephrotic facies, evidence of renal replacement therapy/transplantation, CABG (coronary artery bypass graft) or venous harvest scars, peripheral neuropathy, overriding toes, ulcers, atrophic toes, amputation, etc.
- RA
- Addisonian pigmentation: but the patient should be eu-adrenal and thus not pigmented (see Pigmentation below)
- Pernicious anaemia: peripheral neuropathy
- Alopecia areata
- Morphoea
- Hypoparathyroidism: the patient should be eucalcaemic.

SCENARIO 18. PIGMENTATION

There is generalised skin pigmentation, which is particularly noticeable over the knuckles, at other sites of pressure on the skin such as the knees and elbows, in the palmar creases and over scars. This indicates adrenocorticotrophic hormone (ACTH) excess and is most commonly a result of Addison's disease.

A good candidate

Will consider the matter further and not just think that pigmentation = Addison's disease, thus:

- **Addison's disease** (in MRCP the patient should be appropriately replaced with both glucocorticoids and mineralocorticoids and as such will have neither 'addisonian' pigmentation nor a postural drop in their blood pressure):
  - ask to take a lying and standing blood pressure
  - vitiligo suggests autoimmune Addison's disease; other aetiologies to consider are TB and X-linked adrenoleukodystrophy.
- Rarer causes of ACTH excess:
  - ectopic ACTH syndrome causing Cushing syndrome: very rare, look for signs of hypercortisolaemia (see page 635); consider the proximal myopathies of Cushing syndrome and hypokalaemia, consider Cushing syndrome with cachexia from an underlying malignancy, eg small cell lung cancer.
- **Cushing's disease:** numerically not as rare as ectopic ACTH syndromes, but, as the clinical picture is dominated by hypercortisolaemia leading to treatment, they are often not (or not as) pigmented.
- **Nelson syndrome:** extremely rare but the signs can be quite stable:
  - look for the roof top incision scar on the anterior abdominal wall of a bilateral adrenalectomy or bilateral loin incisions – the scar will most probably be pigmented
  - look for a evidence of pituitary pathology – frontal or transethmoidal craniotomy; bitemporal hemianopia, optic atrophy, loss of acuity; cavernous sinus syndrome
  - the patient should be eu-adrenal.

There is generalised pigmentation with no particular preponderance for sites of trauma or the palmar creases. There are signs of chronic liver disease (see page 27), injection marks indicating diabetes mellitus, clinical evidence of arthritis and hypogonadism, which all indicate that the patient has **haemochromatosis**.

Patches of reddish/brown pigmentation on the upper trunk in a pale-skinned individual is most likely to be pityriasis versicolor, caused by *Malassezia furfur*.

SCENARIO 19. VASCULITIS/PURPURA

There is a non-blanching rash – this is purpura.

Purpura represents extravasation of red blood cells, it is either palpable or not and best classified on this basis.

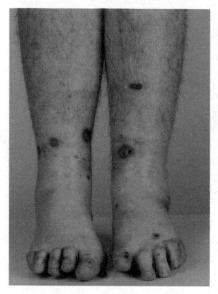 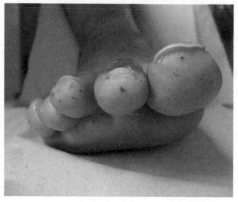

Figure 5.6   Vasculitis.

Causes of purpura

Non-palpable

- Primary cutaneous disorders:
  - trauma
  - solar purpura
  - steroid purpura
- Systemic diseases:
  - coagulation abnormalities:
    - clotting factor defects
    - thrombocytopenia
    - abnormal platelet function
    - warfarin reaction
    - disseminated intravascular coagulation
  - vascular fragility:
    - amyloidosis
    - Ehlers–Danlos syndrome
    - scurvy

  – emboli:
  – fat
  – cholesterol.

Palpable

The lesions are palpable because of localised swelling, which occurs with an inflammatory infiltrate of the vessel wall, leading to extravasation of red blood cells, as in infection or vasculitis.

- Vasculitis:
  - small-vessel vasculitis
  - cryoglobulinaemia type 2 or 3
  - Henoch–Schönlein purpura
  - antineutrophil cytoplasmic antibodies (ANCA)-positive disease:
    - Wegener's granulomatosis
    - Churg–Strauss syndrome
    - microscopic polyangiitis
  - connective tissue disease
    - SLE
    - rheumatoid arthritis
    - Sjögren syndrome
    - Behçet's disease
  - cryoglobulinaemia type 1
  - polyarteritis nodosa
- Infection:
              –acute meningococcaemia
              –disseminated gonococcal infection
  - bacterial endocarditis
  - Rocky Mountain spotted fever
  - group A haemolytic streptococci
  - *Staphylococcus aureus*
  - mycobacteria
  - hepatitis B and C
- Drugs:
  - penicillin
  - sulphonamide
  - thiazides.

SCENARIO 20. NEUROFIBROMATOSIS

A good candidate

● Will collate the signs and justify categorising the disease into type I or type II.

Type 1

NF1 (peripheral; von Recklinghausen's disease). The diagnosis requires a minimum of two of the following:

● Café-au-lait spots (six or more; > 15 mm in adults or > 5 mm in children)
● Two or more skin neurofibromas:
   – subcutaneous, soft, often pedunculated tumours
   – plexiform neurofibromas may form in deeper tissues
● Freckling – in the groin or axilla
● Lisch nodules: two or more; pigmented iris hamartomas seen on slitlamp examination
● Bone dysplasia
● Optic pathway gliomas
(● First-degree relative with NF1).

This is an autoimmune condition caused by a loss of a tumour suppressor gene ($p21^{ras}$) on chromosome 17; it has an incidence of 1 in 2500 live births.

Important complications to be aware of are:

● Hypertension:
   – phaeochromocytoma (< 5% of cases)
   – renal artery stenosis
   – coarctation of aorta
● Nerve root compression from neurofibromas
● Epilepsy.

Mutation analysis of the NF gene can be performed and is available for prenatal diagnosis.

Patients with severe disease should probably be under a specialist clinic; those with milder disease, or who are asymptomatic, may choose not to be but should be fully conversant with the problems that they might face.

Adult patients should:

● have at the least a yearly blood pressure check
● be told to report any unusual symptoms in case they might be related to NF1
● be specifically told the features of:
   – malignant peripheral nerve sheath tumours
   – spinal cord compression.

Type 2

NF2 (central). Any one of the following four sets of manifestations is sufficient for the diagnosis:

- Bilateral vestibular schwannomas
- First-degree relative with NF2 plus unilateral vestibular schwannoma or two of meningioma, schwannoma, glioma, neurofibroma and posterior subcapsular lens opacity
- Unilateral vestibular schwannoma plus two of meningioma, schwannoma, glioma, neurofibroma and posterior subcapsular lens opacity
- Multiple meningiomas plus unilateral vestibular schwannoma or two of schwannoma, glioma, neurofibroma and posterior subcapsular lens opacity.

Skin abnormalities are less common, but café-au-lait patches can occur.
NF2 is an autosomal dominant condition caused by the loss of a tumour suppressor gene on chromosome 22; it has a birth incidence of 1 in 25 000.

SCENARIO 21. PALMAR ERYTHEMA

There is red flushing on the thenar and hypothenar eminences and on the palmar tips of the fingers and thumbs. A similar appearance is seen on the soles of the feet.

It is characteristic of cirrhosis.

A good candidate

Will consider that chronic liver disease (see page 27) is the most likely underlying condition, and look for:

- Dupuytren's contracture
- Leukonychia
- Spider naevi
- Clubbing
- Jaundice
- Ascites
- Hypogonadism
- Caput medusae
- Asterixis
- Bruises
- Pellagra
- Depressed consciousness.

Palmar erythema may also be seen in pregnancy, thyrotoxicosis, RA, polycythaemia, chronic febrile illness, chronic leukaemia, shoulder–hand syndrome or psoriasis and eczema. It can be a normal finding in some; it is attributed to high oestrogen levels.

SCENARIO 22. DUPUYTREN'S CONTRACTURE

There is thickening of the palmar fascia (maybe) with flexion contractures of the ring and little fingers.

It usually occurs in males (10:1) and starts after the age of 25 years. At its very early stages one or more nodules may be apparent in the palm or a dimple may be seen when the fingers are extended; this indicates that the fascia is attached to the skin. Typically it affects the ring finger and years later the little finger; in a third it will affect the ring finger primarily.

In 5% of patients the plantar fascia of one or both feet may be affected.

It is associated with liver disease, especially alcoholic cirrhosis and epilepsy.

It is occasionally familial and may be associated with knuckle pads and Peyronie's disease.

'Congenital' contracture of the little finger, which develops during early childhood, may cause some diagnostic confusion. However, there is no thickening of the palmar fascia and involvement of the ring finger is rare.

SCENARIO 23. CHEILOSIS

This is the appearance of deep cracks or splits at the side of the mouth. If severe these can bleed when the mouth opens and shallow ulcers or a crust may form. It is common in children, who often get temporary relief by licking the affected areas – ultimately making it worse – and in adults during winter – chapped lips. It is also known as perlèche, angular stomatitis or angular cheilitis. It is frequently seen in elderly people who are malnourished when it suggests deficiency of the following:

- Vitamin B
  - vitamin B_2 – riboflavin
  - vitamin B_3 – niacin (nicotinic acid and nicotinamide)
  - vitamin B_{12}
- Folate
- Iron.

It usually coexists with glossitis, except in riboflavin deficiency.

In adults consider the presence of pernicious anaemia, coeliac disease, sprue or inflammatory bowel disease.

SCENARIO 24. HERPES ZOSTER

In a dermatomal distribution there are clustered vesicles with crusting. There is systemic upset with fever, malaise and lymphadenopathy.

In elderly people, during a mild viraemia, it is not unusual for scattered lesions to occur outside the involved dermatome but more severe dissemination with visceral involvement is seen in immunocompromised patients. Patients with Hodgkin's disease are particularly susceptible, especially during chemotherapy.

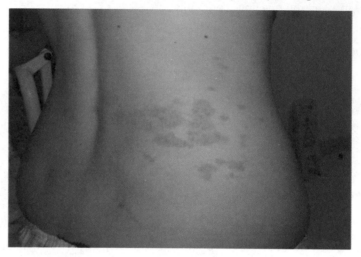

Figure 5.7   Herpes zoster.

Ophthalmic shingles

This is shingles in the ophthalmic division of cranial nerve V. The eye can be damaged directly by the virus or by secondary bacterial infection.

Question

1. What is the natural history?

Varicella-zoster virus, after causing chickenpox, remains latent in the cranial nerve and dorsal root ganglia where it frequently reactivates, decades later, to cause shingles.

Often there is initially severe pain in the affected dermatome (or two associated dermatomes); after 1–3 days the eruption begins, which is exactly the same as in chickenpox, namely a rapid progression through macule, papule, vesicle, pustule and then scab. Often the first visible lesions are vesicles with a little clear fluid and surrounding erythema but pustules are reached within 24 hours. The skin heals over 2–3 weeks but there is often residual pain for several weeks; rarely the pain can be intractable for several years – postherpetic neuralgia; this is more common after ophthalmic shingles or in the immunocompromised host.

SCENARIO 25. PEUTZ–JEGHERS SYNDROME

There are discrete bluish-black macules about the lips, oral mucosa and digits. This is suggestive of Peutz–Jeghers syndrome.

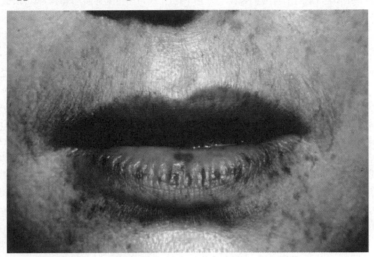

Figure 5.8   Peutz-Jeghers syndrome.

A good candidate

- Will know that this is an autosomal dominant disease characterised by multiple GI hamartomatous polyps, particularly in the jejunum, and an increased risk of various neoplasms. The main symptoms are intussusception and bleeding.
- Will know that these patients have very high relative risks of developing cancer of:
  - oesophagus
  - stomach
  - small bowel
  - colon
  - pancreas
- And less so for cancer of the:
  - lung
  - breast
  - uterus
  - ovary.

The cumulative risk for all cancers is about 90% by 65 years and 2-yearly endoscopic surveillance, plus barium follow-through series at frequent intervals are recommended. The 78-year surveillance of Peutz's original family showed that survival was reduced by obstruction and the development of malignant disease.

SCENARIO 26. LIPODYSTROPHY

Lipodystrophy in HIV-infected patients

This patient has peripheral loss of fat, evident on the face and limbs, with central fat accumulation, evident in the abdomen and neck.

This is most suggestive of lipodystrophy in an HIV-1-infected patient taking protease inhibitors and nucleoside reverse transcriptase inhibitors. It develops in 40% of patients taking protease inhibitors for more than a year and as such is (by far) the most common form of lipodystrophy.

Most patients are healthy but insulin resistance, hypertriglyceridaemia and low levels of HDL cholesterol may occur alongside the development of diabetes mellitus and an increase in cardiometabolic risk. Despite the hyperinsulinaemia, acanthosis nigricans is extremely rare. The mechanisms of insulin resistance are unclear. Stopping protease inhibitors does not seem to improve lipohypertrophy.

There is a suggestion that those patients who develop lipodystrophy during treatment with nucleoside analogues do not develop hyperinsulinaemia or hyperlipidaemia. Sustained improvements in lipoatrophy are seen after switching from a thymidine nucleoside analogue – mainly stavudine.

Acquired partial lipodystrophy

This is very rare. There is loss of fat from the face, neck, arms and trunk with sparing of the lower limbs.

This is suggestive of acquired partial lipodystrophy (very rare, male:female ratio 1:4). The fat loss starts in childhood or adolescence, progressing caudally, affecting the face, neck, arms, thorax and upper abdomen; excess fat may be deposited in the hips and legs, particularly in women. On investigation one would expect to find a low level of serum C3 and a circulating polyclonal IgG autoantibody – C3 nephritic factor. In about 20% of patients type II mesangio-capillary (membranoproliferative) glomerulonephritis develops about 8 years after the lipodystrophy (see page 12).

SCENARIO 27. CAPILLARY HAEMANGIOMA

A dark-red/purplish macular naevus – sometimes called a port wine stain – affecting the face, trunk or limb; naevi are usually unilateral, variable in size and will have been present from birth.

A capillary haemangioma in the distribution of the ophthalmic (Va) or maxillary (Vb) division of the trigeminal nerve may be part of Sturge–Weber syndrome. (see page 372)

A good candidate

- Will know that Sturge–Weber syndrome is the association of a facial port wine stain with underlying vascular anomaly of the brain and/or leptomeninges – classically it is the association of port wine stain and contralateral (often intractable) focal fits; hemiplegia, spasticity or learning disability can also occur. Various ocular anomalies can occur, especially glaucoma; other ophthalmic manifestations are exophthalmos, strabismus or optic atrophy.

Skull radiograph may show vascular calcification although angiography is usually normal.

Capillary haemangioma can be successfully treated by camouflage or dye laser. Sturge–Weber syndrome is sometimes termed the 'fourth phakomatosis' alongside:

- Tuberous sclerosis
- Neurofibromatosis
- Von Hippel–Lindau disease.

Unlike the other phakomatoses Sturge–Weber syndrome has no clear pattern of inheritance.

An excellent candidate will know that a port wine stain on the limb with associated hypertrophy of the related bones and soft tissues is called Klippel–Trenaunay–Weber syndrome.

SCENARIO 28. PSEUDOXANTHOMA ELASTICUM

The skin on the side of the neck, and in the axillae and antecubital fossae is soft, lax, relatively inelastic and wrinkled with a yellowish reticulated pattern or plaques, giving a chicken skin or peau d'orange appearance.

A good candidate

- Will know that on fundoscopy you would expect to find (in 85%) angioid streaks – breaks in Bruch's membrane; they are jagged orange to slate-grey streaks radiating from the disc and represent calcification of the elastic fibres in Bruch's membrane, with subsequent cracking and fissuring. It is symmetrical and usually noted several years after the skin lesions. It is important because it may identify the underlying disease and is a warning that new vessels may grow into the macula, bleed and, devastatingly, lead to blindness. The patient must undergo periodic ophthalmological assessment, and be warned to report any sudden blurring or warping of vision immediately.
- Will know that the other systemic manifestations of pseudoxanthoma are:
  - calcification of the elastic media and intima of the vessels leading to:
    - poorly palpable peripheral pulses
    - hypertension from renal artery involvement
    - ischaemic heart disease from coronary artery involvement
    - intermittent claudication
  - mitral valve prolapse leading to regurgitation
  - fragility of submucosal vessels leading to:
    - GI blood loss: 10% of patients have a revealed GI haemorrhage at some point in their lives; it can occur early in the disease – typically in the second to fourth decades and often without warning; even without revealed loss, anaemia necessitating investigation and transfusion is common
    - haematuria, which is less common
  - intracerebral haemorrhage, which is rare but potentially fatal.

Questions

1. *In what other conditions do angioid streaks occur?*

- Ehlers–Danlos syndrome
- Paget's disease
- Sickle cell disease.

2. Outline the management

- Cutaneous lesions: amenable to cosmetic surgery if required, eg excision of redundant skinfolds.
- Ocular lesions: must be kept under surveillance; Amsler grid examination may allow detection of early subretinal membrane formation, which precedes retinal haemorrhages – facilitating judicious use of retinal photocoagulation:
  - avoid heavy lifting, straining and head trauma, which may increase the risk of retinal haemorrhage
  - adolescents should not participate in weight lifting or contact sports
  - vitamins A, C, E and zinc supplements may reduce the risk of haemorrhage.
- Cardiovascular: yearly blood pressure, peripheral pulses and cardiac examination. Any abnormal finding warrants review by a cardiologist. Mitral prolapse needs consideration for infective endocarditis prophylaxis.
- Laboratory: FBC, ferritin, lipids and urinalysis (low threshold in children, yearly in adults) – refer to a gastroenterologist or a urologist as appropriate.
- Medication: avoid NSAIDs and warfarin. Judicious use of aspirin in high-risk patients; treat hypercholesterolaemia.
- Diet: low cholesterol and moderate calcium (hypocalcaemia has been reported).
- Avoid smoking: tobacco aggravates the disease course.
- Pregnancy: aside from an increase in first trimester miscarriages, pregnancy is well tolerated but perineal tears and abdominal striae are more likely to occur. Multiple pregnancies do aggravate the disease course.
- Genetic counselling: the usual pattern of inheritance is autosomal recessive.

SCENARIO 29. ERYTHEMA MULTIFORME

There are dull, flat, maculopapules with a cyanotic centre (the centre may be purpuric, bullous or necrotic) – target lesions – symmetrically involving the periphery, the hands (both palms and dorsae) and feet mainly, but also the knees, elbows and forearms.

Erythema multiforme (as the name suggests) can present with a variety of patterns – it is a localised form of vasculitis.

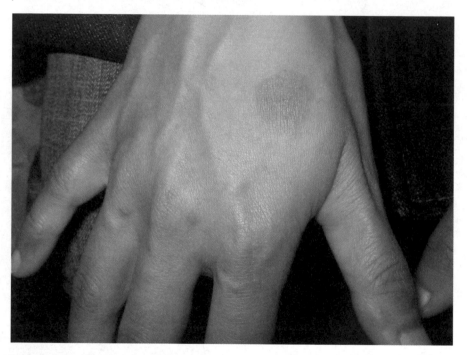

Figure 5.9   Erythema multiforme.

A good candidate

● Will look in the mouth – the mucous membranes can also be affected.

Stevens–Johnson syndrome is a severe, bullous form of erythema multiforme particularly involving the mucous membranes – oral, ocular and genital lesions – with associated pyrexia and malaise.

Causes of erythema multiforme

● Infections:
  – herpes simplex (implicated in 75% cases)

- – *Mycoplasma* sp. (next most common)
- – orf
- – streptococci
- – typhoid
- – diphtheria
- Drugs: sulphonamides
- Pregnancy
- Systemic diseases:
  - – AIDS
  - – RA
  - – SLE
  - – ulcerative colitis.

It can occur at any age, often after a prodromal illness, with an acute eruption lasting for about 3 weeks. Any identified cause should be removed and systemic steroids prescribed if the patient is toxic or very uncomfortable. Recurrent attacks should be treated by eliminating the cause, eg treating the earliest stages of herpes simplex with aciclovir.

SCENARIO 30. SCLERODERMA

The skin is hard and tightly bound down.

Localised morphoea

There are one or a few circumscribed plaques, which can be hypo- or hyperpigmented with an inflamed violaceous border.

They often need no treatment because the prognosis is good but the patient should have serial measurement to see if they are progressing.

Generalised morphoea

There are widespread, (often) itchy, symmetrical lesions following the distribution of the superficial veins.

Raynaud's phenomenon is sometimes associated.

Involvement of the internal organs is very rare but treatment is recommended; inflammation can be suppressed with oral or intravenous steroids and maintained with d-penicillamine or methotrexate, although it is often disappointing.

Linear scleroderma

There are asymmetrical linear lesions on the limbs that follow dermatomal distributions.

It is the most common form of scleroderma occurring in childhood and can lead to serious growth defects on affected limbs. Serial measurement of muscle bulk and limb length is essential.

The treatment is the same as for generalised morphoea with the addition of regular good physiotherapy in childhood-onset disease.

En coup de sabre

There is linear scleroderma affecting the face or scalp. It involves the underlying subcutaneous tissues, muscles, periosteum and bone.

For further discussion on systemic sclerosis see page 552.

SCENARIO 31. LEUKONYCHIA

The nails are white and opaque, the lanula is obliterated; this is leukonychia and is associated with any cause of hypoalbuminaemia, most commonly chronic liver disease; it also occurs in the nephrotic syndrome and malnutrition.

SCENARIO 32. PEMPHIGOID

In this elderly patient there are tense blisters filled with clear fluid (occasionally blood stained). Where lesions have burst, you can see evidence of healing.

It is usually preceded by an itchy, erythematous rash that can be mistaken for urticaria or eczema. The blisters can be localised for weeks before becoming generalised.

The treatment is with prednisolone, and azathioprine to allow subsequent steroid withdrawal. The prognosis is reasonable.

SCENARIO 33. PEMPHIGUS

There are flaccid blisters on the skin and erosions indicating burst blisters that are also present on the mucous membranes.

This is characteristic of pemphigus vulgaris, which you would diagnose on skin biopsy, showing the pemphigus antibody on the keratinocytes. Treatment is with high doses of corticosteroids, prednisolone about 80 mg daily together with azathioprine to allow eventual reduction in the steroid dose.

It is uncommon and most common in middle age, particularly in Ashkenazi Jews. The prognosis is often poor despite treatment – up to a quarter of patients die from the disease or the consequences of treatment.

THE LOCOMOTOR EXAMINATION

This station commonly begins with the instruction 'Please examine this patient's hands …'. RA, scleroderma, gout and psoriatic arthritis are common cases. Alternatively, you may be required to pick up on more subtle cues and be asked the more vague instruction: 'Please examine this patient …'. Ankylosing spondylitis, Marfan syndrome, osteogenesis imperfecta and Paget's disease are common scenarios.

The key principle in all cases is to have a pre-prepared method of examination once you suspect a particular diagnosis. Do not obsess over the presence or absence of minor signs when the diagnosis is obvious.

Examination of the hands

It is important to ensure the patient is comfortable and to rest the hands on a pillow. Expose the hand and forearms up to and including the elbows. A large proportion of the patients may have painful and tender joints and it is imperative therefore to ask about this before palpating the joints, which should be done after careful inspection.

Inspection

General
- Peripheral accessories, eg walking stick
- Peripheral arthropathies, eg knees, ankles.

Face
- Systemic sclerosis (SS): tight, shiny, stretched skin with beaked nose ± telangiectasia
- Cushingoid appearance: steroid treatment
- Horner syndrome: T1 lesion (see Neurological Examination, page 294)
- Ears for evidence of psoriasis, or gouty tophi in helix of ear.

Hands
Approach the examination of the hands themselves in a logical and ordered manner:

- Nails: pitting, onycholysis, clubbing, nailfold infarcts, Beau's lines
- Skin: tight shiny skin over dorsum of hand or fingers (scleroderma); tissue paper thin ± purpura (steroid therapy); surgical scars (joint replacement); tar staining

- Muscles:
  - bilateral wasting of the small muscles with dorsal guttering (RA, syringomyelia, motor neuron disease [MND])
  - unilateral wasting of the small muscles of the hand (C8–T1 root lesion, eg cervical rib, Pancoast's tumour)
  - unilateral wasting involving thenar eminence (median nerve, eg carpal tunnel syndrome)
  - unilateral wasting sparing thenar eminence (ulnar nerve, eg elbow trauma)
- Joints (in order to describe the location of the abnormality accurately, candidates should know the names of the bones and joints)
- Distribution of any abnormalities: symmetrical (eg RA) or asymmetrical (eg seronegative arthritides); proximal or distal joints
- Specific deformities, eg 'swan neck', 'Boutonniere', Z-shaped thumb, subluxation, ulnar deviation, Heberden's nodes, gouty tophi
- Inflammation: calor, rubor, dolor, tumour and loss of function; note that rubor is replaced with shininess of the skin in those with dark skin

Elbows

The elbows should then be examined for psoriatic plaques or rheumatoid nodules.

Function

- Flexion and extension deficits in second to fifth digits are the strongest predictors of actual hand function. Ask the patient to:
  - make a fist, then put the hand together as in prayer.
  - do up a button on the shirt or hold a pen.

Palpation (with caution)

- Palm: Dupuytren's contracture
- Elbow nodules
- Joints: palpate any swelling to determine whether it is soft and boggy (RA) or hard and bony (Heberden's nodes or gouty tophi)
- Skin: tightness or calcinosis in finger pulps (scleroderma/CREST).

It is highly likely that by now the abnormality will have become apparent, but, if not, you should proceed to perform a neurological assessment, focusing particularly on the median and ulnar nerve. Single nerve lesions are occasionally encountered in this station.

The spondyloarthropathies

Classification and PACES

The classification of these conditions is in flux. The following are currently considered 'spondyloarthropathies':

- Psoriatic arthropathy
- Ankylosing spondylitis
- Inflammatory bowel disease (IBD)-associated arthropathy
- Reactive arthritis
- Undifferentiated spondyloarthropathy.

Opinion remains divided as to whether these represent differing expressions of the same underlying disease or separate entities. In PACES, the most commonly encountered cases are psoriatic arthropathy and ankylosing spondylitis. These have obvious signs that lend themselves to the clinical examination setting. It is important, however, not be thrown by overlapping signs.

Each condition shares the following clinical features, albeit expressed to different degrees:

- Axial involvement and/or sacroiliitis
- Peripheral arthritis: asymmetrical and large lower limb joints
- Enthesitis and dactylitis
- Skin involvement, especially psoriasis
- Uveitis/conjunctivitis
- Mucosal inflammation/ulceration/IBD.

Locomotor Scenarios

1. Rheumatoid arthritis
2. Scleroderma
3. Crystal arthropathies
4. Psoriatic arthropathy
5. Ankylosing spondylitis
6. Marfan syndrome
7. Osteogenesis imperfecta
8. Paget's disease

SCENARIO 1. RHEUMATOID ARTHRITIS

Examination

Inspection

Look for characteristic joint, skin, nail and muscle abnormalities and then scan for extra-articular manifestations of the disease.

Joints

- Symmetrical deforming arthropathy affecting the wrist, proximal interphalangeal (IP) and metacarpophalangeal (MCP) joints; sparing of the terminal IP joints
- 'Swan-neck' or 'Boutonniere' deformities; subluxation of the wrist and MCP joints
- Z-shaped deformity of the thumb
- Ulnar deviation at wrist and MCP joints.

Skin

- Rheumatoid nodules (especially on extensor surface of forearm)
- Olecranon bursitis at the elbows
- Steroid purpura
- Vasculitic rash
- Scars of previous surgery.

Nails

- Nailfold infarcts of vasculitis.

Muscles

- Wasting of the small muscles of the hand.

EXTRA-ARTICULAR SIGNS

- Anaemia
- Eyes: scleritis/scleromalacia or keratoconjunctivitis sicca (Sjögren syndrome)
- Abdomen: splenomegaly (Felty syndrome)
- Respiratory: fibrosing alveolitis/pleural effusion
- Cardiac: pericarditis/effusion
- Neurological: carpal tunnel syndrome/peripheral neuropathy/mononeuritis multiplex.

Assess and comment on **function**.

Use **palpation** (cautiously) to determine if joints are actively inflamed – boggy, warm and tender joints imply active disease.

A good candidate

- Will assess the stage of disease and identify active inflammation
- Will estimate the level of functional impairment
- Will identify signs of extra-articular disease and interpret their significance
- Will demonstrate knowledge of treatment modalities and their side effects.

Assess the stage of disease and identify active inflammation

Although the staging of RA is partly radiological, most of the criteria are clinical and can be determined by the examination.

Stage I	Stage II	Stage III	Stage IV
No clinically evident joint destruction or limitation of movement Early osteoporosis on radiology	Some limitation of joint mobility but without deformity Some muscle atrophy Soft tissue extra-articular lesions, such as nodules or tenosynovitis Radiological features of: – periarticular osteoporosis – subchondral bone destruction – minor cartilage destruction	Stage II +: Joint deformity Extensive muscle atrophy	Stage III +: Fibrous or bony ankyloses

Although recognition of an established joint deformity is usually straightforward, diagnosing RA in its early stages is more difficult. The treatment of RA is rapidly advancing, and combination therapy with methotrexate and anti-TNF-antibody therapy can halt joint destruction and functional impairment or prevent its occurrence as long as patients are referred promptly to a specialist.

Questions

1. What are the criteria for urgent referral to a rheumatologist for evaluation?

Clinical guideline (British Society for Rheumatology 2006)

- Morning joint stiffness lasting 30 min or more
- Swelling of three or more joints
- Involvement of the MCP joints or metatarsophalangeal (MTP) joints.

Only 12–15% of those who fulfil these criteria will be given a final diagnosis of RA. The American College of Rheumatology criteria for the diagnosis of RA are complex and their usefulness is somewhat limited to the specialist setting and clinical trials.

---

2. How do you assess the RA patient for active disease?

At each visit to a clinician (including non-specialists) patients should be evaluated for active disease.

Key clinical indicators are:

- Worsening joint pain by visual analogue scale
- Increased duration of morning stiffness
- Increased duration of fatigue
- Inflamed joints on examination
- Worsening limitation of function
- New radiological progression.

Such symptoms in a known patient with RA should prompt rapid reassessment by a specialist.

3. What are the common radiological features of RA?

Joint space narrowing, erosions, periarticular cysts, periarticular osteoporosis, dislocation, subluxation and soft tissue swelling.

Estimate level of functional impairment

Class I	Class II	Class III	Class IV
Able to perform all activities of daily living	Able to perform vocational activities but limited in other activities	Able to perform self-care tasks but limited in vocational and other activities	Limited in all tasks or activities

Identify signs of extra-articular disease and interpret their significance

Extra-articular disease occurs in about 30% of all patients with RA. Look for clues of other organ involvement and state that you would wish to examine the system in question more thoroughly.

System	Signs	Potential diagnoses
Pulmonary	Cyanosis, tachypnoea, clubbing, oxygen, chest deformity	Fibrosing alveolitis Pneumoconiosis Methotrexate pneumonitis Bronchiolitis obliterans Pneumonia (all infections more common in RA)
Cardiac	Raised jugular venous pressure (JVP), pulsus paradoxus	Pericardial effusion
Vascular	Nailbed infarcts, purpuric rash, digit loss, cutaneous ulceration, evidence of renal impairment	Vasculitis
Eye	Episcleritis and scleritis	Keratoconjunctivitis sicca Vasculitis Rheumatoid serositis Scleromalacia perforans
Neurological	Foot drop Wrist drop Wasting of small muscles of hand Signs of compression radiculopathies	Mononeuritis multiplex Carpal tunnel syndrome Cervical spine disease
Abdominal	Splenomegaly	Felty syndrome (RA, splenomegaly, neutropenia)
Other	Rheumatoid nodules Anaemia	Rheumatoid factor positive Anaemia has several causes in RA, including: • Anaemia of chronic disease • GI bleeding from NSAIDs • Felty syndrome • Marrow suppression from gold • Folate deficiency from methotrexate • Associated pernicious anaemia

Questions

1. *What are poor prognostic factors in RA?*

- Extra-articular manifestations and rheumatoid factor (RF) positivity are both poor prognostic factors. The development of extra-articular disease is linked to HLA status. In particular, the HLA-DRB1*04 alleles 01 and 04 are over-represented in patients with vasculitis, Felty syndrome and

rheumatoid nodules. Strangely, the HLA-DRB1*01 alleles that predispose to joint disease do not contribute to the risk of extra-articular disease.
- Anti-citrullinated protein antibodies.
- Male gender.
- Erosive joint disease at 3 years.
- Higher functional disability score at 1 year.
- Inflammatory markers (ESR and CRP) in early disease predict later functional status and health assessment questionnaire scores.
- Multiple joint involvement at presentation also, unsurprisingly, predicts poorer functional status at 5 years.

2. *What clinical emergencies may occur in the patient with RA?*

- **Systemic rheumatoid vasculitis** (SRV): this can occur at any stage of disease (even after many decades of remission) yet the incidence is falling, probably as a result of greater use of disease-modifying anti-rheumatic drugs (DMARDs). The Scott and Bacon criteria define SRV as the presence of one or more of the following in a patient with RA:
  - mononeuritis multiplex or peripheral neuropathy
  - peripheral gangrene
  - biopsy evidence of acute necrotising arteritis plus systemic illness (eg fever, weight loss)
  - deep cutaneous ulcers or extra-articular disease associated with typical nailbed infarcts or biopsy evidence of vasculitis.
- **Atlantoaxial joint subluxation**: acute traumatic atlantoaxial rotatory subluxation is usually easily reduced and then treated with prolonged external immobilisation for 6 weeks. In RA, recurrent or irreducible subluxation may require open reduction and posterior atlantoaxial fusion.

Demonstrate knowledge of treatment modalities and their side effects

The key point in the treatment of RA is that NSAIDs have effective analgesic and anti-inflammatory effects but do not delay disease progression. A good response to NSAIDs in early RA is not a reason to defer therapy with DMARDs.

It is increasingly recognised that early treatment with a combination of DMARDs is more effective than successive monotherapies. Methotrexate in combination with TNF-α inhibitors appears to be particularly efficacious although current British Society for Rheumatology (BSR) guidelines suggest use of biologic therapies only if the response to methotrexate has been suboptimal.

The Tight Control of Rheumatoid Arthritis (TICORA) study showed that using conventional agents (non-biologic) more intensively with protocol-driven escalation resulted in 65% remission rates vs 16% with standard therapy.

3. What are the principal DMARDs and what is their mechanism of action?

- Methotrexate/azathioprine: inhibits purine metabolism and therefore immune cell turnover
- Leflunomide: inhibits pyrimidine metabolism and therefore immune cell turnover
- Ciclosporin: calcineurin inhibition (preventing interleukin 2 [IL-2] production and T-helper cell recruitment)
- Corticosteroids: inhibit all stages of T-cell maturation and activation; they also prevent IL-1 and IL-6 production by macrophages
- Sulfasalazine: precise mechanism unknown
- Azathioprine: reduces DNA and RNA synthesis, thus limiting immune cell turnover
- Infliximab: a chimaeric human/mouse monoclonal anti-TNF-α antibody; abrogates the inflammatory actions of TNF-α
- Adalumimab: human monoclonal anti-TNF-α antibody
- Etanercept: soluble TNF-α receptor
- Rituximab: anti-CD20 monoclonal antibody targeting B cells (currently being evaluated in large randomised controlled trials).

4. What risks are associated with NSAID use and how could they be attenuated?

Peptic ulcer disease

Gastric ulcers occur secondary to a decrease in protective prostaglandin synthesis resulting from cyclo-oxygenase (COX) inhibition. NSAID-induced gastric ulcers account for around a quarter of all cases. The risk of ulceration is not reduced with parental or rectal administration of NSAIDs.

Up to 10% of patients may develop duodenal ulceration within 3 months of starting NSAIDs. The minority of these present with bleeding, yet overall NSAID-induced ulcers are around five times more likely to bleed than *Helicobacter pylori*-associated ulcers. Old age, high doses, long-term use and female gender are all associated with greater risk.

H. pylori infection and NSAIDs are synergistic in ulcer causation, so eradication in *H. pylori*-positive individuals will reduce the risk of GI bleeding.

The risk of peptic ulceration can also be reduced in high-risk patients by:

- Selective COX-2 inhibitors (although many now withdrawn because of an increased risk of myocardial infarction and stroke)
- Misoprostol or other gastroprotective agents
- Concomitant proton pump inhibitors (PPIs).

Cardiovascular events

Cardiovascular disease is one of the principal causes of reduced life expectancy in RA. The increased risked of cardiovascular disease (approaching the level of risk in diabetes) remains even after controlling for traditional cardiovascular risk factors. Inflammation seems to be the principal mechanism by which increased risk is conferred – the chronicity and magnitude of the inflammatory response have been show to correlate directly with the degree of carotid atherosclerosis. Dyslipidaemia is also more common in RA and, furthermore, HDL-cholesterol has less ability to prevent oxidation of LDL-cholesterol in RA.

NSAIDs and COX-2 inhibitors have both been show to increase cardiovascular risk further. Both interfere with the anti-platelet function of aspirin, whereas COX-2 inhibitors specifically inhibit prostacyclin production (which is vascular protective). Prostacyclin is also vasodilatory, so COX-2 inhibitors demonstrate a dose-dependent hypertensive effect.

The BSR guidelines suggest that NSAIDs should not be used in patients at high risk of cardiovascular disease unless it is the only effective analgesia (in which case it should be used at the lowest effective dose).

SCENARIO 2. SCLERODERMA

Examination

Principal signs are in the hands and face, which should be examined carefully.

Hands

- Sclerodactyly: the skin is shiny, smooth and tight over the fingers
- Erosive arthritis with or without deformity
- Telangiectasia
- Nailfold infarcts
- Raynaud's phenomenon: digital ischaemia, red, blue or white fingers
- Calcinosis.

Face

- Beaked nose
- Perioral puckering
- Telangiectasia
- Small mouth
- Sclerosis of the frenulum limiting tongue mobility and affecting speech
- Tight, shiny skin.

State that you would like to examine other systems to exclude the following.

Respiratory

- Evidence of interstitial lung disease: oxygen therapy, cyanosis, short of breath (SOB) at rest
- Pulmonary hypertension: tricuspid regurgitation, raised jugular venous pressure (JVP).

Cardiac

- Signs of restrictive cardiomyopathy: pulmonary oedema, raised JVP, quiet heart sounds
- Arrhythmias.

Abdominal

- Percutaneous endoscopic gastrostomy (PEG; oesophageal dysmotility), previous abdominal surgery scars
- Malabsorption: low BMI, vitamin D deficiency/hypocalcaemia, anaemia
- Evidence of renal replacement therapy/chronic renal impairment (see page 12).

Other

- Hyper- or hypothyroidism
- Hoarse voice from vocal fold involvement.

A good candidate

- Will differentiate between disease phenotypes and demonstrate understanding of the associated complications and prognosis
- Will estimate the level of functional impairment
- Will demonstrate awareness of multisystem complications and their management.

Differentiate between disease phenotypes and demonstrate understanding of the associated complications and prognosis

The cardinal feature of scleroderma is sclerosis of the skin, which begins at the fingers, hands and face, particularly the lips and frenulum of the tongue. In some, disease remains limited to these acral areas but in others it ascends progressively to the trunk, eventually affecting all skin areas. Such patients invariably suffer from internal organ involvement and have a poor prognosis.

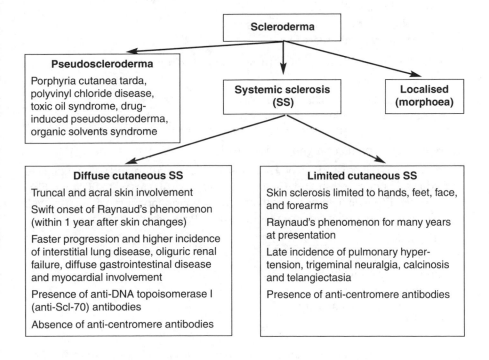

Limited and diffuse conditions are thus distinguished clinically by the degree of skin involvement. It is therefore crucial to demonstrate during the examination that you are assessing this. Be seen to pinch the skin gently between finger and thumb from the hands up the arm towards the trunk, to demonstrate the extent of cutaneous disease.

Questions

1. What are the diagnostic criteria for SS?

Clinical guideline

The American College of Rheumatology has devised criteria that identify SS with > 95% sensitivity and specificity. The major criterion or two of three minor criteria are required:

- Major criterion: truncal (proximal) skin sclerosis
- Minor criteria:
  - sclerodactyly
  - digital pitting scars or pulp loss
  - bilateral pulmonary fibrosis.

In addition to these 1980 criteria, two further minor criteria are commonly accepted:

- Abnormal nail capillary microscopy
- Anticentromere antibody positivity.

---

2. What factors predict prognosis in scleroderma?

Thee is a 4.6-fold increased risk of death in scleroderma compared with unaffected individuals. In one Swedish study, 5- and 10-year survival rates were 86% and 69% respectively. The main causes of death are cardiopulmonary or renal disease, with a significantly increased incidence of lung cancer. Poor prognostic factors include:

- Male gender
- Truncal skin disease
- Internal organ involvement
- Proteinuria
- Low CO diffusion capacity
- High ESR.

3. What is the prevalence of Raynaud's phenomenon in SS compared with the general population?

Raynaud's phenomenon is episodic digital ischaemia, often provoked by cold. Characteristically fingers change colour through three phases – pallor (caused by vasoconstriction), cyanosis (resulting from ischaemia) and finally reactive hyperaemia with redness and swelling.

Raynaud's phenomenon almost invariably accompanies SS. In two-thirds of patients it is the presenting symptom. It is also common in the general population, occurring as a transient benign phenomenon in around a third of young women.

Estimate level of functional impairment

As in RA a multitude of scoring systems exist to monitor functional impairment. Such systems tend to assess either actual movement limitation (physical impairment) or ability to perform the activities of daily life (functional impairment). Their use is mostly limited to clinical trials.

For the purposes of PACES, impaired fist closure or inability to spread the hands completely is strongly associated with higher scores on functional assessment scales.

Demonstrate awareness of multisystem complications and their management

Internal organ involvement determines the prognosis in SS. Without internal organ involvement, the 5-year survival rate is usually around 90%.

System involved	Common manifestations	Prevalence in SS	Survival impact
Gastrointestinal	Oesophageal dysmotility Small bowel bacterial overgrowth and malabsorption Association with primary biliary cirrhosis	About 80%	Minimal
Lung	Pulmonary fibrosis Pulmonary hypertension	About 40–80%	Pulmonary hypertension reduces 5-year survival by about 40%
Cardiac	Ischaemic heart disease Pericarditis	About 20–25%	Reduces 5-year survival by 20%
Renal	Sclerodermal renal disease (onion-skin hypertrophy of glomerular arteries)	About 20%	Reduces 5-year survival by about 80% untreated, 40% treated
Musculoskeletal	Myositis Arthritis, often resembling rheumatoid disease	15–20%	Minimal
Neurological	Trigeminal neuralgia Carpal tunnel syndrome	About 5%	Minimal

Question

1. *What treatments are available for the various manifestations of SS?*

Raynaud's phenomenon: vasoactive substances

- Calcium channel antagonists inhibit endothelial smooth muscle contraction and have an anti-platelet aggregation effect. They reduce the frequency and severity of attacks of Raynaud's phenomenon and the number of digital ulcerations after 6 weeks of therapy in double-blind randomised controlled trials (RCTs).
- Prostacyclin analogues: intravenous infusion for 5–10 days has a beneficial effect on Raynaud's phenomenon for several weeks.
- ACE inhibitors/angiotensin II antagonists reduce the severity and frequency of attacks of Raynaud's phenomenon.
- α-Receptor blockers induce vasodilatation but relieve Raynaud's phenomenon only at high doses (thus leading to orthostatic hypotension).
- Pentoxyphyllin reduces digital infarction but does not reduce the frequency of attacks.

Skin sclerosis

- Benzylpenicillin/d-penicillamine: both these agents probably improve skin softening but side effects are common and their efficacy has yet to be proved in large RCTs.
- Methotrexate may be of benefit in improving skin sclerosis.

Renal failure/hypertension

ACE inhibitors are the treatment of choice for renal failure or hypertension in SS. They should be started early and have a powerful protective effect on further decline in renal function.

Pulmonary fibrosis

Cyclophosphamide in addition to prednisolone seems to slow the progression of fibrosis in SS.

Pulmonary hypertension

Bosentan, an endothelin-receptor antagonist, is of benefit in both primary and scleroderma-associated pulmonary hypertension. Traditional therapies such as iloprost infusion are also beneficial.

GI dysmotility

- PPIs for gastro-oesophageal reflux disease
- Antibiotics for small bowel bacterial overgrowth
- Enzyme supplements for exocrine pancreatic insufficiency
- Metoclopromide and other prokinetics for bowel dysmotility. Botulinum toxin may be of benefit in dysphagia. Electrical gastric stimulation is a promising new therapy for severe gastroparesis.

SCENARIO 3: CRYSTAL ARTHROPATHIES

Examination

The patient may have her or his feet and hands exposed.

Acute gout

Erythema, warmth, swelling, limitation of movement and extreme tenderness of affected joints.

Typically:

- First MTP joint (podagra) in 90%
- Inflamed Heberden's or Bouchard's nodes
- Bursitis at olecranon or patellar bursa.

Chronic tophaceous gout

More common in PACES. Hard, painless nodular calcified swellings typically affecting:

- Pinnas of ears
- Joints of hands and feet
- Ulnar surface of forearm (resembling RA)
- Achilles' tendon.

Be sure to look for the following:

- Signs of chronic renal failure/renal replacement therapy (see page 12)
- Metabolic syndrome (hypertension, obesity, diabetes).

A good candidate

- Will differentiate between acute and chronic inactive gout
- Will venture possible underlying causes
- Will demonstrate understanding of important differential diagnoses
- Will demonstrate knowledge of basic management.

Differentiate between acute and chronic gout

Chronic tophaceous gout is the consequence of chronic hyperuricaemia. Tophi nearly always develop in joints that have been acutely affected and also in relatively avascular areas (the pinnas and pressure points such as the olecranon). When tophi form close to bone they can cause erosions and joint deformity. This is becoming increasingly rare, however, with the widespread availability of xanthine oxidase inhibitors (eg allopurinol) and uricosurics (eg probenecid).

Acute gout is sometimes encountered in PACES. It can be monoarticular (90%) or polyarticular (10%) and is frequently accompanied by:

- Fever (up to 50%)
- Cellulitis and desquamation of overlying skin
- Bursitis and joint effusions.

Distinguishing the two is usually straightforward – acute gout is exquisitely painful, whereas tophi are painless.

Question

1. What can precipitate an attack of acute gout in the hyperuricaemic patient?

The common pathway for development of acute gout is the deposition of urate microcrystals in the synovial fluid and phagocytosis by macrophages, followed by neutrophil recruitment and amplification of the inflammatory response.

Precipitant	Mechanism
Sepsis	Catabolic state leading to raised urate levels Lactic acidosis favouring crystal deposition
Surgery/trauma	Catabolic state and increased urate production
Trauma to joint	Release of microcrystals from larger stable deposits
Starvation/crash dieting/ alcohol binge	Catabolic state and increased urate production Ketoacidosis favouring crystal deposition
Nocturnal onset	Intra-articular dehydration and raised urate concentration
Allopurinol	Sudden lowering of urate levels encourages break-off of microcrystals from larger stable deposits

Possible underlying causes

Hyperuricaemia results from impaired excretion in 90% of cases and increased production in 10%. Note that about three-quarters of patients with elevated serum urate levels never develop gout.

Principal mechanisms and predisposing conditions are summarised below.

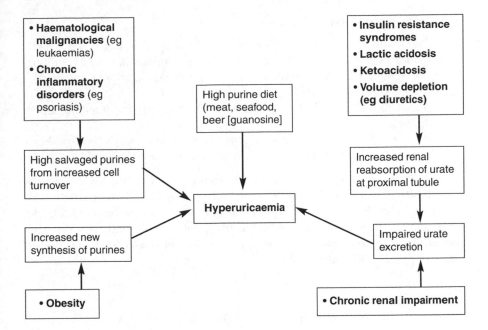

Question

1. What is the role of alcohol in gout?

Consumption of alcohol has been shown to proportionally increase the risk of developing gout. Drinking over 50 g ethanol a day (around 6 units or 3 pints of beer) corresponds to a 150% increased risk of an acute episode. Alcohol contributes to the development of gout by several disparate mechanisms:

- Highly absorbable, guanosine-rich alcoholic beverages (especially beer) increase urate levels
- Volume depletion and subsequent increased resorption of urate with sodium
- Ethanol accelerates the degradation of ATP → AMP → urate
- Impaired gluconeogenesis and subsequent ketoacidosis stimulate both urate resorption at the proximal tubule and crystal deposition in the joint.

Demonstrate understanding of the important differential diagnoses

The clinical picture in acute gout is often indistinguishable from septic arthritis. If you suspect acute gout in PACES, it is crucial to make examiners aware that you would wish to exclude septic arthritis immediately. **The key point is that there is no single diagnostic test that reliably excludes infection in the acute setting.**

Note that the risk of joint infection is not increased in gout (unlike RA in which septic arthritis is more common), but the two conditions can occur concurrently.

Synovial fluid aspiration and analysis:

- Urate crystals are negatively birefringent, needle-shaped crystals on polarised light microscopy. Their presence does not exclude concomitant septic arthritis.
- Synovial fluid leukocyte counts are raised in both septic arthritis and acute gout (as are peripheral inflammatory markers).
- Synovial fluid Gram stain has only about 60% sensitivity for detecting septic arthritis.
- Synovial fluid culture has a higher sensitivity (about 80%) but this is negligible if antibiotics have already been given and much lower in gonococcal infections.

Chronic tophaceous gout is sometimes indistinguishable from RA. Plain radiographs are useful here. In gout, erosions are usually 'punched out' with sclerotic margins and distant from the joint and sometimes outside the joint capsule. Rheumatoid erosions are always within the joint capsule and near the joint margin. Furthermore, joints affected by gout do not develop narrowed joint space or periarticular osteopenia.

Questions

1. *What is the optimum strategy for managing a hot swollen joint?*

Clinical guideline (British Society of Rheumatology 2006)

Evaluating symptoms and signs:

- A short history of swollen, hot and tender joint(s) with impaired movement is septic arthritis until proved otherwise
- It is imperative to treat with antibiotics even in the absence of fever.

Key investigations:

- Blood cultures and synovial fluid: Gram stain and culture must be performed before commencing antibiotics. If the hip is involved, ultrasound-guided aspiration is recommended
- A negative Gram stain or culture does not exclude septic arthritis
- Polarising microscopy must always be carried out.

Other investigations:

- Serum urate level is of no diagnostic value
- White cell count (WCC), ESR and CRP are useful for monitoring response to treatment but have no diagnostic value
- Plain radiographs may show chondrocalcinosis (pseudo-gout) or punched-out erosions and are a useful baseline investigation in septic arthritis
- MRI is the investigation of choice where osteomyelitis is suspected.

Treatment:

- Intravenous antibiotics are required for at least 2 weeks if sepsis in confirmed
- The presence of a prosthesis requires immediate referral to an orthopaedic surgeon.

Exception: solitary involvement of the first MTP (podagra) in the absence of systemic features of sepsis can be assumed to be gout and treated accordingly.

2. *Which organisms most commonly cause septic arthritis?*

- Most common: staphylococci and streptococci
- Young adults: consider gonococci
- Elderly and immunocompromised individuals: consider Gram-negative organisms
- Penetrating trauma: consider anaerobic organisms.

3. *What is pseudo-gout?*

Pseudo-gout is a metabolic arthropathy characterised by episodes of acute monoarthitis and polyarthritis very similar to gout and secondary chronic osteoarthritis. It is caused by deposition of calcium pyrophosphate crystals (positively birefringent) in and around joints.

Clinical presentations vary:

- Most cases are asymptomatic and detected by chance finding of chondrocalcinosis on a plain radiograph
- An acute pseudo-gout is indistinguishable clinically from septic arthritis or gout
- Pseudo-osteoarthritis: resembles osteoarthritis on plain radiograph but with chondrocalcinosis. It affects joints rarely affected by osteoarthritis (MCPs, wrists, elbows, shoulders); a similar picture is encountered in haemochromatosis
- Pseudo-RA (rare): resembles RA but RF is negative and chondrocalcinosis present
- Pseudo-neuropathic arthritis (rare): this is a severe destructive arthropathy, most commonly affecting the knee.

Demonstrate knowledge of basic management

- Identification of urate crystals in synovial fluid or soft tissue aspirates establishes the diagnosis of gout.

- Acute gout attacks can be terminated with the use of colchicine, NSAIDs, corticosteroids or corticotrophin.
- When recurrent attacks occur, a urate-lowering agent should be prescribed.
- Urate-lowering therapy should be life-long.
- Low-dose colchicine or NSAID should be prescribed in a prophylactic manner before initiating urate-lowering therapy and continued for up to 3 weeks thereafter.

SCENARIO 4. PSORIATIC ARTHROPATHY

Examination

Psoriatic arthropathy (PsA) occurs with equal frequency in men and women (unlike RA). Once you have spotted the skin and/or nail lesions, pay particular attention to the pattern of joint involvement.

Skin

The degree of skin involvement does not correlate with the severity of arthritis. After looking at the extensor surfaces of the arms and legs, say that you would like to examine the 'hidden sites' where psoriasis can be missed: the scalp, intergluteal cleft, perineum and umbilicus.

Nails

- Onycholysis
- Transverse ridging
- Pitting.

Dactylitis

Also known as sausage digits.

Enthesitis

This refers to inflammation of tendons at their insertion, giving rise to tenderness superseded by calcification and sometimes ossification. Common sites are:

- Plantar fasciitis
- Achilles' tendonitis
- Costochondritis.

Joints

There are five main patterns of joint involvement:

1. Asymmetrical oligoarticular arthritis (about 45%)
2. Polyarticular RA like (about 35%)
3. Distal IP arthropathy (about 15%, mostly men)
4. Spondylitis (about 5%, mostly men)
5. Arthritis mutilans (< 2%, mostly women).

Extra-articular features:

- Conjunctivitis and uveitis more common than scleritis or sicca syndromes
- Amyloidosis (rare).

A good candidate

- Will use the available signs to distinguish PsA from other arthritides (especially RA) or spondyloarthropathies
- Will demonstrate a basic knowledge of treatment and prognosis.

Use the available signs to distinguish PsA

Beware the patient without skin lesions but diagnostic nail changes! Several clinical features help distinguish PsA from RA with incidental psoriasis.

Feature	PsA	RA
Gender	Males = females	Females > males
Joint involvement pattern	Asymmetrical (even in polyarticular disease)	Symmetrical
Joint tenderness	Low	High
Extra-articular manifestations	Rare	Common
Enthesitis	Common	Rare
Dactylitis	Common	Rare
Spondylitis	Common	Rare
Rheumatoid factor	13%	75%

Questions

1. Are there any diagnostic criteria for PsA?

Clinical guideline: CASPAR study group 2006

The recent international CASPAR (**Clas**sification criteria for **P**soriatic **Ar**thritis) criteria provide 99% specificity and 91% sensitivity for the diagnosis of PsA:

A diagnosis of PsA requires 3 or more points (in addition to arthropathy) scored by the following criteria:

- Current psoriasis (2)
- History of psoriasis (1)
- Family history of psoriasis only (1)
- Dactylitis (1)
- Juxta-articular new bone formation (1)
- Rheumatoid factor negative (1)
- Nail dystrophy (1).

---

2. What are the characteristic radiological features of PsA?

- Osteolysis, resulting in:
  - resorption of the tufts of the distal phalanx
  - 'pencil-in-cup' deformity in the MTP, MCP and distal IP joints
  - complete dissolution of the small bones (as in arthritis mutilans)
- Juxta-articular new bone formation
- Normal joint space and absence of juxta-articular osteopenia (as found in RA).

3. What is arthritis mutilans?

This is the severest form of PsA in which osteolysis results in complete disso-lution of many of the small bones of the hand and wrist. Finger shortening or 'telescoping' is a characteristic feature.

Demonstrate a basic knowledge of treatment and prognosis

Treatment

PsA is a potentially destructive arthropathy, yet there is currently insufficient trial evidence to determine optimum treatment. Traditionally, treatment is based around a programme of regular exercise (to reduce stiffness) in combination with:

- First-line therapy: NSAIDs
- Second-line therapy: sulfasalazine and ciclosporin.

There is no clear evidence that these treatments halt radiological or clinical progression of disease. Systemic steroid therapy is usually avoided if there is florid skin disease because of the risk of rebound exacerbations.

TNF-α inhibitors (etanercept, infliximab, adaluminab) do arrest disease progression and are now licensed for use in PsA. However, the BSR's current guidelines recommend use of anti-TNF-α agents only when patients have failed to respond or are intolerant to first- or second-line therapy.

Prognosis

This is usually better than in RA but a 20-year cohort study has recently revealed an increased mortality ratio in patients with PsA (1.6), mostly attributable to cardiovascular disease. Men and those with fewer affected joints at presentation tend to enjoy longer periods of remission.

SCENARIO 5. ANKYLOSING SPONDYLITIS

Examination

On suspicion of ankylosing spondylitis (AS), the following examination routine should stage disease and detect associated signs.

Establish restricted spinal movement

- Lumbar spine: modified Shober's index – with the patient standing upright, place two marks 10 cm apart on the lumbar spine in the midline. The lower mark is at the level of the posterosuperior iliac spines. The patient then flexes forward (ask him or her to touch the toes) and at maximal flexion the distance is re-measured. In normal individuals there is an expansion of at least 5 cm between the two marks. Lower values indicate decreased mobility of the lumbar spine.
- Thoracic spine: occiput-to-wall distance – the patient stands with the back against a wall (both heels and buttocks must be touching the wall) with a horizontal gaze. In normal individuals the occiput will touch the wall. Any wall-to-occiput gap is a measure of restriction of the thoracic and cervical spines.

Examine for sacroiliitis/enthesitis

Examine (carefully) for tenderness over the sacroiliac (SI) joints. Palpate for evidence of other enthesitides over the heels, costochondral joints and iliac crest.

Tell the examiner that you would like to perform the FABERE (**f**lexion, **ab**duction, **e**xternal **r**otation and **e**xtension) test. The patient places one ankle on the opposite knee and allows the ipsilateral knee to fall outwards (external rotation at the hip) to form the shape of a figure 4. If this causes pain over the sacroiliac joint, sacroiliitis should be suspected.

Examine for peripheral arthritis

But note dactylitis is uncommon in primary AS and suggests PsA or reactive arthritis.

Exclude extra-articular manifestations from head to toe

- Eyes: acute uveitis
- Mouth: mucosal inflammation manifesting as oral ulceration is common
- Chest: apical fibrobullous disease (1%)
- Cardiac: aortic root dilatation and associated aortic valve incompetence, arrhythmias

- Abdomen: 15–20% will develop symptomatic Crohn's disease (stoma present?). Evidence of amyloidosis (hepatomegaly, evidence of renal failure or replacement therapy).

A good candidate

- Will reach the diagnosis of AS, demonstrate knowledge of/detect extra-articular manifestations and comment on the stage of disease
- Will demonstrate knowledge of effective treatments and prognosis.

Reach the likely diagnosis of AS

Following the above system, this should be straightforward. Important points to observe include:

- The characteristic kyphotic 'question mark' posture is usually immediately evident unless the patient is lying down with the head supported by pillows.
- Men are affected three times more frequently than women.

The prevalence of extra-articular features: the 'A's

Feature	Prevalence (%)
Aortitis ± aortic valve incompetence	2–10
Anterior uveitis	25–40
Apical fibrosis	About 5
Aphthous ulcers	About 30
'Abdominal': IBD	70% microscopic evidence of bowel inflammation 6% prevalence of Crohn's disease
Amyloid (secondary)	About 1

Other important complications

Osteoporosis of the vertebral column

This is the result of both immobility of the spine and local inflammation. A vertebral fracture should always be excluded in patients with AS presenting with new back pain, even without a history of trauma.

Cord compression/cauda equina syndrome

Patients with AS are at greater risk of **atlantoaxial subluxation, cervical vertebral fracture** and **adhesive arachnoiditis**. The first two can result in devastating quadraparesis. Arachnoiditis describes fibrous entrapment of the lumbar and sacral nerve roots, resulting in a cauda equina syndrome.

Patients with ankylosis of the cervical spine are at great risk of fracture during intubation for anaesthesia.

Questions

1. What are the key radiological findings in AS?

The hallmark lesion of AS is inflammation at ligament or tendon insertions (entheses), progressing to calcification and then ossification. This process usually begins at the sacroiliac joint and then involves the lumbar spine before progressing cranially and involving other large joints. Disease is almost always bilateral and symmetrical.

Early   **SI joint: indistinct/widened/joint**
- Enthesiopathy: ill-defined erosions with adjacent sclerosis at the sites of ligament and tendon insertions
- Squaring of the vertebral bodies caused by corner erosions and periosteal new bone formation anteriorly.

SI joint: subchondral erosions progressing to sclerosis
- Syndesmophyte formation (ossification of the annulus fibrosus) resulting in bridging across the corners of vertebrae.

SI joint: ankylosis (fusion)
- Bamboo spine: complete fusion of the vertebral bodies by syndesmophytes and ossified paravertebral ligaments
- Vertebral osteoporosis ± chalk-stick fractures: transverse

Late   anteroposterior fractures of the verterbral column.

---

2. In the absence of radiological evidence of sacroiliitis, how is the diagnosis of AS made?

Radiological changes may appear many years after the onset of symptoms, resulting in a delay in diagnosis of up to 10 years. With ever-increasing emphasis on early aggressive treatment to halt disease and limit disability, it is crucial to recognise the disease before radiological changes and disability occur. The high prevalence of chronic lower back pain makes this extremely difficult. The following key signs and symptoms are useful in differentiating a true axial spondyloarthropathy from simple chronic lower back pain.

Sign/symptom	Approximate likelihood ratio of AS
Chronic back pain	1.05
Elevated CRP/ESR	2.5
Heel pain	3
Peripheral arthritis	4
Responds to NSAID	5
Positive family history	6
Anterior uveitis	7
HLA-B27 positive (in white people)	9
Abnormal MRI of sacroiliac joint	9
Grade 3 sacroiliitis on radiograph	20

In the absence of radiological evidence, it has been suggested that having four or more of these criteria should be sufficient for a diagnosis of 'axial undifferentiated spondyloarthropathy'. Such patients should be considered for early therapy.

Demonstrate knowledge of effective treatments and prognosis

Treatment

NSAIDs have been the bedrock of therapy in AS for many years. These provide useful symptomatic relief but do not halt disease progression. A recent Cochrane Review (2006) emphasised the importance of **regular supervised physiotherapy**.

TNF-α inhibitors are the only treatments to have been shown in to halt disease progression as measured by clinical indices of symptoms (Bath Ankylosing Spondylitis Disease Activity Index or BASDAI), histopathological markers of inflammation, bone densitometry and MRI assessment of inflammation (more sensitive than plain radiography). There are no long-term data as yet on whether these drugs are effective at preventing ankyloses.

Prognosis

Life expectancy is reduced with a standardised mortality ratio of 1.5. This is mostly attributable to aortic valve disease, amyloidosis and complications of fractures.

Most morbidity results from **hip arthritis** and **osteoporosis**.

Question

1. What criteria must be fulfilled for use of anti-TNF therapy in AS?

Clinical guideline (BSR 2006)

- Before treatment with infliximab or etanercept patients should:
  - fulfil the modified New York diagnostic criteria for AS
  - have active disease
  - have failed NSAID therapy.

The modified New York criteria (1986) are as follows:
- Sacroiliitis, grade 2 bilaterally or grade 3/4 unilaterally + at least one of the following:
  - lower back pain for more than 3 months which improves with exercise and is not relieved by rest
  - limitation of motion of the lumbar spine in sagittal and frontal planes
  - limitation of chest expansion relative to normal age and sex-adjusted values.

Some would argue that anti-TNF agents should be used much earlier in the disease process to prevent patients from fulfilling the New York criteria, ie in undifferentiated spondyloarthropathies.

SCENARIO 6. MARFAN SYNDROME

Examination

If you suspect Marfan syndrome, expose the patient to the waist and ask him or her to stand with arms stretched out to the side. Start by looking for skeletal abnormalities (the most obvious will be overgrowth of the long bones).

Skeletal manifestations
- Pectus carinatum or excavatum
- Reduced upper segment:lower segment ratio > 1.05
- Arm span exceeds height by a ratio > 1.05
- Arachnodactyly (see figure on next page)
- Walker–Murdoch sign: the distal phalanges of the thumb and fifth finger fully overlap when wrapped around the contralateral wrist (see figure on next page)
- Steinberg sign: the distal phalanx of the thumb fully extends beyond the ulnar border of the hand when folded across the palm (see figure on next page)
- Scoliosis of > 20°
- Hyper-extension at the elbows
- Flat feet
- High arched palate and crowding of teeth
- Joint hypermobility (see figure on next page).

It may be prudent at this point to state: 'This patient has several skeletal manifestations of Marfan syndrome. To complete my examination I would like to examine the eyes, cardiopulmonary system, abdomen, skin and take a full history focusing on the family history.'

The examiner may stop you and ask a few questions, or ask you to carry on.

Eyes
- Ectopia lentis
- Flat cornea
- Hypoplastic iris.

Cardiopulmonary
- Aortic regurgitation
- Mitral valve prolapse
- Scar from previous aortic root surgery
- Evidence of previous video-assisted thoracoscopic surgery (VATS) and pleurodesis for recurrent spontaneous pneumothorax.

Abdomen
- Hernia and/or scars from previous hernia repair.

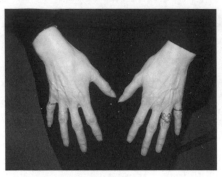

Arachnodactly

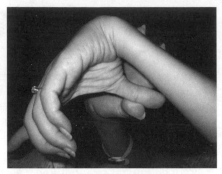

Joint hypermobility

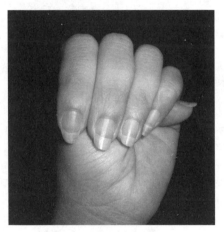

Steinberg's sign

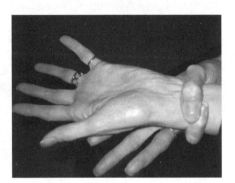

Walker Murdoch sign

Figure 5.10 Marfan syndrome

Skin

- Stretch marks.

A good candidate

- Will identify the key features associated with Marfan syndrome
- Will demonstrate knowledge of potential complications and their prevention/management.

Identify the key features of Marfan syndrome

These are outlined above. Note that many features are detected only after specific imaging, eg lumbrosacral dural ectasia, pulmonary apical blebs, aortic root dilatation and protrusio acetabulae.

Demonstrate knowledge of potential complications and prevention/management

Skeletal system

Craniofacial features are often present (but not with sufficient specificity to be included in diagnostic criteria). These include a long, narrow skull (dolicocephaly), a high arched palate, retrognathia (a recessed lower mandible), micrognathia (a small chin), downward slanting palpebral fissures and tooth crowding. Patients may request corrective cosmetic surgery for some of these features.

Pectus excavatum may sometimes cause restrictive lung disease and require surgical correction.

Severe scoliosis is normally beyond correction with bracing and surgical correction is often required.

Eyes

Ectopia lentis (dislocation of the lens, usually in an upward direction) may require surgical removal of the lens and implantation of an artificial lens at a later date. Often the condition can be managed with glasses or contact lenses.

Retinal detachment, **cataracts** and **glaucoma** are common so yearly assessment by an ophthalmologist is important.

Cardiovascular

Aortic root dilatation: the rate of acute aortic dissection is directly proportional to the maximum diameter of the aorta. When the diameter > 5 cm the risk of dissection is great enough to warrant elective surgery, and such surgery to repair the aortic root is recommended when the maximum aortic diameter reaches 5 cm. Yearly assessment is therefore needed with echocardiography (and occasionally CT if chest deformity means that adequate images cannot be obtained with echocardiography). The rate of growth of the aortic root is equally important in determining the timing of surgery. More frequent surveillance is necessary during pregnancy.

Avoidance of isometric exercise and β blockers (or ACE inhibitors) are indicated to reduce the risk of aortic root dilatation.

If dissection occurs it is usually a type A that either remains confined to the aortic root (type II) or propagates along the descending aorta (type I).

Mitral valve dysfunction is found in approximately half of patients with confirmed Marfan syndrome. About a quarter of these will progress to mitral valve regurgitation by adulthood.

Pulmonary

Spontaneous pneumothorax occurs in up to 15% of patients. Pleurodesis may be necessary to prevent recurrence.

Restrictive lung disease caused by thoracic cage or sternal abnormalities can also occur. Restrictive lung function tests are rare, however.

Risks to relatives

Marfan syndrome is inherited in an autosomal dominant manner and couples should be counselled of the 50% risk of passing the disease on to children. After diagnosis of the proband, examination of family members is usually necessary. However, 25% of patients have a spontaneous mutation rather than hereditary disease.

Questions

1. What is the pathogenesis of Marfan syndrome?

Deficiency in fibrillin-1 – the principal component of the extracellular matrix microfibril – is found in all tissues where the Marfan syndrome phenotype is manifest.

Mutations in one allele for the fibrillin-1 gene (*FBN1*) – of which over 500 have been identified to date – produce a mutant protein that is non-functional and quickly degraded. Furthermore, the mutant fibrillin protein may interfere with function and breakdown of the normal allele, resulting in less than half normal fibrillin-1 levels.

Fibrillin-1 not only is important in extracellular matrix strength but also regulates the activity of cytokines, in particular transforming growth factor β (TGF-β). This seems crucial to the pathogenesis of Marfan syndrome. Indeed, mutations in the type II TGF-β receptor (*TGFBR2*) gene result in the classic Marfan syndrome phenotype.

2. What other conditions may mimic Marfan syndrome?

Homocystinuria can phenotypically mimic Marfan syndrome. Such patients have tall stature with long bone overgrowth and ectopia lentis. Aortic root abnormalities are not a feature of homocystinuria and inheritance is recessive. Furthermore, individuals often have learning disability, recurrent thromboembolic disease and ischaemic heart disease.

Familial thoracic aortic aneurysm syndrome, similar to Marfan syndrome, is inherited in an autosomal dominant trait.

MASS phenotype (standing for mitral, aortic, skin and skeletal manifestations) has many of the features of Marfan syndrome but does not meet the strict diagnostic criteria. Similar to Marfan syndrome it is an inherited fibrillinopathy but follows a more benign course, eg aortic root dilatation tends to be non-progressive.

SCENARIO 7. OSTEOGENESIS IMPERFECTA

Examination

Look for the following features:

- Blue sclera
- Dentinogenesis imperfecta (discoloured, translucent teeth)
- Evidence of multiple previous fractures (may be in a wheelchair or have walking aids nearby)
- Bowing of long bones
- Scoliosis of spine
- Joint hypermobility (eg the ability to oppose the thumb to the ipsilateral forearm by wrist flexion)
- Skin hyperlaxity.

A good candidate

- Will successfully identify the features of osteogenesis imperfecta (OI)
- Will demonstrate a basic knowledge of the phenotypic variants of OI.

Successfully identify the features of OI

These are outlined above. Radiological features of OI include:

- Fractures
- Excessive callus formation
- Wormian bones in the skull and enlargement of frontal and mastoid sinuses
- Fractured and beaded ribs, pectus carinatum
- Narrow pelvis, compression fractures and protrusio acetabulae.

Demonstrate basic knowledge of the phenotypic variants of OI

OI is usually caused by an autosomal dominantly inherited defect in type I collagen production and/or function. There are seven classifications of OI (according to Sillence et al. 1979) organised according to clinical and histopathological features rather than the nature of the underlying genetic mutation.

- **Type I** is the most common form and mildest phenotype. It is non-deforming and a normal height is usually achieved. Fractures normally occur during childhood and become less frequent in adolescence and adulthood.
- **Type II** is the most severe form of disease and is usually fatal in the perinatal period.

- **Type III** is the most severe form of disease compatible with survival into adulthood. Deformity progresses rapidly and the incidence of fractures remains high into adult life. Patients usually suffer from very short stature and severe disability. Dentinogenesis imperfecta is common.
- **Type IV** encompasses all those individuals who do not fulfil criteria for types I–III. Clinical signs are diverse but moderate deformity is usually present.
- **Types V–VII** are defined by specific bony and histological abnormalities. On the whole these are moderately deforming types of OI.

Question

1. *What treatments are available for OI?*

Cyclical intravenous bisphosphonates are now the mainstay of treatment. Unopposed osteoblast activity allows cortical thickening of bone and reduces the risk of fracture.

Orthotics and surgical intervention can help stabilise lax joints and correct bony deformities.

Before the bisphosphonate era structured activity was discouraged as a result of the risk of injury but is now increasingly recognised as an effective means of increasing bone density and reducing disability.

SCENARIO 8. PAGET'S DISEASE

The patient is usually over 50. Look for the following features:

- Bony deformity:
  - bowing of the tibia and/or femur
  - kyphosis
  - facial deformity
  - frontal bossing
  - enlarged maxilla
- Warm to palpation over affected bones
- Neurological complications:
  - hearing aid (nerve VIII compression and/or cochlear dysfunction)
  - paraplegia, suprapubic catheter (cord compression/spinal stenosis)
- Other:
  - scars from previous orthopaedic operations (commonly pinning of femoral fracture)
  - tophi indicating concomitant gout
  - congestive cardiac failure (rare).

A good candidate

- Will identify the key features suggestive of Paget's disease.
- Will demonstrate a basic knowledge of diagnosis and treatment.

Identify the key features of Paget's disease

Some candidates have reported being asked questions about a radiograph of a long bone or skull with pagetian changes. Classic radiological features of Paget's disease include:

- Osteoporosis circumscripta (osteolytic lesions) in the occipital bones of the skull
- V-shaped border between healthy and pagetian bone in the long bones
- Thickened iliopectineal line in the pelvis: 'brim' sign
- Mixed sclerotic areas and osteolytic areas in the skull: the 'cotton-wool' sign.

You should comment on whether deformity has led to functional impairment (be sure to examine the gait).

Question

1. What causes Paget's disease?

Paget's disease is a curiously British disease – it is most prevalent in countries with migrant British ancestry (eg Australia, New Zealand, North America). This probably reflects the strong genetic component – one in five cases has a first-degree relative with the disease. The cause of increased osteoclast bone resorption (followed by compensatory osteoblastic bone deposition) is unknown but there may be a viral trigger such as paramyxovirus infection. The incidence is declining rapidly (50% in the past 20 years) and patients tend to have less severe deformity at presentation.

Demonstrate a basic knowledge of diagnosis and treatment

Diagnosis is based on clinical features, imaging and serum biochemistry. The first two are outlined above. Alkaline phosphatase (ALP) is the most useful marker of disease activity, but a normal value does not exclude the diagnosis. Vitamin D levels should always be requested; this helps differentiate the disease from osteomalacia (which also presents with a high ALP and bone pain) and ensures that it is safe to treat the condition with bisphosphonates (which may cause severe hypocalcaemia in the context of vitamin D deficiency)

Treatment is with second- and third-generation bisphosphonates, which dramatically reduce osteoclast activity. This is always given with calcium and vitamin D supplements to prevent hypocalcaemia. Usually only symptomatic Paget's disease requires treatment. However, treatment of asymptomatic base-of-skull disease may avert irreversible deafness and, if joint surfaces are involved, therapy may reduce the risk of secondary arthritis.

Treatment regimens:

- Pamidronate (up to four infusions over several weeks)
- Risendronate (a weekly dose for 3 months)
- Alendronate (a weekly dose for 2 months).

The efficacy of treatment is measured by the ALP level and relief of symptoms. Upper GI symptoms (especially oesophagitis and heartburn) are common side effects of oral bisphosphonates; patients should be instructed to take tablets in an upright position (not before bed) with plenty of water. A PPI may be necessary to alleviate symptoms.

EXAMINATION OF THE EYES

It is almost certain that you will be asked to examine the eyes and, in particular, the fundus in the PACES examination. There must be no confusion that fundoscopy is a core skill for a practising clinician and MRCP candidate but it is one with which many have considerable difficulty. It is essential to practise the technique until it is fluent and, by doing so, you will become increasingly confident in your competence to diagnose the relatively few possibilities.

This section should be read in conjunction with the section on examination of the cranial nerves (page 276).

Appearance

Look carefully for symmetry involving the eyelids, pupils and general eye movements. In particular, check for signs such as ptosis, lid retraction or irregular pupils.

Look for clues suggesting decreased visual acuity, eg white stick, adjacent Braille books, or for evidence of other systemic diseases such as diabetes, eg glucose testing sticks, diabetic drinks, foot ulcers or evidence of coexistent dialysis.

Visual acuity (VA)

You assess acuity with the patient wearing his or her normal spectacles.

Ask the patient if he or she can see from each eye, and then assess individually by use of a Snellen chart. Visual acuity is defined as $V = d/D$ where d is the distance at which numbers are read and D the distance at which they should be read.

Visual fields

Visual fields should be assessed by confrontation with you sitting about 1 m from the patient and with your eyes at the same level. When assessing the patient's right eye, ask him or her to cover up the left eye and, after covering your right eye, slowly bring an object in from the periphery in a plane equal between you and the patient.

What should the object be? A moving finger is commonly used but it is very insensitive; it may be fine for a screening test if examining the cranial nerves. The top of a pen, placed in the quadrants in turn, is better, but do not bring it in too quickly, because the patient must have the time to say when he or she first sees it.

A red pin can be used for assessing central colour vision, which is located around the macula and, indeed, when it is first visible gives a good indication of peripheral vision also.

Eye movements

Fundoscopy

This should be performed in a dark room; if it is not dark ask to turn the lights off.

A mydriatic, such as tropicamide, will usually have been used. It is essential that you examine the patient's right eye with your right eye and the left eye with your left eye. The latter is a routine with which many candidates have difficulty, but failure to do this, for whatever reason, is frowned upon.

Find the red reflex, keep it in view and get in close!

Although the temptation and tendency are to go straight to the retina, you should get into the routine of gradually racking down through the lens strengths, examining first the front of the eye and gradually, by reducing the strength of the lens, move to the retina, which is usually observed with a zero or slightly negative lens, depending on whether the patient is myopic.

The disc and each quadrant of the retina should be identified and studied in turn.

Disc: note its shape, colour (pale in optic atrophy), margins and if there is papilloedema.

Retinal blood vessels: examine the vessels noting their diameter (arteries are narrower than veins) and the point at which they cross. Is there AV nipping?

Look for arterial emboli (arteries become much thinner or thread like) or venous thrombosis (veins become engorged with surrounding haemorrhages).

Each retinal quadrant should be examined for the presence of

- Haemorrhages
  - dot, blot or flame shaped
- Microaneurysms
- Pigmentation
  - Exudates, distinguish between:
  - hard – white/yellow and shiny with well-defined edges
  - soft ('cotton-wool spots')
- The presence of new vessels should be identified and any previous photocoagulation scars.

The macula

It should be specifically examined because the surrounding area is, as the name suggests, the site of diabetic maculopathy.

Examine the peripheries of the retina, looking particularly for evidence of retinitis pigmentosa.

Considering the cases that you might be asked to see, look around the bedside for clues.

Eye Scenarios

1. Diabetic retinopathy
2. Ophthalmoplegia
3. Visual field defect
4. Ptosis
5. Horner syndrome
6. Proptosis
7. Optic atrophy
8. Internuclear ophthalmoplegia
9. Argyll Robertson pupil
10. Papilloedema
11. Retinitis pigmentosa
12. Holmes–Adie syndrome
13. Choroidoretinitis
14. Age-related macular degeneration
15. Hypertensive retinopathy
16. Nystagmus

SCENARIO 1. DIABETIC RETINOPATHY (DR)

You will be attuned to look for clues whenever and wherever you consult a patient; this is never more important than in PACES.

When asked to perform fundoscopy look specifically for:

- White stick
- Diabetes book
- Diabetic drinks
- Glucometer or marks on the fingertips from glucose testing
- Complications of diabetes:
  - amputation
  - Charcot's joints
  - ulcers.

Classification of diabetic retinopathy

Non-proliferative:
- Mild non-proliferative DR
  - microaneurysms
  - 'dot-and-blot' haemorrhages
  - hard exudates
- Moderate-to-severe non-proliferative
  - the above, usually with exacerbation, plus:
  - soft exudates – 'cotton-wool spots'
  - venous beading or loops
  - intraretinal microvascular abnormalities (IRMAs)
  - is there evidence of treatment – laser photocoagulation scars?
- Proliferative retinopathy:
  - neovascularisation of the retina, optic disc or iris
  - preretinal fibrosis and/or tractional retinal detachment
  - preretinal or vitreous haemorrhage.

Maculopathy:
- Suggested by a drop in acuity to 6/12 or below; it is difficult to diagnose on direct fundoscopy; the following suggest it:
  - exudate within 1 disc diameter (DD) of the fovea
  - circinates or groups of exudates within the macula
  - any microaneurysm or haemorrhage within 1 DD of the macula if associated with a best VA of = 6/12
  - greyish reflection/discoloration at the macula, suggesting retinal oedema near/at the macula
- Diagnosis rests with stereoscopic assessment of retinal thickness using a slitlamp. Fluorescein angiography might also be carried out.

Cataracts: look anteriorly in the eye; you may not see a red reflex.

Consider the postural blood pressure – orthostatic hypotension can worsen retinopathy.

Question

1. *What are the principles of management of the eye in diabetes?*

The aim is to prevent visual loss with central visual loss being the most devastating. At diagnosis and at least yearly each patient aged over 12 with diabetes mellitus (of any cause – in practice people with type 1 diabetes do not need formal screening until they have had diabetes for 5–10 years, but it is prudent to look in the eyes yearly, eg for cataracts, so younger patients know that their retinas are important) should have their acuity checked and, with pupillary dilatation, have their retinas examined. Increasingly, this is done by a network of retinal screeners although the diabetologist and general physician do have a role.

The main risk in type 1 diabetes is retinopathy, of which the devastating endpoint is pre-retinal or vitreous haemorrhage with subsequent retinal traction and detachment. Visual loss is preventable with meticulous care, which will delay progression of DR to sight threatening; before it gets to that stage pan-retinal photocoagulation can be performed to reduce progression or directed to treat new vessels.

The main risk in type 2 diabetes is maculopathy, which causes loss of central acuity.

Maculopathy should be suspected if there is impairment in central acuity, often with no obvious changes on fundoscopy.

Central acuity is checked using a Snellen chart, with the patient wearing normal prescription spectacles. Normal acuity is 6/6; if it is impaired, check with a pinhole; if the corrected acuity is = 6/12 without an obvious cause, an ophthalmologist ought to be consulted; he or she will perform stereoscopic retinoscopy with a slitlamp ± fluorescein angiography to look for maculopathy.

Diabetes-related risk factors

- Duration of disease.
- Glycaemia:
  - DCCT or Diabetes Control and Complications Trial (type 1 diabetes mellitus) – intensive treatment reduces the risk of development and progression of DR
  - UKPDS or UK Prospective Diabetes Study (type 2 diabetes mellitus) – intensive treatment reduces the risk of progression of DR.
- Blood pressure: UKPDS (type 2 diabetes) – tight blood pressure control reduces progression of DR.

- Lipids: epidemiological data suggest a link between elevated lipids and the severity and progression of DR.
- Proteinuria: there is a strong relationship between DR and nephropathy independent of blood pressure.
- Pregnancy:
  - can accelerate the progression of established retinopathy
  - in those with no DR at conception, about 10% will develop DR
  - those with proliferative DR do poorly unless treated with panretinal photocoagulation; treated proliferative DR does not worsen in pregnancy
  - women who begin pregnancy with poor control often have a worsening of the DR when the glycaemia is brought under strict control
  - severe DR is an indicator of a higher congenital abnormality risk in type 1 diabetes.

SCENARIO 2. OPHTHALMOPLEGIA

A good candidate

- Will examine and comment on the presence/abscence of ptosis, abnormalities of the pupil, eye movements.

This scenario may occur in the neurology station.

Third nerve palsy

In the position of primary gaze there is a left complete ptosis, the left eye is deviated down and out, the pupil is dilated and unresponsive to light and accommodation; this indicates a complete third nerve palsy.

The intact fourth nerve may be demonstrated by observing intorsion of the eyeball on attempted accommodation. The comparative weakness of the medial rectus compared with the lateral rectus (innervated by the sixth nerve) leads to abduction.

In diabetes mellitus there is characteristically sparing of the pupil.

A good candidate

- Will know what the significance of pupillary sparing is.

The explanation is thought to be that the parasympathetic fibres, which supply the sphincter pupillae muscles of the iris, lie on the outside of the oculomotor nerve. With an ischaemic or toxic injury to the nerve the outside of the nerve is usually spared, and as such constriction is preserved. In surgical third nerve palsies, usually suggesting extrinsic compression disruption of the nerve, these fibres are not spared. It is not a completely reliable guide.

Consider the causes (the causes of an *isolated* nerve III lesion are in bold):

- **Posterior communicating artery aneurysm**: usually painful
- **Diabetes mellitus**
- Chronic meningitis: malignant or infective
- **Raised intracranial pressure** (ICP)
- Cavernous sinus lesions (see page 371): check sensation in the ophthalmic and mandibular divisions of the trigeminal nerve
- Tumour at the superior apex of the orbit: check VA
- Strokes or tumours in the midbrain affecting either the nucleus or the nerve as it leaves the brain stem, eg Weber syndrome (see page 372)
- Inflammation: **Tolosa–Hunt syndrome**
- **Syphilis**: a historical cause.

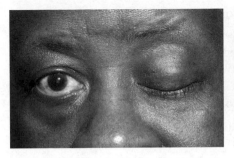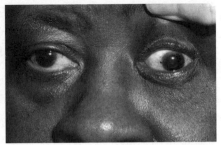

Figure 5.11   3rd nerve palsy on the left

Abducens palsy

There is a failure of abduction of one eye with no other ocular findings. This indicates weakness of the lateral rectus muscle, most commonly resulting from an abducens nerve palsy.

The abducens nerve nucleus is in the pons and in close relation to the facial nerve and the pyramidal tract, so consider the presence of an ipsilateral facial palsy or ipsilateral hemiparesis (see figure above).

Causes

- Diabetes
- Hypertension
- Raised ICP
- Cavernous sinus lesions (see page 371)
- Inflammatory, eg demyelination, giant cell arteritis or sarcoid.

Often no cause is found.

Trochlear palsy

Right trochlear palsy

On attempted lateral gaze the right eye rides up; on vertical gaze the right eye will depress when abducted but not when adducted, ie it will not look towards the tip of the nose. The head is tilted to the left.

It most commonly occurs after head injury. It also occurs secondary to diabetes and hypertension. Tumours and aneurysms may present with an isolated trochlear palsy but they usually progress to cause other nerve lesions or signs.

Internuclear ophthalmoplegia

See page 599.

Conjugate lateral gaze palsy (uncommon)

There is failure of conjugate gaze to the right (or left), which usually suggests a destructive lesion (stroke or tumour) in either the contralateral (palsy away from) prefrontal area or the ipsilateral (palsy towards) pons.

Loss of downward gaze (uncommon)

In an elderly patient this might be caused by Steele–Richardson–Olszewski syndrome (progressive supranuclear palsy), a Parkinson's plus syndrome.

Proceed to demonstrate the anatomy as follows: there is failure of voluntary vertical gaze and pursuit but the presence of normal reflex movements demonstrates that the nerves and nuclei are intact, ie the lesion is supranuclear. If you ask the patient to fix on a distant point and then you tilt the head back the eyes will depress.

Parinaud syndrome (rare)

On attempted upgaze the eyes flicker towards each other rapidly with a rhythmic retraction–convergence–retraction nystagmus. Pupillary responses to light (not accommodation), convergence and downgaze may all be affected. The usual cause is compression of the midbrain by a pinealoma and consequent hydrocephalus (which may feature in the history) and headache. Patients have a tendency to fall backwards. It can occur with stroke, demyelination, encephalitis and brain-stem toxoplasmosis.

SCENARIO 3. VISUAL FIELD DEFECT

Homonymous hemianopia

There is a left homonymous hemianopia. Say what side the lesion is on – a left homonymous hemianopia indicates a lesion on the right.

Where is the lesion?

The underlying lesion must be behind the chiasma on the right-hand side, anywhere from the optic tract to the visual cortex in the occipital lobe. If there is macular sparing it implies a vascular lesion in the occipital lobe.

A good candidate

- Will go on immediately to describe the site of the lesion and its likely cause before proceeding to consider any associated signs – see below.
- Will consider:
  - dominant parietal lobe lesions – evidence of dysphasia, hemisensory loss or inattention
  - non-dominant parietal lobe function – ask the patient to draw a clock, put a cross in the middle of a line and copy a cube; the presence of hemisensory loss or inattention
- Will look quickly for hemiparesis in large lesions.

Stroke or tumour is the most common lesion.

Homonymous quadrantanopia

There is a right upper quadrantanopia: the lesion is likely to be in the left temporal lobe.

There is a left lower quadrantanopia: the lesion is likely to be in the right parietal lobe.

Bitemporal hemianopia

There is a bitemporal hemianopia.

All candidates will be expected to state that the lesion is at the chiasma.

- The most likely cause is a pituitary adenoma and it is important immediately look for the changes of acromegaly and/or hypopituitarism. The soft tissue changes of acromegaly will revert almost to normal on treatment, whereas the bony changes persist. The only features of hypopituitarism that might be present are those of growth hormone deficiency where the skin is fine and vertical lines surround the mouth – simian facies.

- Look for a frontal craniotomy scar or very unusually a scar just under the eyebrow – this approach is used for suprasellar tumours, eg craniopharyngioma or meningioma.

A pointer for a craniopharyngioma might be a young patient with evidence of hypothalamic damage, the most noticeable of which may be morbid obesity.

The clinical history will dictate matters somewhat but diabetes insipidus that is not postsurgical must lead you to consider the following causes:

- Pituitary metastasis
- Germ-cell tumour: very rare but worthy of mention because recognition may allow prompt chemo- and radiotherapy to which they are often exquisitely sensitive
- Craniopharyngioma: craniotomy scar or the habitus of hypothalamic damage?
- Gliomas: often not bitemporal. Is there evidence of neurofibromatosis?

Blindness – cause is in the history

Unilateral: sudden onset:	– retinal artery emboli
	– retinal vein thrombosis
	– retinal detachment
	– temporal arteritis
	– optic neuritis
	– migraine – occasionally
Bilateral: sudden onset:	– bilateral occipital lobe infection or trauma
	– bilateral optic nerve damage, eg methyl alcohol
	– pituitary apoplexy
	– hysteria
Unilateral/bilateral: gradual onset:	– cataract
	– glaucoma
	– macular degeneration
	– retinitis pigmentosa
	– diabetic retinopathy
	– optic nerve or chiasmal compression
	– nerve damage, eg tobacco amblyopia
	– scotoma
	– tunnel vision.

SCENARIO 4. PTOSIS

You might be asked to examine the cranial nerves; examine the eyes or take a look at this patient.

Bilateral ptosis

When it is mild, bilateral ptosis can be difficult to recognise. Consider the following cases:

- Myotonic dystrophy (see page 310)
  - frontal balding
  - furrowed brow
  - haggard face
  - thin neck
  - myotonia
- Myasthenia gravis
  - furrowed brow
  - fatigability
  - diplopia on sustained gaze (see page 350)
- Ocular myopathy:
  - ophthalmoplegia
  - facial/neck weakness
  - furrowed brow
- Intrinsic cord lesions, eg syringomyelia: bilateral Horner syndrome
- Syphilis: Argyll Robertson pupils.

Unilateral ptosis

Complete nerve III palsy

There is a complete ptosis. On inspection of the eye there is pupillary dilatation on the affected side (the pupil may be normal in a 'medical' nerve III – diabetes mellitus being the most common cause), and there is a divergent strabismus (the eye is looking down and out); there is diplopia in the position of primary gaze and it is maximal on adduction. The other eye is normal.

If the ptosis is complete a complete nerve III palsy is the likely diagnosis (see page 586).

A good candidate

Will consider the following:

- Is there proptosis? If so – suspect an orbital tumour or vascular anomaly; listen for a bruit over the eye.

- Will test pupillary reflexes, acuity, fields, perform ophthalmoscopy, look for facial weakness and, if he or she suspects disease in the cavernous sinus, facial sensation.
- Is there a contralateral hemiparesis to suggest Weber syndrome? Rare (see page 372).

Partial nerve III palsy

There is a partial ptosis with a large pupil on the affected side.

Horner syndrome

There is a partial ptosis with a small pupil on the affected side. The pupils are normally reactive and the movements normal (see page 278).
Any cause of bilateral ptosis may cause unilateral disease.

Questions

1. How would you investigate ptosis?

- Plasma glucose to consider the presence of diabetes mellitus (see page 626)
- Consider other causes of mononeuritis: RA, SLE, PAN, Wegener's granulomatosis, sarcoid, so check ESR/CRP and consider the following: ANA, ANCA, RF and anticholinesterase
- Anticholinesterase antibodies are 100% specific and 90% sensitive for myasthenia gravis (see page 350)
- Chest radiograph: apical malignancy or cervical rib, ± CT of chest
- Syphilis serology: usually a TPHA (*Treponema pallidum* haemagglutination assay) or a specific treponemal antigen test is performed rather than a Venereal Disease Reference Laboratory (VDRL) test
- MRI of the brain ± cervical spine and brachial plexus ± MR angiography (MRA): in the investigation of nerve III palsy of uncertain aetiology; note that a posterior communicating artery aneurysm is usually painful
- Electromyography (EMG): see page 311.

2. How does ptosis occur?

Ptosis is a result of weakness of levator palpebrae superioris. Nerve III is the efferent limb. The lower part of the levator is connected to the tarsus by Muller's muscle – smooth muscle fibres – supplied by the cervical sympathetic chain. Ptosis results from damage to these nerves, or from disorders of the muscles or the neuromuscular junction.

Note the following:

- Mechanical ptosis may occur in an elderly patient as a result of dehiscence of the levator palpebrae superioris; there are no associated signs, and it is unlikely to appear in the MRCP.

- In a complete nerve III palsy there may be mild proptosis when the patient sits up as a result of loss of tone in the extraocular muscles; it disappears on lying down.
- Ptosis with a big pupil: oculomotor palsy, best seen in the light.
- Ptosis with a small pupil: Horner syndrome, best seen in the dark.

SCENARIO 5. HORNER SYNDROME

There is unilateral miosis, partial ptosis and enophthalmos: the pupillary reflexes and external ocular movements are normal. On the same side of the face there is (maybe) anhidrosis.

In congenital ptosis the affected iris remains blue, ie heterochromia.

A good candidate

- Will localise the lesion
  - preganglionic
  - post ganglionic
- Will look for signs of causative
  - Loss of the corneal reflex ipsilaterally: suggesting an orbital or retro-orbital tumour
  - Weakness, wasting and hypo-/areflexia in the ipsilateral upper limb: suggesting an avulsion injury to the brachial plexus or Pancoast's tumour
  - Ipsilateral loss of pain and temperature: brain-stem lesion (bilateral signs may be present).

Anatomy

The fibres originate in the ipsilateral hypothalamus, run down through the midbrain and descend to the cervical cord, where they synapse on ipsilateral preganglionic sympathetic fibres before emerging via the anterior roots of C8/T1–2.

From here they pass into the cervical sympathetic trunk, and thence upwards to the superior cervical ganglion.

From here the postganglionic fibres enter the skull with the sympathetic chain around the internal carotid artery, before terminating in the eye.

Horner syndrome indicates that this pathway is interrupted.

Preganglionic lesion

Central: unilateral loss of sweating of head and trunk. The fibres for sweating leave the ascending cervical sympathetic trunk before the ganglion.

- Syringomyelia: bilateral wasting of the small muscles of the hand, dissociated sensory loss, dysarthria, nystagmus, bulbar palsy and reduced reflex in arms (see page 345)
- MS: signs dissociated in space, eg optic atrophy, cerebellar and pyramidal signs. Is there anything in the history to suggest lesions dissociated in time (see page 303)?
- Cord lesion

- Pancoast's tumour:
  - primary tumour at the lung apex interrupting T1
  - clubbing, unilateral wasting of the small muscles of the hand, apical lung signs
- Cervical rib
- Cervical lymphadenopathy: disrupting the preganglionic fibres
- Neck surgery and trauma: scars.

Postganglionic lesion

No unilateral loss of sweating:

- Carotid aneurysm
- Retro-orbital tumours.

Question

1. *What do you conclude from the presence of anhidrosis?*

It is a good lateralising sign but (as you will appreciate from the above description) it is a poor localising sign.

SCENARIO 6. PROPTOSIS

Bilateral proptosis

There is bilateral symmetrical proptosis, which is most probably a result of Graves' disease.

Comment on the following:

- Closure: is it complete?
- Conjunctival suffusion: indicating activity and pressure in Graves' disease
- Ophthalmoplegia: usually a result of fibrosis within inflamed muscles rather than weakness as such
- Acuity and visual fields: compression at the orbital apex can lead to decreased central acuity and concentric field loss
- Fundi: papilloedema or consecutive optic atrophy
- Check the thyroid status of the patient (see page 609) and consider the other features of Graves' disease – dermopathy, acropachy and a diffuse goitre.

If the signs are not symmetrical, even if the patient has Graves' disease, consider the possibility of a retro-orbital tumour.

Unilateral proptosis

There is unilateral proptosis, which is most probably a result of Graves' disease.

Everything is the same as above except that you must exclude a retro-orbital tumour with the appropriate imaging, usually an MRI of the orbits.

SCENARIO 7. OPTIC ATROPHY

There is a pale disc with well-demarcated margins.

The direct pupillary light reflex is absent but the consensual reflex is present; this indicates that the afferent limb of the reflex (the optic nerve) is damaged but the efferent limb (the oculomotor nerve) is intact.

In very early disease you may see the Marcus–Gunn pupil, ie a relative afferent pupillary defect.

Is there papilloedema in the other eye? This is the Foster–Kennedy syndrome, indicating a unilateral frontal lobe tumour that causes ipsilateral optic atrophy and contralateral papilloedema.

A good candidate

- Will look for other signs of underlying cause or explain what they would look for
- Hazard a diagnosis of the underlying cause.

Questions

1. What are the causes of optic atrophy?

MS (the most common cause)
- nystagmus
- cerebellar signs
- pyramidal weakness
- sphincter dysfunction

Optic nerve compression: pituitary tumour or aneurysm
Glaucoma: cupping of disc margins
Ischaemic, eg central retinal artery occlusion:
- look for cherry red macula
- temporal arteritis

Friedreich's ataxia:
- cerebellar signs
- pes cavus

Paget's disease: large skull, bowing of the long bones
Vitamin B_{12} deficiency:
- glossitis
- dementia
- subacute degeneration of the cord (very rare)

Retinitis pigmentosa and panchoroidoretinitis
Leber's optic atrophy: especially in males
Toxins: tobacco, methyl alcohol, lead
Neurosyphilis
DIDMOAD or Wolframm syndrome
- **d**iabetes **i**nsipidus
- **d**iabetes **m**ellitus
- **o**ptic **a**trophy
- **d**eafness.

2. *What investigations might you do?*

- MS:
  - MRI of brain and brain stem
  - visual evoked potentials
  - LP (lumbar puncture)
- Compression within the eye (glaucoma): intraocular pressures
- Compression behind the eye:
  - pituitary disease:
    - MRI of the pituitary
    - Goldmann perimetry
  - Paget's disease (rarer):
    - skull radiograph
    - ALP
    - bone scan
- Ischaemia:
  - glucose
  - ESR
  - fasting lipids
  - carotid Doppler ultrasonography
- Miscellaneous:
  - serum vitamin B_{12}
  - syphilis serology
  - HIV test.

3. *How might you classify optic atrophy*

Three types of optic atrophy:

1. Primary: without preceding visible change to the disc
2. Secondary: to papilloedema from increased ICP
3. Consecutive: after widespread retinal damage, eg retinitis pigmentosa/choroidoretinitis.

Note that the pupil size is normal in optic nerve disease because the direct and consensual reflexes are equal.

SCENARIO 8. INTERNUCLEAR OPHTHALMOPLEGIA

Internuclear ophthalmoplegia in isolation

On attempted gaze to the right, the right eye abducts normally but the left eye fails to cross the midline.

Note that, in a recovering internuclear ophthalmoplegia, the eye may just be slow to adduct or hold momentarily before adducting normally!

The third cranial nerve is intact because the rest of the external ocular movements controlled by it are perfectly normal. The medial rectus itself is functioning normally because there is normal accommodation. The normal abduction tells you that the pathway from the right motor cortex to the abducens nucleus in the pontine horizontal gaze centre is intact, as are nerve VI and lateral rectus. Therefore the lesion lies between the abducens nucleus and the oculomotor nucleus. This is an internuclear ophthalmoplegia, and you suspect that the cause is ????.

Internuclear ophthalmoplegia bilaterally

On attempted lateral gaze the adducting eye fail fails to cross the midposition, whereas the abducting eye abducts normally.

This is usually caused by MS because bilateral stroke is rare.

Internuclear ophthalmoplegia with ataxic nystagmus

Ataxic nystagmus is so closely allied, anatomically, to an internuclear ophthalmoplegia that they usually appear together. On attempted gaze to the right, the right eye, having passed the midposition, goes into a fine well-sustained nystagmus; the left does not pass the midposition, failing to adduct, and remains more or less fixed, possibly with barely perceptible dancing movements, more or less vertically.

Question

1. What is the likely cause?

Gradual onset, bilateral, internuclear ophthalmoplegia with ataxic nystagmus is most probably the result of MS, particularly in a young female from a temperate clime. Look for other features to suggest MS. Bilateral internuclear ophthalmoplegia is usually caused by MS because bilateral stroke is rare.

A sudden onset of a unilateral internuclear ophthalmoplegia with ipsilateral hemiparesis suggests that stroke is the cause. Does the age of the patient give any clues to the diagnosis? Are there lesions dissociated in space to suggest the diagnosis of MS? Was the history of the hemiparesis gradual because this suggests MS rather than stroke?

- Euphoria
- Nystagmus
- Cerebellar speech or gait
- Wheelchair or spastic paraparesis
- Bladder catheterisation
- Scotoma
- Optic atrophy.

Sudden-onset, unilateral internuclear ophthalmoplegia with ataxic nystagmus, in an older patient with a hemiparesis on the side that fails to adduct, or facial numbness is indicative of a brain-stem stroke.

SCENARIO 9. ARGYLL ROBERTSON PUPIL

The left pupil is small and irregular, there may be or is depigmentation of the iris on the same side; it does not respond to light but is reactive on accommodation. It is often found in tabes dorsalis and general paralysis of the insane; occasionally it is seen in longstanding diabetes mellitus.

The causes of prolonged constriction of the pupil are:

- Argyll Robertson pupil
- Horner syndrome
- Parasympatheticomimetic drugs (eg pilocarpine) used in the treatment of glaucoma.

SCENARIO 10. PAPILLOEDEMA

The disc is pink and the border ill defined. The veins are engorged and some disappear as they cross into the disc and cannot be traced down into the cup. There are haemorrhages and exudates on and around the disc. The visual acuity is (maybe) normal (at least in the early stages) but the blind spot is enlarged.

A good candidate

Will present a quick and thorough differential:

- Any intracranial tumour or space-occupying lesion within the CNS, eg brain tumour, subdural haematoma
- Benign intracranial hypertension: pseudotumour cerebri
- Decreased CSF (cerebrospinal fluid) resorption, eg venous sinus thrombosis, inflammatory processes, meningitis, subarachnoid haemorrhage
- Increased CSF production: tumours
- Obstruction of the ventricular system, eg subacute and chronic meningitis
- Craniosynostosis.

Accelerated hypertension can cause papilloedema but there are characteristic arterial changes and the haemorrhages and exudates extend far beyond the region of the disc.

SCENARIO 11. RETINITIS PIGMENTOSA

There is symmetrical and widespread peripheral spiculated black pigment in the both retinas. This is retinitis pigmentosa.

Retinitis pigmentosa is a phenotypic description of several distinct, yet related dystrophies of the retinal pigment epithelium; the underlying genetic abnormalities are being teased out but most cases are still idiopathic.

A good candidate

Will mention that it is associated with the following conditions and have considered if any of these features are present:

- Refsum's disease: autosomal recessive, treatable with a chlorophyll-free diet:
  - cerebellar syndrome (see page 347)
  - peripheral neuropathy (see page 312)
  - cardiomyopathy
- Laurence–Moon–Biedl syndrome: autosomal recessive:
  - obesity
  - hypogonadism
  - short stature
  - learning disability
- Usher syndrome: congenital deafness
- Kearns–Sayer syndrome:
  - progressive external ophthalmoplegia
  - heart block
- Bassen–Kornzweig syndrome (also known as hereditary acanthocytosis or abetalipoproteinaemia):
  - malabsorption
  - spinal cerebellar ataxia.

Question

1. *What are the symptoms of retinitis pigmentosa?*

Initially there is loss of night vision; the rods are affected more than cones because they are peripheral. With progressive disease, the pigmentation advances towards the centre of the retina with consequent increasing tunnel vision. The macula is spared until very late. Most patients are registered blind by the age of 40 years.

Although the pattern of retinitis pigmentosa should present no diagnostic difficulties the other conditions with retinal pigmentation are:

- Choroidoretinitis (posterior uveitis)
- Retinal photocoagulation
- Age-related macular degeneration.

SCENARIO 12. HOLMES–ADIE SYNDROME

The patient is often a young woman. The right (or left) pupil is large and regular and does not respond (or at best responds sluggishly) to a very bright light. It constricts slowly on accommodation, and may constrict excessively before recovering slowly (hence, also described as a tonic pupil).

In time the pupil may become small, and the age of the patient and the regularity of the pupil should enable the correct diagnosis to be made.

The ankle and knee jerks can be depressed or absent.

It is a result of degeneration of the ciliary ganglion in the orbit.

SCENARIO 13. CHOROIDORETINITIS

There are asymmetrical, well-defined areas of black pigmentation occurring randomly throughout the retina, with pale areas resulting from retinal atrophy. It can be unilateral.

A good candidate

- Will state the diagnosis and correctly identify the most common cause, which is prior asymptomatic toxoplasma choroidoretinitis.

What are the possible causes of choroidoretinitis?

- TB: constitutional symptoms
- Sarcoidosis: lupus pernio, lymphadenopathy, erythema nodosum
- Syphilis
- Beçhet's disease: oral and genital ulcers.

What is the differential diagnosis of retinal pigmentary change?

- Old choroidoretinitis
- Laser-treated diabetic retinopathy
- Retinitis pigmentosa
- Macular degeneration.

SCENARIO 14. AGE-RELATED MACULAR DEGENERATION (ARMD)

Early ARMD

There are small drusen on the retina. Some may coalesce to form small confluent spots of hypo- or hyperpigmentation.

A history of subtle visual impairment must be present otherwise one would just have drusen.

Late ARMD

Dry ARMD (Geographical atrophy)

Usually there is a large, well-demarcated, perifoveal spot in which large choroidal vessels are visible.

The first symptom is usually gaps occurring in an image or it can appear as if letters have dropped out of a line of text.

Wet ARMD

Serous or haemorrhagic fluid causes the neuroretina of the pigment epithelium to detach from Bruch's membrane – this gives a much less distinct area on the retina. The symptoms are usually more rapidly progressive and, as the detachment disturbs the photoreceptors, it causes an image distortion called metamorphopsia. Initially it can be present in just one eye before rapidly spreading to the other eye where, if untreated, it will rapidly cause legal blindness (acuity = 1/60).

SCENARIO 15. HYPERTENSIVE RETINOPATHY

- Grade 1: narrowing of retinal arteries
- Grade 2: increased light reflex caused by atherosclerosis ('silver wiring') and AV nipping
- Grade 3: flame haemorrhages and cotton-wool spots
- Grade 4: papilloedema.

Grades 3 and 4 lead to an accelerated/malignant condition.

The grading of hypertensive retinopathy is in some respects a historical nicety. It was developed before effective treatment for hypertension and was a way, albeit imprecise, of staging the condition.

In practical terms now, the presence or absence of grade 3 or 4 hypertension is what is important – it signifies accelerated or malignant hypertension and is evidence of ongoing end-organ damage visible to the naked eye.

A good candidate

Will, on discussion, be able to cover the following matters:

- Consider the other systemic features of hypertension:
  - renal microvasculature – dip the urine and if there is blood you would want to perform microscopy to look for casts and, if there is protein, quantify it
  - heart – are there signs of congestive cardiac failure? You would want an ECG and an echocardiogram
  - cerebral microcirculation – if there are any abnormalities on examination or a severe headache suggesting hypertensive encephalopathy, you might consider an MRI to document matters
- And consider other important macrovascular considerations:
  - signs of dyslipidaemia:
    - xanthelasma
    - presenile arcus
    - palmar xanthomas
    - tar staining on the fingers
  - features to suggest an underlying cause, eg Cushing's disease, acromegaly, neurofibromatosis, polycystic kidney disease, radiofemoral delay or renal bruit.

SCENARIO 16. NYSTAGMUS

The direction of nystagmus is defined by the direction of the fast phase. However, the slow phase is the pathological component, and fast phase the correction.

Nystagmus usually results from dysfunction of the labyrinth of the ear (peripheral) or of the vestibular connections of the brain stem and cerebellum (central).

Those with peripheral lesions will usually complain of deafness, tinnitus, rotationary vertigo, often with nausea and vomiting, but have few other signs and by contrast those with nystagmus from the brain stem often have other signs. As such peripheral nystagmus is unusual in PACES and central is common.

The cases that you may see are:

- A few beats of horizontal nystagmus only present on the extremes of lateral gaze. This is physiological nystagmus.
- Fine horizontal nystagmus only present on looking to the left:
  - in a peripheral lesion the fast phase is away from the lesion

The important physiology is that each labyrinth slowly 'pushes' the eye to the opposite side and the cortex quickly corrects it; in health this is obviously balanced. Thus, on looking to the left, as the right labyrinth is 'weak' the eyes are pushed to the right (the slow phase) and the correction is to the left (the fast phase). It may be present in the primary direction of gaze but characteristically it worsens when the eyes are turned in the direction of the fast phase (Alexander's law).

  - in a central lesion the fast phase is towards the lesion:
  - test hearing (see examination of the vestibulocochlear nerve): it might be impaired in a peripheral lesion such as Ménière's disease or in a cerebellopontine angle lesion (see page 354). If it is impaired perform Rinne's and Weber's tests, and if doubt remains request a pure-tone audiogram
  - test facial and corneal sensation and look for facial weakness: cerebellopontine angle tumour or pontine lesion
  - look for cerebellar signs – dysarthria, intention tremor, ataxic gait (see page 347)
  - look for a hemiparesis.
- These signs suggest a brain-stem or cerebellar lesion, eg tumour, stroke, MS or hereditary causes such as Friedreich's ataxia (see page 349).
- Sustained horizontal nystagmus on lateral gaze in both directions is commonly seen in drug toxicity with phenytoin, benzodiazepines or

barbiturates, where there is dysarthria or limb ataxia. It can also occur with disease of the cerebellum or brain stem above.

- Vertical nystagmus usually signifies a central lesion but it can be caused by the above drugs. There are two types:
  - upbeat – the fast phase is up; lesions at the medulla or anterior vermis of the cerebellum such as MS, stroke, tumour or Wernicke's encephalopathy
  - downbeat – the fast phase is down; less common and associated with lesions at the foramen magnum or the medulla at the cervicomedullary junction, eg Arnold–Chiari malformation
- Nystagmus confined to one eye: ataxic nystagmus invariably associated with an internuclear ophthalmoplegia
- Convergence nystagmus suggests a lesion at the midbrain centre for convergence and vertical gaze in the roof of the midbrain. It may be damaged by stroke, MS, encephalitis or thiamine deficiency.

A tumour at this region (eg a pinealoma) obstructs CSF flow, causing headaches; there is paralysis of upgaze, downgaze and convergence and, as with other tumours at this area, the patient often has an uncontrollable tendency to topple backwards – Parinaud syndrome.

- Pendular nystagmus has no recognisable fast or slow phase; the movements are sinusoidal. It may be congenital or acquired, eg loss of macular vision.

Question

1. *What symptoms might the patient have?*

- Oscillopsia
- Dizziness and vertigo may be associated with vestibular or central abnormalities

Investigations
- Pure-tone audiogram and caloric tests for peripheral nerve VIII function
- MRI: if lesions at the cerebellopontine angle (CPA), brain stem or cerebellum, or demyelination is suspected
- Phenytoin level
- Blood alcohol, γ-glutamyltransferase (GGT), liver function tests (LFT)
- Red cell transketolase for Wernicke's encephalopathy, although practically it is not performed.

EXAMINATION OF THYROID STATUS

The assessment of the thyroid status of a patient is an absolutely basic clinical skill and one that should not present any difficulties provided that the following scheme is followed. The most likely cases that you might meet are goitre and euthyroid Graves' disease. For obvious reasons, patients with hyper- or hypothyroidism are unlikely to appear, although it is essential to be competent in demonstrating these. (Note that patients who are being followed up for differentiated thyroid cancer may be investigated for recurrence while off thyroid medication [often liothyronine]; as the time of their assessment is totally predictable they *might* appear in the examination and be clinically hypothyroid.)

General observations

Look for signs of thyroid dysfunction:

- Hypothyroidism:
  - pale dry skin
  - peaches and cream complexion
  - dry hair: loss of the outer third of the eyebrows is unreliable and non-specific
- Hyperthyroidism:
  - anxious, fidgety patient
  - staring eyes (lid retraction)
  - sweating.

Hands

Shake the patient's hand:

- Warm and sweaty or cool and dry?
- Fine tremor: hands outstretched with a piece of paper resting on fingers
- Pulse:
  - rate
  - rhythm (atrial fibrillation often occurs in thyrotoxicosis)
  - volume (typically large volume and collapsing in hyperthyroidism)
- Thyroid acropachy: a rare feature of Graves' disease
- Tar staining: Graves' ophthalmopathy is worse in smokers.

Eyes

Look closely at the eyes, because there is a wealth of information there.

Lid retraction

This is indicated by visible sclera above the superior limbus of the cornea.

This results from sympathetic stimulation of levator palpebrae superioris of *any* aetiology, eg thyrotoxicosis, anxiety, β agonists.

Lid lag

Ask the patient to follow the slow downward movement of your finger at a distance of about 50 cm. The upper lid lags behind the descending eyeball.

Graves' disease

Exophthalmos

The sclera is visible below the inferior limbus of the cornea with the patient sitting at the same level as yourself and looking straight ahead.

This sign is independent of thyroid status but suggest an aetiology i.e. Graves' disease; the term is synonymous with proptosis; it can be unilateral, although a retro-orbital tumour should always be excluded.

Other features

- Periorbital oedema
- Chemosis
- Conjunctival injection
- Ophthalmoplegia.

If Graves' ophthalmopathy is present on inspection it is necessary to perform a more detailed examination (be aware, however, that if the thyroid is not the focus of the case and the patient is elderly with a small nodular goitre, to go on to perform a theatrical examination of the eyes irritates certain examiners – with good reason).

- Are the eyes painful in any way? Are they gritty or dry? And ask if any part of the subsequent exam causes pain or discomfort.
- Is eyelid closure adequate? With exophthalmos there is a greater volume of eye to be covered with each blink, the frequency of blinking is reduced and the time of each blink is increased.
- Ask patient to follow your finger (and to say if he or she experiences diplopia) as you test all directions of gaze (see page 279):
  - limitation of upward gaze is the most common abnormality in Graves' ophthalmopathy
  - however, the combination of enlarged ocular muscles ± subsequent fibrosis may lead to complex ophthalmoplegia that is not explained by either single nerve or muscle disease.

- Ptosis: a very rare occurrence in either Graves' disease or hyperthyroidism. Its presence should raise the possibility of coexistent myasthenia gravis.
- Acuity: as the most important concern of Graves' ophthalmopathy is a threat to the sight it is critical to assess vision in the following fashion (should the examiner wish you to – in routine clinical practice you should):
  - acuity using a Jaeger or Snellen chart (+ pinhole)
  - colour vision – either using Ishihara plates or a red pin to look for desaturation
  - fields – compression of the nerve head at the orbital apex can cause constriction of the fields
  - ophthalmoscopy:
  - Is there papilloedema or consecutive optic atrophy?
  - if closure is poor or you have concerns about the cornea you may want an ophthalmologist to perform slitlamp examination to look for corneal scars or ulcers. You can get a reasonable view with a direct ophthalmoscope but not good enough to preclude a proper examination.

Goitre

Follow the sequence observation, palpation, percussion, auscultation (see Goitre below).

Neuromuscular manifestations

Reflexes

Slow, relaxing in hypothyroidism and brisk in thyrotoxicosis.

Proximal myopathy

Thyrotoxicosis – ask the patient to stand from a chair unaided.

Legs

Graves' disease dermopathy
- Sheet-like myxoedema: coarse diffuse skin with non-pitting oedema
- Nodular localised: violaceous, infiltrative, waxy area on the shin, resembling erythema nodosum
- Horny: papilliform, irregular, firm, red dermopathy on shin/upper foot.

Endocrine Scenarios

1. Goitre
2. Graves' disease
3. Hypothyroidism
4. Acromegaly
5. Diabetes mellitus
6. Addison's disease
7. Nelson syndrome
8. Haemochromatosis
9. Gynaecomastia
10. Pseudo-hypoparathyroidism
11. Turner syndrome
12. Cushing syndrome
13. Klinefelter syndrome

SCENARIO 1. GOITRE

The *presence* of the goitre usually rests on observation and the character on palpation; percussion has some bearing on size and auscultation can define one particular aetiology.

Is the thyroid nodular or symmetrical? If it is nodular is it a discrete nodule or multinodular?

Ask the patient to swallow a sip of water and look for upward movement of the thyroid gland. Note that a thyroglossal cyst will move upwards on both swallowing and protrusion of the tongue, and can be transilluminated.

Is there any evidence that the thyroid is compressing any of the following:

- Trachea: monophonic syncope (rare), but the history may have suggested some dyspnoea, particularly on lying flat
- Recurrent laryngeal nerve: hoarseness
- Oesophagus: dysphagia, very rarely odynophagia
- Venous return from the head: superior vena cava obstruction (very rare).

Scar – previous hemi-/total thyroidectomy.

Palpation

Stand behind the patient and gently palpate the gland, located two finger-widths below the thyroid cartilage, with one hand on each side and the neck gently flexed.

- If a goitre is present, comment on the following:
  - size
  - consistency:
    - soft – like the lips
    - firm – like the tip of the nose $\left.\right\}$ do not say these, obviously!
    - hard – like the forehead
  - diffuse or nodular: if nodular – multinodular or a single nodule
  - tender – suggests thyroiditis
- Lymphadenopathy
- Does the thyroid move freely; is it tethered? This suggests cancer.

Percussion

Percuss very gently for retrosternal extension.

Auscultate

Bruit – classically occurs in Graves' disease thyrotoxicosis.

A good candidate

- Will comment on the thyroid status, either having examined it formally or from general observation if the instruction was just to palpate the thyroid
- Will also comment on the likely aetiology.

Question

1. How will you manage the patient?

Is there a possibility of cancer? Books are written on the problem of finding the 750 cases of thyroid cancer a year in the UK when palpable nodules are present in 1 and 5% of men and women, respectively.

- Define the aetiology
- Determine the thyroid status and manage appropriately
- Exclude cancer if palpable nodules present.

SCENARIO 2. GRAVES' DISEASE

This woman is sitting comfortably, has warm dry palms and no tremor; there is no lid retraction or lag and as such she is clinically euthyroid.

In the neck there is a moderate, diffuse, fleshy goitre, which does not have a bruit; it is not tender and moves freely on swallowing, there is no retrosternal extension.

There is bilateral symmetrical exophthalmos, the conjunctivae are not inflamed and, although blink is prolonged, it is adequate. There is modest limitation of upgaze and adduction symmetrically and diplopia on abduction, indicating tethering of the lateral rectus bilaterally. There are no other extra-thyroidal signs on examination such as pretibial myxoedema or acropachy. There is tar staining on the fingers indicating that the patient is a smoker.

In conclusion this patient has Graves' disease; she is currently euthyroid. There is thyroid eye disease (*synonym* ophthalmopathy) which is currently quiet. Ask whether could you examine visual acuity, test the visual field and perform fundoscopy.

There are no features of other autoimmune disease, eg vitiligo, diabetes mellitus.

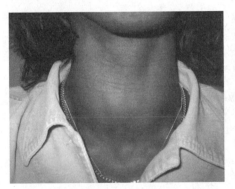 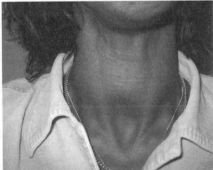

Figure 5.12 Goitre–movement with swallowing

The good candidate

- Will make a clear unequivocal statement of the thyroid status, the aetiology and if there is Graves' ophthalmopathy try to classify it somewhat into active or quiet and be able to describe any worrying features.

What is the aetiology?

Graves' disease is caused by IgG antibodies stimulating the thyroid-stimulating hormone (TSH) receptor.

Questions

1. *When a patient presents with thyrotoxicosis what is the differential diagnosis?*

- Thyroid:
  - Graves' disease – most common cause
  - toxic multinodular goitre
  - single toxic adenoma
  - thyroiditis
  - factitious ingestion of thyroxine
  - amiodarone therapy
  - exogenous iodine (Jod–Basedow effect)
- Non-thyroid:
  - psychiatric disorders, eg anxiety states
  - phaeochromocytoma
  - malignancy
  - alcohol withdrawal
  - excess caffeine intake.

Presenting symptoms of thyrotoxicosis

- Weight loss
- Anxiety
- Palpitations
- Fatigue
- Tremor
- Sweating
- Heat intolerance
- Staring eyes.

Presenting features of Graves' disease

Any or none of the above and:

- Neck swelling
- Gritty eyes
- Staring or protruding eyes.

Investigations in thyroid disease

	Free T$_4$	Free or total T$_3$	TSH
Hyperthyroidism	Usually ↑ or →	Usually ↑ or →	Always undetectable
Hypothyroidism	Usually ↓ or →	↓ or →	Always ↑
Sick euthyroid	↓ or usually →	↓ or →	↓ or low →
Pituitary disease	↓ or usually →	Usually ↓ or →	Usually ↓ or low →
Amiodarone	Usually ↑	Usually ↓	Usually modestly ↑
TSH-oma	Usually ↑ or →	Usually ↑ or →	Detectable or modestly ↑
Thyroid hormone resistance	→	→	Elevated

- Thyroid antibodies: usually microsomal or peroxidase are measured: they become increasingly detectable with age (like most antibodies), but where they are present in a high titre with thyrotoxicosis they suggest autoimmunity.
- Uptake scan: usually ^{99}Tc (technetium-99) or more rarely ^{123}I (iodine-123):
  - the definitive investigation to demonstrate a single functioning toxic adenoma, the presence of which often changes the management, strongly favours ^{131}I treatment – the toxic nodule takes up the iodine whereas the normal gland does not, ideally rendering the person euthyroid with a low chance of subsequent hypothyroidism
  - otherwise its role is quite limited, but opinions on that matter vary a great deal.
- Ultrasonography:
  - not necessary to diagnose nodularity unless taken in the context of the prevalence of nodularity in the general population and the antibody results
  - in reality quite a limited role: useful investigation in skilled hands for assessing dominant nodules or dominance within nodules when considering neoplasia and to guide fine-needle aspiration (FNA).

Questions

1. How do you manage thyrotoxicosis?

- Carbimazole or propylthiouracil: first-line medical treatments (see page 396). Either titrate dose by biochemical response or use 'block-and-replace' regimen. Warn patients of side effects (rash about 1 in 200; agranulocytosis about 1 in 2000. Patients to seek urgent FBC if they develop a sore throat or other infection).
- β-Adrenergic blockers (eg propranolol): provide symptomatic relief until euthyroid. Often require large doses.
- ^{131}I –labelled radioiodine:
  - useful for long-term treatment although 50% will become hypothyroid; contraindicated in pregnancy and breastfeeding
  - may worsen ophthalmopathy, especially in smokers.
- Surgery: total or subtotal thyroidectomy depending on local practice.

2. What do you know about management of thyrotoxicosis in pregnancy?

The management of hyperthyroidism in pregnancy requires specialist advice.

The fetus is at risk of either hyperthyroidism (passage of thyroid-stimulating antibodies across the placenta) or hypothyroidism as a result of transfer of anti-thyroid drugs. Monitoring of fetal heart rate is the best measure of disease activity.

SCENARIO 3. HYPOTHYROIDISM

The patient has pale skin ('peaches-and-cream' complexion), puffiness of the face, particularly round the eyes, cool, dry hands, coarse, dry hair with a hoarse, croaky voice.

There is bradycardia and slow relaxing reflexes. If severe, cerebellar ataxia may be present.

A good candidate

Will consider the following:

- The aetiology: a small, firm, diffuse goitre may suggest Hashimoto's thyroiditis.
- In severe hypothyroidism the patient may collect effusions within the body cavities – pleural, cardiac
- Erythema ab igne on the legs or abdomen
- Depression or psychosis ('myxoedema madness')
- Features of other autoimmune disease (eg pernicious anaemia, Addison's disease)
- Symptoms, signs or evidence of treatment of carpal tunnel syndrome.

Loss of outer third of eyebrows is an unreliable and non-specific sign.

Investigations

- TSH and free T_4 (see Graves' Disease, page 617)
  - the pattern whereby the TSH is elevated outside the normal range – (usually > 10 mU/l) with a low normal or frankly low T_4 level is characteristic of primary hypothyroidism; the elevated TSH is the key thing to note
  - in the rarer, secondary hypothyroidism, the TSH is inappropriately normal or low for a low free hormone level (low normal free T_4 and low normal TSH are perfectly compatible with secondary hypothyroidism!).
- 09:00 cortisol: mandatory: Addison's disease can cause the biochemical picture of hypothyroidism or it can coexist as another organ-specific autoimmune disease or as part of a polyglandular autoimmune syndrome. In the latter an adrenal crisis can be precipitated by rendering the patient euthyroid and increasing the metabolic 'demand' for cortisol from the failing adrenals. Adrenal failure must be treated first.
- Antibodies: thyroid peroxidase or microsomal, will help delineate the aetiology.
- Ultrasonography: may reveal a goitre, though by no means a necessary test.
- Fasting lipids: raised LDL-cholesterol.
- FBC.

Questions

1. *What are the symptoms of hypothyroidism?*

- Fatigue
- Sleepiness
- Weight gain
- Cold intolerance
- Puffy face
- Hoarse, croaky voice
- Snoring
- Aches and pains
- Dry skin
- Hair loss
- Constipation
- Menorrhagia
- Deafness
- Psychosis – 'myxoedema madness'
- Cerebellar disturbance (see page 347).

2. *What are the complications of hypothyroidism?*

- Carpal tunnel syndrome
- Hyperlipidaemia
- Ischaemic heart disease.

3. *What is the aetiology?*

- In the UK, and in any iodine-replete area, the most common cause is autoimmune thyroiditis, either atrophic or Hashimoto's thyroiditis.
- Worldwide the most common cause is iodine deficiency. Iatrogenic hypothyroidism occurs in a third of people after radioiodine or surgery.
- Hypothyroidism occurs secondary to pituitary or hypothalamic disease.

The other causes to consider are the following drugs:

- Amiodarone (but more often causes thyrotoxicosis)
- Excess iodine: the Wolff–Chaikoff effect. This is used occasionally to prepare people for urgent thyroid surgery
- Poor compliance with thyroxine replacement
- Lithium.

4. *How would you manage someone with hypothyroidism and IHD?*

Treat coexisting ischaemic heart disease (IHD) first then cautious replacement, often as an inpatient. There is a compelling argument for starting with a very modest dose of liothyronine, ie 5 mg once daily alongside a daily ECG, slowly building up, in stages to 20 mg twice daily, before a 5-day crossover with 100 mg T$_4$, which will continue.

SCENARIO 4. ACROMEGALY

Features resulting from excess growth hormone

The patient has large hands and feet. There are prominent supraorbital ridges, macroglossia, prognathism, interdental separation, broad nose, coarse facial features and the skin is thick. (The signs of acromegaly are clear to see and quite stable, so the case is over-represented in PACES. The case is also a good example of endocrine principles.)

Examine for carpal tunnel syndrome, hypertension and a multinodular goitre (found in 10–20%)

A good candidate

- Will identify and comment on the key diagnostic features (above)
- Will look for signs of a pituitary tumour
- Will look for signs of associated disease (or explain what they would like to examine).

Look for signs of a pituitary tumour

Optic chiasma

There is a visual field defect – classically bitemporal upper quadrantanopia or hemianopia. If there is severe longstanding pressure on the optic chiasma there may be a reduction in central acuity and optic atrophy.

Cavernous sinus involvement

Ophthalmoplegia and pain or sensory loss in the ophthalmic and maxillary divisions of the trigeminal nerve may be present.

Caused by compression of adjacent normal pituitary

Hypopituitarism.

Look for signs of associated disease

- Cardiovascular disease:
    - hypertension
    - ischaemic heart disease
    - cardiomyopathy
- Respiratory disease: upper airway obstruction caused by macroglossia, goitre and soft tissue enlargement results in obstructive sleep apnoea
- Colorectal adenomas and cancer
- Glucose intolerance and diabetes mellitus.

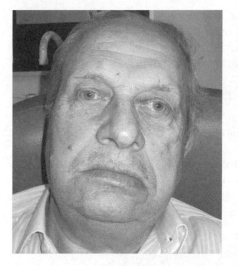

Acromegalic facies

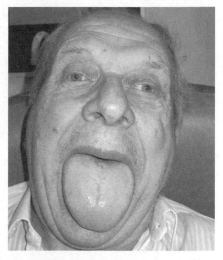

Large tongue

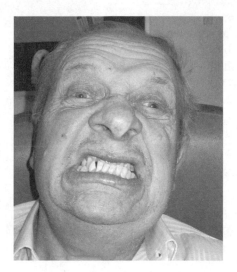

Increased interdental spacing

Figure 5.13   Acromegaly

Questions

1. How do you assess the activity of the disease clinically?

Active disease is usually accompanied by two things – sweaty or greasy skin and headache (which is often out of proportion to the size of the tumour); as soon as the growth hormone is controlled the sweating (and often the headache) ceases; subsequently over the coming days the marked puffiness of the skin reduces and over the coming months to years the thick skin slowly returns towards normal – as do the cardiometabolic effects. The bony changes remain with some minimal remodelling.

2. *What is the aetiology?*

● Of cases 99% are the result of a pituitary growth hormone (GH)-secreting adenoma.
● About 5% of patients are part of multiple endocrine neoplasia type 1 (MEN-1).
● Very rarely ectopic growth hormone-releasing hormone (GHRH) from a neuroendocrine carcinoid tumour (gut, pancreas, lung).

3. *How might the patient present?*

● General coarsening of facial features
● Enlargement of hands and feet
● Increasing ring and shoe sizes
● Sweating
● Musculoskeletal abnormalities/osteoarthritis
● Carpal tunnel syndrome
● Local effects of pituitary tumour: headache, visual deterioration
● Symptoms of hypopituitarism:
    – fatigue
    – decreased libido
    – secondary hypothyroidism
    – amenorrhoea.

4. *How will you investigate the patient?*

1. Make the diagnosis:
    – Demonstrate the failure of GH to suppress to undetectable levels after an oral glucose tolerance test
    – Elevated serum insulin growth factor I (IGF-I).
2. Establish the aetiology:
    – Image the pituitary, ideally with MRI – demonstrates tumour size, local invasion and avoids ionising radiation
    – Anterior pituitary function:
        – corticotrophic – 09:00 cortisol: if < 500 nmol/l perform a dynamic test, ie insulin or glucose tolerance test
        – thyrotrophic – T_4, T_3 and TSH
        – gonadotrophic – LH, FSH, testosterone and sex hormone-binding globulin (SHBG) or estradiol
        – lactotrophic – prolactin

- Posterior pituitary function: U&Es, serum and urine osmolality
- Bone profile – hyperparathyroidism suggests MEN-1
- GHRH – very rare, ectopic source from neuroendocrine tumours.
3. Look for complications:
   - Visual perimetry
   - ECG/echocardiography
   - Chest radiograph
   - Fasting lipids
   - Oral glucose tolerance test – from diagnosis
   - Colonoscopy
   - ± Sleep studies
   - ± Nerve conduction studies.
   Note that a plain skull radiograph, done for some other reason, may show enlargement of pituitary fossa and thickening of skull vault but is not routine or necessary.

5. *How will you manage the patient?*

Surgical

Trans-sphenoidal surgery remains the initial treatment of choice in most patients. Success depends on operator skill and the size of the tumour.

Medical

- Somatostatin analogues (eg octreotide or lancreotide) reduce serum GH in 90% of patients and to a safe GH level in about 50% of patients. Side effects are abdominal discomfort and gallstones (approximately 50% by 5 years).
- Dopamine agonists (eg bromocriptine, carbergoline) are effective in only 10% of patients.
- Pegvisomant – a newly developed growth hormone receptor antagonist; is very effective, normalising serum IGF-I in >90% of patients.

Radiotherapy

Pituitary external irradiation is indicated for patients unfit for or not cured by surgery. It results in a 50% decline in GH levels by 2 years but with a continuing exponential decline thereafter. Significant risk of late hypopituitarism.

Stereotactic focused radiosurgery is currently second-line therapy.

SCENARIO 5. DIABETES MELLITUS

There are often clues around the bed or on general examination that a patient has diabetes mellitus.

Look for: injection marks; lipohypertrophy or lipoatrophy on the abdomen, thighs or in the flesh of the arms; marks on the fingertips from capillary monitoring; white stick; special footware; sugar stains on the shoes (precipitated glucose); dextrose tablets; home glucose monitoring diary; necrobiosis lipoidica diabeticorum (see page 492); xanthelasma or xanthomas (see page 494).

Diabetic foot

There is a large variety of cases that can be found; however, there are some specific things to look for and comment on.

A peripheral sensorimotor neuropathy (see page 312) is usual.

A good candidate

- Although in many patients sensory features predominate, will take the case further with a detailed description of the salient features of the case
- Will consider the following aspects to the diabetic foot, which usually coexist in varying degrees:.

Sensory neuropathy

- The small diameter pain and temperature fibres are affected first and thus the susceptibility to trauma or pressure damage is increased.
- The small diameter fibres are best tested asking the patient to distinguish between the blunt and sharp end of a neuro-pin.
- The larger fibres are most purely tested by proprioception.
- Light touch is mostly large fibres but partially smaller fibres too.

Motor neuropathy

This affects the longer fibres that affect the foot, in turn affecting the intrinsic foot muscles and muscles of the leg. With atrophy of the intrinsic muscles of the foot the strong flexors draw the toes into a clawed position (see figure on next page), causing pressure on the tips of the toes and across the metatarsal heads.

Autonomic neuropathy

The skin is dry through loss of sweat and oil gland function; the dry skin has a susceptibility to breakdown and fissuring, creating portals of entry for bacteria:

- Ischaemia
- Ulcers
- Infection/osteomyelitis
- Amputations.

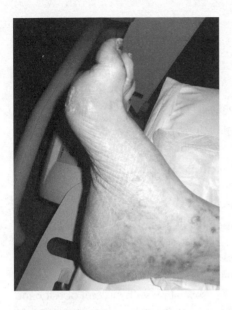

Figure 5.14
Diabetic foot, advanced sensory motor neuropathy. Clawing of the toes from motor neuropathy affecting the small muscles of the foot. Note also ischaemic pressure area on the proximal IPJs, callus under the first metatarsal head, dry skin of autonomic neuropathy and probable necrobiosis on the ankle.

Charcot's joint

This usually occurs at the ankle and/or the midfoot. The contour of the foot is grossly abnormal with disorganisation of the bones/joints. It is not painful as a result of the sensory neuropathy. which usually affects deep proprioception alongside pain/temperature, vibration sense and light touch; autonomic neuropathy often leaves the foot dry with bounding pulses. If it is active, the foot will be hot compared with the other one, reflecting active inflammation and destruction within the foot.

Amyotrophy

The patient complains of pain and weakness in the legs and is unable to walk. The findings are usually of wasting and weakness of the quadriceps with loss of the knee jerk (see Proximal Weakness in the Lower Limb, page 366). The muscles below the knee are less often affected. The cause is vascular damage to a large nerve trunk or root (radiculopathy); the femoral nerve is most often involved. It is usually acutely painful and presents during a period of poor control; slow recovery is usually the rule especially if the glycaemia is well controlled.

Miscellaneous conditions

Diabetic cheiroarthropathy

Ask the patient to place the hands together, as in prayer. The palms do not oppose and the fingers remain flexed at the IP and MTP joints.

Mononeuritis

- Oculomotor palsy (see page 279)
- Abducens palsy (see page 279)
- Ulnar nerve palsy (see page 332)
- Median nerve palsy (see page 331)
- Common peroneal nerve palsy (see page 318).

In any of the above cases, where complications of diabetes are evident, it is always reasonable to ask to examine a few specific things:

- Pulse and blood pressure: resting tachycardia and postural hypotension from autonomic neuropathy; hypertension
- Urinalysis: proteinuria.

It may be too much in these instances specifically to consider the aetiology of the diabetes but be aware of the causes of secondary diabetes, eg Cushing's disease, acromegaly, haemochromatosis, etc.

Any discussion on the complications of diabetes must be taken in the context of the prevailing burden of type 2 diabetes, its association with visceral obesity and the important complication of early cardiovascular death. Thus you need to attend to the other macrovascular risk factors, eg smoking, lipids (LDL-cholesterol concentration, particle size and density, HDL concentration) and blood pressure.

SCENARIO 6. ADDISON'S DISEASE

There is generalised pigmentation of the skin; it is particularly noticeable in recent scars or sites of skin trauma, in the buccal mucosa and in the palmar creases. There may be areas of vitiligo, (an associated organ-specific autoimmune disease, see page 518), which suggests autoimmune adrenalitis. Check for postural hypotension and consider the presence of other organ-specific and non-organ-specific autoimmune conditions.

In practice, a patient with Addison's disease will have both glucocorticoids and mineralocorticoids replaced; despite this the ACTH may still be modestly elevated, especially overnight, but clinically obvious pigmentation tends to suggest inadequate replacement.

Thus in PACES Addison's disease is unlikely to occur; a patient would have to have presented with Addison's disease in the days leading up to the exam; to appear as a case with the presence of pigmentation indicates excess ACTH which could occur in only the context of under-treatment. Clues that might suggest Addison's disease would be a very thin patient, vitiligo or a history of other organ-specific autoimmune diseases.

SCENARIO 7. NELSON SYNDROME

Pigmentation is again the result of ACTH but in this particular case the patient will have had a bilateral adrenalectomy to cure persistent hypercortisolaemia after pituitary surgery for Cushing's disease; after adrenalectomy a proportion of these patients get aggressive regrowth of the pituitary tumour – and may have signs of such – with hyperpigmentation and raised plasma ACTH. The association of hyperpigmentation with elevated ACTH (after the morning dose of replacement hydrocortisone) ± a regrowth of the pituitary tumour is Nelson syndrome.

If the glucocorticoid and mineralocorticoid replacement is adequate the patient will have signs of neither Addison's nor Cushing's disease.

SCENARIO 8. HAEMOCHROMATOSIS

This is generalised pigmentation with no predilection for scars, buccal mucosa or palmar creases; there may be signs of chronic liver disease, arthritis, hypogonadism or diabetes mellitus.

SCENARIO 9. GYNAECOMASTIA

Gynaecomastia is benign enlargement of the male breast as a result of proliferation of ductal tissue. It is distinct from pseudo-gynaecomastia where the enlargement is the result of an increase in adipose tissue. The key clinical finding is distinct, tender, subareolar masses, which can be, although not necessarily, confirmed by distinct mammographic findings.

A good candidate

Will consider the associated signs:

- Chronic liver disease: cirrhosis and/or spironolactone
- AF: digitalis
- Heart failure: spironolactone
- Loss of secondary sexual hair: hypogonadism of any cause, eg pituitary tumour or Klinefelter syndrome.

And will give a differential diagnosis (see below).

It is normal in neonates (about 90%) as a result of the transplacental passage of oestrogens and so common in puberty (about 25%) and old age (> 40%) as to be physiological.

Physiological

- Puberty
- Neonatal
- Old age
- Refeeding after starvation.

Pathological

- Primary hypogonadism
- Cirrhosis
- Testicular tumour
- Secondary hypogonadism: Klinefelter syndrome – XXY
- Thyrotoxicosis
- Hypothyroidism: structural homology between TSH and gonadotrophins, which are not being released
- Tumours:
  - human chorionic gonadotrophin (hCG) secreting
  - Leydig cell
  - adrenal
- Steroid disorders:
  - 17β-hydroxysteroid oxidoreductase deficiency
  - testicular feminisation

- Renal disease
- Idiopathic.

Pharmacological

- Spironolactone
- Digitalis
- Cannabis
- Cyproterone acetate
- Oestrogen ingestion
- Alcohol.

Question

1. What treatment is available?

Treat or remove the underlying cause; if that is not possible and the underlying gynaecomastia causes sufficient pain, embarrassment or emotional discomfort to affect the patient's daily life then there are two options: medical therapy or surgical removal. The high rate of spontaneous regression must be borne in mind when considering treatment and the fact that medical therapy is most effective in the active, proliferative phase of the development of gynaecomastia. Of the medical treatments available, a 3-month course of tamoxifen is reasonable because it has an acceptable safety, efficacy and side-effect profile but rarely leads to complete resolution. Surgery is the favoured treatment for severe gynaecomastia.

SCENARIO 10. PSEUDO-HYPOPARATHYROIDISM

The patient is short with short fourth and fifth metacarpals and metatarsals. The history may suggest learning difficulties. Biochemically you will expect an elevated parathyroid hormone (PTH) and hypocalcaemia because the defect is caused by partial or complete failure to respond to PTH.

If hypocalcaemia is not present this may be pseudo-pseudo-hypoparathyroidism

SCENARIO 11. TURNER SYNDROME

The usual case is a short female with a history of primary amenorrhoea, more rarely secondary amenorrhoea or infertility and (again rarely) coarctation of the aorta.

The following are other features and their frequencies:

- **General**: short stature 100%, hypertension 25+% increasing with age
- **Gonad**: ovarian dysgenesis 90+%
- **Lymph**: lymphoedema – puffiness over the fingers and toes may be all that remains in adulthood 80+%
- **Thorax**: shield chest with widely spaced nipples, these may be hypoplastic, inverted or both; often mild pectus excavatum 80+%
- **Ear**: anomalous auricles, most commonly prominent 80+%; otitis media in childhood 40+%
- **Facies**:
  - narrow maxilla and/or high arched palate 80%
  - small, wide mandible 70+%
  - inner canthal folds 40+%
  - ptosis 16%
- **Neck**:
  - low posterior hairline, appearance of short neck 80+%
  - webbed posterior neck 50%
- **Extremities**:
  - cubitus valgus or other deformity at elbow 70+%
  - knee anomalies, eg medial tibial exostosis 60+%
  - short fourth metacarpal and/or metatarsal 50+%
- **Nails**: narrow, hypoplastic and/or hyperconvex and/or deep set nails 70+%
- **Skin**
  - excessive pigmented naevi 50+%
  - distal palmar axial triradii 40+%
  - loose skin, especially around the neck in infancy

- **Renal**: most commonly horseshoe kidney, double or cleft renal pelvis and minor alterations 60+%
- **Cardiac**: bicuspid aortic valve 10+% or coarctation 15+%; they are four times more common in patients with webbing of the neck
- **CNS**: hearing loss 50+%.

The most serious, life-threatening consequence of chromosome X haploinsufficiency involves the cardiovascular system. During fetal development major defects in cardiac and aortic development result in a very high mortality for fetuses with a 45,X karyotype. In those fetuses that survive clinically occult bicuspid aortic valve may become a site of infective endocarditis. Those with a bicuspid valve and/or coarctation are at risk of aortic dilatation and dissection and must receive appropriate diagnostic imaging (often MR and echocardiography) at suitable intervals.

SCENARIO 12. CUSHING SYNDROME

Various historical and less favourable terms are shown in parentheses. The patient has central obesity with thin legs and arms (lemon on sticks); there are supraclavicular and intrascapular fat pads (buffalo hump); the face is rounded (moon face) and plethoric (often) and hirsute; the skin is thin with purpura and bruises. Patients have evidence of a proximal myopathy in that they cannot rise from a squat and they are hypertensive.

A good candidate

Will look for the following less common features:

* Short stature: either from a kyphosis resulting from osteoporotic collapse, or growth failure if Cushing syndrome occurred in childhood
* Agitation: if the hypercortisolaemia is severe
* Injection marks suggesting insulin therapy
* Infections, eg tinea or thrush.

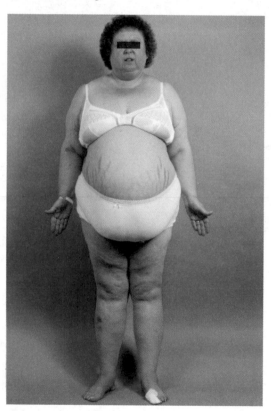

Figure 5.15   Cushing syndrome

Features suggesting the cause

- Pigmentation: this suggests elevated ACTH and is particularly seen in ectopic ACTH secretion or severe Cushing's disease
- Scars from pituitary surgery or adrenalectomy scars on the abdomen (rooftop scar of transabdominal bilateral adrenalectomy or loin incisions from unilateral or bilateral adrenalectomy)
- Cushing's disease
  - bitemporal hemianopia
  - hypogonadism in males (although may occur with any cause of Cushing syndrome).

Signs suggesting the underlying condition

- COPD (chronic obstructive pulmonary disease)
- Renal transplantation
- Eczema
- RA.

Symptoms of Cushing syndrome

- Weight gain, particularly centrally
- Change in appearance
- Growth delay
- Loss of height
- Weakness
- Hirsutism
- Acne
- Bruising and thin skin
- Mood change
- Purple stretch marks
- Nocturia/polyuria
- Decreased libido, impotence in men
- Oligo-/amenorrhoea in women
- Infections
- Headaches
- Visual disturbance.

Questions

1. *What is the likely cause of Cushing syndrome?*

- Iatrogenic: the most common cause, eg:
  - RA
  - psoriasis – topical steroid cream
  - asthma – inhaled and oral steroids
  - post-transplantation – renal

- Spontaneous Cushing syndrome (and approximate percentage of cases):
  - ACTH-dependent disease: 80% of total
    - Cushing's disease (pituitary dependent): 70%
    - ectopic ACTH syndrome: 12%
  - ACTH independent: 18% of total
    - adrenal adenoma: 10%
    - adrenal carcinoma: 7%
    - rare causes
- Pseudo-Cushing syndrome:
  - alcoholism
  - depression.

2. *What are the principles of establishing the diagnosis?*

- **Screen** with tests that are easy to perform with high sensitivity at the expense of some specificity, eg an overnight dexamethasone suppression test.
- **Confirm the diagnosis** with a test that is highly specific and sensitive, eg a 48-hour low-dose dexamethasone suppression test or midnight cortisol.
- **Establish the aetiology**: highly specialist care: plasma ACTH, inferior petrosal sinus sampling, MRI of the pituitary; CT of the chest and abdomen.

SCENARIO 13. KLINEFELTER SYNDROME

Tall, thin male patient with long limbs and increased arm span:height ratio. The musculature is poorly developed with an accumulation of subcutaneous fat around the hips (there is a tendency to become obese as adults); virilisation is poor (in practice the patient should be treated with testosterone) and gynaeco-mastia is present (in 40%). If you were to examine the external genitalia you would find small testes. Scoliosis occurs during adolescence in a minority, as does diabetes mellitus (< 10%) in adulthood.

The group of patients has a tendency to learning difficulties and behavioural problems, especially shyness, poor judgement, and unrealistically boastful and assertive behaviour.

The cause is XXY or XXY/XY mosaicism. It is the most common single cause of hypogonadism and infertility in males, affecting about 1 in 500. Treatment is with testosterone replacement, ideally starting in adolescence such that normal skeletal and emotional maturity can be achieved.

Mock Examinations

The following are a collection of likely examinations with some brief discussion around the clinical cases.

THE POTENTIALLY EASY EXAM

Station 1 Abdominal: Chronic Liver Disease

There are a plethora of signs. Think about how you might present the case, striking a balance between mentioning everything and making sure that the examiner knows that you have the important features of the case in hand.
If you are sure of the diagnosis say it; if you suspect a particular aetiology, say it; be prepared to have a discussion about the diagnostic and therapeutic work-up and subsequent management.

Station 1 Respiratory: Chronic Obstructive Pulmonary Disease

You will see one of these patients every time that you are on call. Think about the important information that the examiner needs to know that you know, or want to know, so that you can manage this patient safely overnight, get him or her through a weekend on the wards, set him or her up for discharge with a plan for clinic or the GP practice, and what you would want to do in clinic. Be prepared to discuss diagnostic and therapeutic pitfalls in these patients, such as the differentiation of COPD from asthma, the diagnosis and management of a bullous disease and pneumothorax and oxygen therapy, both in the acute situation and with regard to long-term oxygen therapy (LTOT).

Station 2 History Taking: Haemochromatosis

Take a history from a middle-aged white man with polyuria, polydipsia, fatigue and weight loss. He has a strong family history of type 2 diabetes. He also has arthritis and erectile dysfunction.

Station 3 Cardiovascular: Aortic Stenosis

Your duty to yourself here is not to get the diagnosis. Often it is absolutely clear that it is aortic stenosis. (**Often**, but not always, the diagnosis of aortic stenosis is

639

clear. If the examiner thinks that it is clearly aortic stenosis and you do not think that it is clear, this is a cast iron reason to fail this station.) The age of the patient should give you some clues to a more precise diagnosis, along with the nature of the second sound and whether there is an opening snap; as such what you must want to show in PACES is that you can think beyond the easy and the obvious, and look for precision and accuracy with your clinical skills. Furthermore, you will be expected to be able to discuss the acute (and in outline, the chronic) management of aortic stenosis.

Station 3 Neurological: Dystrophia Myotonica

This has got to be potentially the most predictable neurology case with which you might be faced, the reason being that at the end of the bed you should have the diagnosis and can concentrate on eliciting the signs with casual aplomb. To do justice to your preparation, do not expect it to be good enough to demonstrate percussion myotonia; every candidate will do that. How will you ensure that you get top marks?

Station 4 Communication and Ethics: Breaking Bad News

There are a limitless number of situations that you might face, but often the crux of the case is breaking bad news and you will have to fall back on the skills that you use *every day* in clinical practice and the notes that we have prepared. Every time any news, bad or good, is conveyed, be as objective as possible about how it is done. It is naïve to the diversity of human life to expect one pattern of behaviour to fit every situation, so be flexible, compassionate, honest and certain in your uncertainty.

Station 5 Skin: Necrobiosis Lipoidica Diabeticorum

This diagnosis should be recognised from the end of the bed; you must expect to give a good description of the lesion (often symmetrical) and the associations. Bearing in mind that you will have a non-dermatologist as an examiner you may do well to be completely familiar with the strategies for diagnosing diabetes mellitus.

Station 5 Locomotor: Rheumatoid Hands

Are you going to describe the signs as you go through the case or wait till the end to present the findings? With the legion of signs this is one case where it can be more favourable to present the findings as you see them. Perform a good functional assessment of the patient, comment on the activity of the disease, and be prepared to have a discussion about the therapy of rheumatoid arthritis and/or the differential diagnosis of a symmetrical polyarthropathy affecting the small joints of the hands/feet.

Station 5 Eyes: Laser-treated Diabetic Retinopathy

The peripheral distribution of retinal pigmentation that nevertheless is made of discrete patches should cause no confusion about the diagnosis. Chances are you will not find proliferative diabetic retinopathy alongside this, because that should have been treated! You may expect to find red eye disease and hard exudates, but cotton-wool exudates less so. It is not acceptable to misdiagnose this case as retinitis pigmentosa or old diffuse choroidoretinitis.

Station 5 Endocrine: Graves' Disease

Your patient will most probably be euthyroid (hyperthyroid possible) with a smooth diffuse goitre and ophthalmopathy. The case can be thrown away by not having an examination sufficiently robust to comment on whether the patient is hypo-, hyper- or euthyroid, or not understanding the difference between the signs specific to Graves' disease and the signs of hyperthyroidism of any cause. (If your examination is good and you make a misjudgement on the patient's thyroid status at least that is acceptable; it is in fact better than being correct but on the basis of a bad examination.) You will be expected to be able to discuss the management of common thyroid dysfunction.

THE POTENTIALLY DIFFICULT EXAM

Station 1 Abdominal: A Renal Transplant

Finding the renal transplant should present no problem; you must be able to have a sensible discussion about the probable aetiology of the renal failure, in specific relation to this case and in general in the western world today; furthermore you will have to comment on the specifics of therapy that the patient might be taking. As such there can be a lot to get through.

Station 1 Respiratory: Interstitial Lung Disease (with signs of an underlying cause)

In this case it is not so much the problem of finding fine basal crackles that suggests the diagnosis of interstitial lung disease but of missing the clues to the underlying cause, eg systemic sclerosis or sarcoidosis, and not doing justice to yourself.

Station 2 History Taking: Hypercalcaemia

Some histories can be relatively obvious from the first few sentences about what is required, whereas others are complex because of the broad number of symptoms or a broad differential diagnosis. Hypercalcaemia may have a vague presentation with a wide differential diagnosis and many causes that change with age. Occasionally it can be difficult in the examination to see the wood for the trees.

Station 3 Cardiovascular: Old Fallot's Tetralogy

Patients with Fallot's tetralogy would now have an attempted correction at an early age. The group of patients with corrected Fallot's tetralogy should give you a clue from age and possibly the scars on the chest wall with cyanosis.

Station 3 Neurological: Proximal Myopathy

Difficult in walking is often the lead into the case – here the difficulty is being prepared for this clinical case before the examination and then working through the findings methodically in the short period of time. It will be clear from our description of this clinical problem that there are many causes and your job is to work towards a precise and accurate diagnosis. Should you arrive at proximal myopathy, there is still a diagnostic sieve to go through

Station 4 Communication and Ethics: Do not tell the Patient the Diagnosis

This occurs commonly in PACES and can present some real difficulties. Do not lose your head. Obviously the ideal endpoint is the actor agreeing that it is imperative for the patient to know but, if the actor remains rigid, you might well be tested on your ability to broach the subject and at least move the matter forward to some degree. Never conspire against the patient.

Station 5 Skin: Heliotrope Rash

This sign can be difficult to see, as can some others in this station. You might be told to look at this woman's face and proceed as you see fit. Thinking of possible diagnoses you must not get trapped into making something up. The age of the patient might be a clue; use your wide-angled lens to look elsewhere – Gottren's pads, diffuse erythema, subcutaneous calcification, difficulty in rising from a chair?

Station 5 Locomotor: Diffuse Systemic Sclerosis

The history may give some pointers towards Raynaud's phenomenon and the skin changes should be obvious to see. The extent of the skin changes should provide no problems with regard to the classification of diffuse vs limited but again in this case it is more the discussion around the case that can make or break your performance. There can be a lot to talk about.

Station 5 Eyes: Internuclear Ophthalmoplegia

Do not examine the movements of the eyes from too close or you might miss this important sign. If you do miss it, will the presence of nystagmus, a young patient in a wheelchair or an intention tremor on shaking your hand stimulate you to think again? Beware of a unilateral internuclear ophthalmoplegia (INO) in a patient with a hemiparesis from a stroke – you might be asked to examine the eyes and be convinced that you are looking for a homonymous hemianopia and miss the INO.

Station 5 Endocrine: Turner Syndrome

How might this case be introduced? Perhaps with a comment about congenital heart disease, amenorrhoea or infertility; however, studying the case you can see several other more recherché ways to suggest what is essentially a spot diagnosis, with a lot of potential for discussion. In the unlikely event of you seeing this case, if you did not state that cardiac disease was the most worrisome consideration you might wonder whether you should pass the station.

List of abbreviations

5HIAA	5-hydroxyindole acetic acid
AA	amyloid A or Alcoholics Anonymous
A&E	accident and emergency
ACE	angiotensin-converting enzyme
ACTH	adrenocorticotrophic hormone
ADH	antidiuretic hormone
ADL	activities of daily living
ADM	abductor digiti minimi
ADPKD	autosomal dominant polycystic kidney disease
AF	atrial fibrillation
AFB	acid-fast bacilli
AFP	α-fetoprotein
Ag	antigen
AIDS	acquired immune deficiency syndrome
AIP	acute interstitial pneumonia
ALL	acute lymphoblastic leukaemia
ALP	alkaline phosphatase
ALS	amyotrophic lateral sclerosis
ALT	alanine transaminase
AMA	anti-mitochondrial antibody
AML	acute myeloid leukaemia
ANA	antinuclear antibody
ANCA	anti-neutrophil cytoplasmic antibody
ANF	antinuclear factor
AP	anteroposterior
APB	abductor pollicis brevis
APKD	adult polycystic kidney disease
APS	antiphospholipid syndrome
APTT	activated partial thromboplastin time
AR	aortic regurgitation
ARB	angiotension receptor antagonist
ARDS	acute respiratory distress syndrome
ARMD	age-related macular degeneration
AS	aortic stenosis or ankylosing spondylitis
ASD	atrial septal defect
ASOT	anti-streptolysin O titre
AST	aspartate transaminase
AV	atrioventricular or arteriovenous
AVM	arteriovenous malformation
AVR	aortic valve replacement

AZT	azidothymidine
BAL	bronchoalveolar lavage
BCC	basal cell carcinoma
BHL	bilateral hilar lymphadenopathy
BSH	British Society of Hypertension
BIPAP	bipositive airway pressure ventilation
BMI	body mass index
BP	blood pressure
BTS	British Thoracic Society
CABG	coronary artery bypass graft
CAD	coronary artery disease
CAPD	continuous ambulatory peritoneal dialysis
CF	cystic fibrosis
CHB	complete heart block
CHF	congestive heart failure
CK	creatine kinase
CLL	chronic lymphocytic leukaemia
CML	chronic myeloid leukaemia
CMV	cytomegalovirus
CNS	central nervous system
COA(P)D	chronic obstructive airway (pulmonary) disease
COX	cyclo-oxygenase
CPA	cerebellopontine angle
CRC	colorectal cancer
CRF	chronic renal failure
CRP	C-reactive protein
CSF	cerebrospinal fluid
CT	computed tomography
CTPA	computed tomography pulmonary angiogram
CVA	cerebrovascular accidents
CVP	central venous pressure
DCM	dilated cardiomyopathy
DEXA	dual energy X-ray absorptiometry
DI	dorsal interosseus
DIP	distal interphalangeal
DKA	diabetic ketoacidosis
DMARD	disease-modifying anti-rheumatic drug
DNA	deoxyribonucleic acid
DNAR	do not resuscitate
DPLD	diffuse parenchymal lung disease
DR	diabetic retinopathy
dsDNA	double-stranded DNA
DVLA	Driving and Vehicle Licensing Authority
DVT	deep vein thrombosis

EBV	Epstein–Barr virus
ECG	electrocardiogram
EEG	electroencephalogram/-graphy
EGFR	epidermal growth factor receptor
ELISA	enzyme-linked immunosorbent assay
EMG	electromyogram/-graphy
ENT	ear, nose and throat
ERCP	endoscopic retrograde cholangiopancreatography
ESR	erythrocyte sedimentation rate
ESRF	end-stage renal failure
ETT	exercise tolerance test
FAP	familial adenomatous polyposis
FAPS	functional abdominal pain syndrome
FBC	full blood count
$FEV_1[bl]$	Forced expiratory volume in 1 second
FNA	fine-needle aspiration
FRC	functional residual capacity
FSH	follicle-stimulating hormone
FVC	forced vital capacity
GBM	glomerular basement membrane
GCA	giant cell arteritis
GCS	Glasgow Coma Scale
GFR	glomerular filtration rate
GGT	γ-glutamyl transferase
GH	growth hormone
GHRH	growth hormone-releasing hormone
GI	gastrointestinal
GMC	General Medical Council
GnRH	gonadotrophin-releasing hormone
GORD	gastro-oesophageal reflux disease
GP	general practitioner
GUM	genitourinary medicine
HAART	highly active antiretroviral therapy
HAV	hepatitis A virus
HBV	hepatitis B virus
HCC	hepatocellular carcinoma
hCG	human chorionic gonadotrophin
HCOM	hypertrophic cardiomyopathy
HCV	hepatitis C virus
HDL	high-density lipoprotein
HE	hepatic encephalopathy
HH	hereditary haemochromatosis
HHV8	human herpesvirus 8
HIV	human immunodeficiency virus

HNPCC	hereditary non-polyposis colorectal carcinoma
HPV	human papillomavirus
HRCT	high-resolution computed tomography
HRT	hormone replacement therapy
HS	hereditary spherocytosis
HSMN	hereditary sensorimotor neuropathy
HSP	Henoch–Schönlein purpura
HSV	herpes simplex virus
HZV	herpes zoster virus
ICP	intracranial pressure
ICU	intensive care unit
IBD	inflammatory bowel disease
IBS	irritable bowel syndrome
ICP	intracranial pressure
IFN-a	interferon α
Ig	immunoglobulin
IGF-I	insulin growth factor I
IHD	ischaemic heart disease
IIP	idiopathic interstitial pneumonias
INR	international normalised ratio
IP	interphalangeal
IPF	idiopathic pulmonary fibrosis
IRMA	intraretinal microvascular abnormality
ITP	idiopathic thrombocytopenia purpura
ITU	intensive therapy unit
IU	international units
IVDU	intravenous drug use/user
IVU	intravenous urography
JVP	jugular venous pressure
LBBB	left bundle-branch block
LDH	lactate dehydrogenase
LDL	low-density lipoprotein
LFT	liver function test
LH	luteinising hormone
LMN	lower motor neuron
LMWH	low-molecular-weight heparin
LP	lumbar puncture
LSE	left sternal edge
LV	left ventricular
LVEDP	LV end-diastolic pressure
LVOT	LV outflow tract
MAI	*Mycobacterium avium-intracellulare*
MC&S	microscopy, culture and sensitivity
MCH	mean corpuscular haemoglobin

MCP	metacarpophalangeal
MCV	mean corpuscular volume
MDRTB	multi-drug-resistant TB
MDT	multidisciplinary team
MEN	multiple endocrine neoplasia
MI	myocardial infarction
MLF	medial longitudinal fascicle
MMR	measles, mumps and rubella
MND	motor neuron disease
MR	mitral regurgitation
MRA	magnetic resonance angiography
MRC	Medical Research Council
MRCP	magnetic resonance cholangiopancreatography
MRI	magnetic resonance imaging
MRSA	meticillin-resistant *Staphylococcus aureus*
MS	mitral stenosis or multiple sclerosis
MSU	mid-stream specimen of urine
MTP	metatarsophalangeal
MTS	mental test score
MV	mitral valve
NASH	non-alcoholic steatohepatitis
NHS	National Health Service
NICE	National Institute for Health and Clinical Excellence
NIV	non-invasive ventilation
NMDA	N-methyl-D-aspartate
NNRTI	non-nucleoside reverse transcriptase inhibitor
NRTI	nucleoside reverse transcriptase inhibitor
NSAID	non-steroidal anti-inflammatory drug
NSCLC	non-small cell lung cancer
NSTEMI	non-ST-elevation MI
NYHA	New York Heart Association
OCP	oral contraceptive pill
OCD	obsessive compulsive disorder
OI	osteogenesis imperfecta
OSCE	Objective Structured Clinical Examination
PA	posteroanterior
PACES	Practical Assessment of Clinical Examination Skills
PALS	Patients' Advice Liaison Service
PAN	panarteritis nodosa
PBC	primary biliary cirrhosis
PCOS	polycystic ovarian syndrome
PCP	*Pneumocystis carinii* pneumonia (see PJP)
PCR	polymerase chain reaction
PCT	primary care trust

PDA	patent ductus arteriosus
PE	pulmonary embolus
PEFR	peak expiratory flow rate
PEG	percutaneous endoscopic gastrostomy
PET	positron emission tomography
PFO	persistent foramen ovale
PJP	*Pneumocystis jiroveci* pneumonia
PMR	polymyalgia rheumatica
PND	paroxysmal nocturnal dyspnoea
POP	progestogen-only pill
PPI	proton pump inhibitor
PRV	polycythaemia rubra vera
PS	pulmonary stenosis
PsA	psoriatic arthropathy
PSA	prostate-specific antigen
PSC	primary sclerosing cholangitis
PT	prothrombin time
PTCA	percutaneous transluminal coronary angioplasty
PUVA	psoralen + UVA
PVR	pulmonary vascular resistance
PVS	persistent vegetative state
PVSG	polycythemia vera study group
RA	rheumatoid arthritis
RBBB	right bundle-branch block
RCA	right coronary artery
RCT	randomised controlled trial
RF	rheumatoid factor
rhDNase	recombinant human DNase
RIA	radioimmunoassay
RSV	respiratory syncytial virus
RTA	road traffic accident
RUQ	right upper quadrant
RVH	right ventricular hypertrophy
SAH	subarachnoid haemorrhage
SCC	squamous cell carcinoma
SCDC	subacute combined degeneration of the cord
SCLC	small cell lung cancer
SHBG	sex hormone-binding globulin
SHO	senior house officer
SIADH	syndrome of inappropriate antidiuretic hormone production
SLE	systemic lupus erythematosus
SOB	shortness of breath
SOL	space occupying lesion
SPECT	single photon emission CT

SpR	specialist registrar
SR	sinus rhythm
SS	systemic sclerosis
SSRI	selective serotonin release inhibitor
STI	sexually transmitted infection
SVC	superior vena cava
SVCO	SVC obstruction
T_3	triiodothyronine
T_4	thyroxine
TB	tuberculosis
TFT	thyroid function test
TGF-β	transforming growth factor β
TIA	transient ischaemic attack
TIBC	total iron-binding capacity
TIMI	thrombolysis in myocardial infarction
TIPSS	transhepatic portosystemic shunt
T_{LCO}	transfer factor for carbon monoxide
TNF-α	tumour necrosis factor α
TPHA	*Treponema pallidum* haemagglutination assay
TR	tricuspid regurgitation
TS	tricuspid stenosis
TSH	thyroid-stimulating hormone
TTP	thrombotic thrombocytopenic purpura
TV	tricuspid valve
TVF	tactile vocal fremitus
U&Es	urea and electrolytes
UC	ulcerative colitis
UKPDS	UK Prospective Diabetes Study
UMN	upper motor neuron
UTI	urinary tract infection
UTRI	upper respiratory tract infection
VA	visual acuity
VDRL	Venereal Disease Reference Laboratory
VHL	von Hippel–Lindau
VLDL	very-low-density lipoprotein
VR	vocal resonance
VSD	ventricular septal defect
WCC	white cell count

Index

References

Station 1: Abdominal and Respiratory
Abdominal
Czaja AJ, Freese DK. Hepatology (Baltimore, Md.), 2002 – cat.inist.fr
Diagnosis and treatment of autoimmune hepatitis.

Swash M. *Hutchinson's Clinical Methods*. Oxford: WB Saunders Co Ltd, 2001.

Respiratory
Fletcher CM, Elmes PC, Fairbairn MB et al. The significance of respiratory symptoms and the diagnosis of chronic bronchitis in a working population. *British Medical Journal* 1959; ii: 257–66.

Station 2: History Taking
Hasbun R, Abrahams J, Jekel J et al. Computed tomography of the head before lumbar puncture in adults with suspected meningitis. *New England Journal of Medicine* 2001, Dec. 13th; 345(24): 1727–33.

Jalan R, Hayes PC. British Society of Gastroenterology Gut, 2000. UK guidelines on the management of variceal haemorrhage in cirrhotic patients.

Station 3: Cardiology and Neurology
Cardiology
Bonow RO, Carabello BA, Kanu C et al. ACC/AHA 2006 guidelines for the management of patients with valvular heart disease: a report of the American College of Cardiology/American Heart Association task force on Practice Guidelines (writing committee to revise the 1998 Guidelines for the Management of Patients with Valvular Heart Disease): developed in collaboration with the Society of Cardiovascular Anesthesiologists: endorsed by the Society for Cardiovascular Angiography and Interventions and the Society of Thoracic Surgeons.
Circulation 2006; 114, e84–231.

Brickner ME, Hillis LD, Lange RA. Congenital heart disease in adults. First of two parts.
New England Journal of Medicine 2000; 342: 256–63.
Brickner ME, Hillis LD, Lange RA. Congenital heart disease in adults. Second of two parts.
New England Journal of Medicine 2000; 342: 334–42.

Swanton RH. *Cardiology*. Oxford: Blackwell Science Ltd, 1998.

Neurology
Allen D, Dunn L. Aciclovir or valaciclovir for Bell's palsy (idiopathic facial paralysis). *Cochrane Databases System Reviews* 2003: CD001869.

Gilden DH. Bell's palsy. *New England Journal of Medicine* 2004; 351: 1323–31 and subsequent correspondence in 352: 416–18.

Holland NJ, Weiner GM. Recent developments in Bell's palsy. *British Medical Journal* 2004; 329: 553–7.

McDonald WI, Compton A, Edan G et al. Recommended diagnostic criteria for Multiple Sclerosis. *Ann Neurol* 2001; 50: 121–7.

National Institute for Health and Clinical Excellence. *Multiple Sclerosis*. NICE guideline CG8 26. London: NICE, 2003.

Salinas RA, Alvarez G, Alvarez MI, et al. Corticosteroids for Bell's palsy (idiopathic facial paralysis). *Cochrane Database System Reviews* 2004; 4: CD001942.

Sullivan FM, Swan IRC, Donnan PT et al. New England Journal of Medicine 2007, Oct 18th; 1598–607. PMID: 17942873.

Station 4: Communications Skills and Ethics
Sykes NP. Morphine kills the pain, not the patient. *Lancet* 2007; 369: 1325–6.

Station 5: Skin, Locomotor, Eyes and Endocrine
Skin
Shovlin CL, Guttmacher AE, Buscarini E et al. Diagnostic criteria for hereditary haemorrhagic telangiectasia (Rendu–Osler–Weber syndrome). *American Journal of Medical Genetics* 2000; 91: 66.

Fuchizaki U, Miyamori H, Kitagawa S et al. Hereditary haemorrhagic telangiectasia (Rendu–Osler–Weber disease). *Lancet* 2003; 362: 1490–4.

Jung AC, Paauw DS. Diagnosing HIV-related disease using the CD4 count as a guide. *Journal of International General Medicine* 1998; 13: 131–6.

Locomotor
Sillence D. Classification for Osteogenesis Imperfecta, 1979.